Crossover Designs

Crossover Designs
Testing, Estimation, and Sample Size

Kung-Jong Lui

Department of Mathematics and Statistics
San Diego State University, USA

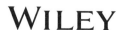

Library of Congress Cataloging-in-Publication Data

Names: Lui, Kung-Jong, author.
Title: Crossover designs : testing, estimation, and sample size / Kung-Jong Lui.
Other titles: Statistics in practice.
Description: Chichester, West Sussex ; Hoboken : John Wiley & Sons, Inc., 2016. |
    Series: Statistics in practice | Includes bibliographical references and index.
Identifiers: LCCN 2016012478 (print) | LCCN 2016013006 (ebook) | ISBN 9781119114680 (cloth) |
    ISBN 9781119114697 (pdf) | ISBN 9781119114703 (epub)
Subjects: | MESH: Cross-Over Studies | Data Interpretation, Statistical | Sample Size |
    Statistical Distributions | Models, Statistical | Clinical Trials as Topic
Classification: LCC R853.S7 (print) | LCC R853.S7 (ebook) | NLM WA 950 | DDC 610.72/7–dc23
LC record available at http://lccn.loc.gov/2016012478

A catalogue record for this book is available from the British Library.

Cover Image: Gettyimages by Nick Koudis

Set in 10/12pt Times by SPi Global, Pondicherry, India
Printed and bound in Malaysia by Vivar Printing Sdn Bhd

1   2016

To
Dan-Yang, Kung-Yi, Kung-Jen, Chieh-Yun and Jen-Mei

Contents

About the author

Kung-Jong Lui is a professor in the Department of Mathematics and Statistics at San Diego State University. He obtained his Ph.D. degree in biostatistics in 1982, M.S. degree in biostatistics in 1979, M.A. degree in mathematics in 1977, all from UCLA, and B.S. degree in mathematics in 1975 at Fu-Jen Catholic University in Taipei, Taiwan. He has had 185 publications in peer-reviewed journals, including *Statistical Methods in Medical Research, Biometrics, Statistics in Medicine, Biometrical Journal, Journal of Biopharmaceutical Statistics, Computational Statistics and Data Analysis, Journal of Applied Statistics, Pharmaceutical Statistics, Contemporary Clinical Trials, Drug Information Journal, Statistical Methodology, Environmetrics, IEEE Transactions on Reliability, Test, Journal of Official Statistics, Journal of Modern Applied Statistical Methods, Communications in Statistics – Theory and Methods, Communications in Statistics – Simulation and Computation, Science, Nature, Proceedings of the National Academy of Sciences, American Journal of Epidemiology, American Journal of Public Health, New England Journal of Medicine, Journal of the American Medical Association,* and *Journal of Safety Research.* He is the sole author of the book *Statistical Estimation of Epidemiological Risk* published by Wiley in 2004 and the book *Binary Data Analysis of Randomized Clinical Trials with Noncompliance* published by Wiley in 2011. He is or has served as an associate editor for *Biometrical Journal, BMC Medical Research Methodology, Enliven: Biostatistics and Metrics, Journal of Epidemiological Research,* and *JP Journal of Biostatistics.* He is a Fellow of the American Statistical Association, a Fellow of the American College of Epidemiology, and a life member of the International Chinese Statistical Association.

Preface

When studying treatments for non-curable chronic diseases, including asthma, epilepsy, angina pectoris, migraine, and hypertension, the crossover design has been often employed to increase power or reduce the number of patients needed for a parallel groups design. In a randomized clinical trial, the patient responses of interest can be on various scales, including continuous data, binary endpoints, ordinal outcomes, or frequency of events. Because different types of data may lead us to consider various statistical methods and modeling, we have organized this book according to the data scale. Furthermore, when the data are categorical, most test procedures and interval estimators discussed elsewhere are derived on the basis of large-sample theory. Because the number of patients in a crossover design is frequently small, asymptotic test procedures and interval estimators based on normal approximation can be inappropriate for use in these cases. Thus, exact test procedures and exact interval estimators for categorical and frequency data presented in this book are desirable and useful in practice.

To avoid the possible loss of substantial efficiency with adjusting carry-over effects and the bias of our estimators derived under models not being able to account for the complicated structure of carry-over effects, we focus our discussions on the situations in which investigators can apply adequate washout periods based on their best knowledge to deal with carry-over effects. If we unexpectedly encounter carry-over effects (which are found and supported by clinical evidence rather than by statistical tests exclusively), however, we still include some discussions on hypothesis tests and estimation in the presence of carry-over effects under the assumed models at the end of some chapters. To account for the intraclass correlation between responses within patients, we assume that the effects due to individual patients are random rather than fixed. Except for the cases of continuous data focused on in Chapter 2, we do not assume the random effects due to patients to follow any specified parametric distribution, such as normal distribution, that is commonly done in random effects models on the basis of the likelihood-based approach. To eliminate these nuisance random effects, we consider use of a conditional approach. Because most test procedures and interval estimators presented here are expressed in closed forms, readers can easily appreciate and calculate them by use of a hand pocket calculator even without the knowledge of any software. This book suggests the use of Agresti's α', also called the generalized odds ratio (GOR), to measure the relative treatment effect when we encounter ordinal data in a crossover trial. When using the GOR, we do not need to assume any specific data structure and parametric distribution for the random effects, as in the use of the normal random effects proportional odds model for the underlying data, nor employ any complicated iterative numerical procedures to obtain parameter estimates. Furthermore, because the GOR depends on the marginal subtotal frequencies, use of the GOR may have less concern than use of the likelihood-based approach in sparse data.

This book is intended to systematically provide biostatisticians and clinicians working in medical and pharmaceutical industries with a useful resource on the commonly encountered crossover designs. To facilitate the utility of the book, the notation and material in each chapter are self-contained. Readers may choose chapters according to their own interests without the need to read through all the preceding chapters, although I must admit that some definitions of notation and notes are repeated between chapters to avoid ambiguities in formulas and discussions. This book is aimed at postgraduates and researchers in universities and research institutes, consultants in consulting firms, and biostatisticians at the FDA and NIH. This book can be also used as a desk reference book or supplemental material for courses relevant to clinical trials.

Key features of the book include (i) models with distribution-free random effects are assumed, and hence our approach is semi-parametric. (ii) Exact test procedures and interval estimators, which are especially of use in small-sample cases, are provided. (iii) Most test procedures and interval estimators are presented in closed forms and thus readers can calculate them by use of a pocket calculator. (iv) Each chapter is self-contained, allowing the book to be used as a reference source. (v) Real-life examples are used to illustrate the practical use of test procedures and estimators. (vi) Many exercises help readers appreciate the underlying theory, learn other relevant test procedures, and calculate the required sample size.

I wish to express my greatest appreciations to Profs. G. P. Herbison and D. R. Taylor at the University of Otago for providing the data regarding the number of exacerbations in a trial comparing treatments salbutamol and salmeterol with placebo in asthma patients. I also want to express my deepest indebtedness to my colleagues Drs. Sam Shen, Kuang-Chao Chang, and Joey Lin, my former classmate Dr. Yin Liu, as well as my three sons, Jeffrey, Steven, and Derek for their editorial corrections and suggestions. As always, I would like to thank my former professors, Drs. W. G. Cumberland and A. A. Afifi, for their teaching and inspiration in biostatistics when I was a student at UCLA. Special thanks are given to my wife Jen-Mei for her patience and understanding that have endured for so many years. Finally, I feel obliged to wholeheartedly thank my parents for their love, advice, and encouragement, which have continued guiding and supporting me throughout my career.

About the companion website

Don't forget to visit the companion website for this book:

www.wiley.com/go/lui/crossover

There you will find valuable material designed to enhance your learning, including:

- SAS Programs

Scan this QR code to visit the companion website:

1

Crossover design – definitions, notes, and limitations

A crossover or change-over design is a trial in which each eligible patient after obtaining his/her informed consent is randomly assigned to receive more than one treatment according to one of the predetermined treatment-receipt sequences. By contrast, a parallel groups design is a trial in which each eligible patient after obtaining his/her informed consent is randomly assigned to receive exactly one of the treatments under comparison. Similar to parallel groups design, the main goal of a crossover design is to study the difference between individual treatments (rather than the difference between treatment sequences). Because each patient serves as his/her own control, the crossover design is a useful alternative to the parallel groups design for increasing power or saving the number of patients needed via elimination of response variation between patients when treatments are compared (Hills and Armitage, 1979; Fleiss, 1986a; Senn, 2002). A review of the history of the crossover design can be found in Jones and Kenward (2014, pp. 5–7).

The simplest crossover design is the AB/BA design, in which patients are randomly assigned to either the AB group, in which patients receive treatment A first and then cross over to receive treatment B, or the BA group, in which patients receive treatment B first and then cross over to receive treatment A. The AB/BA design is also called the simple crossover or 2 × 2 design (Jones and Kenward, 1989). Because of its simplicity, the application of AB/BA design has accounted for a large proportion of crossover trials used in practice (Hills and Armitage, 1979; Senn, 2002, 2006; Mills *et al.*, 2009). As noted in a survey of 12 large pharmaceutical companies in the United States (Fava and Patel, 1986), more than half of the 72 cross-over trials conducted

Crossover Designs: Testing, Estimation, and Sample Size, First Edition. Kung-Jong Lui.
© 2016 John Wiley & Sons, Ltd. Published 2016 by John Wiley & Sons, Ltd.
Companion website: www.wiley.com/go/lui/crossover

over a five-year period by these companies used the AB/BA design (Jones and Kenward, 1989, p. 6). Because of the characteristics of the study design features, there are limitations in use of a crossover design.

1.1   Unsuitability for acute or most infectious diseases

The crossover design is inapplicable for studying acute or most infectious diseases that are likely to be either fatal or curable, such as food poisoning, the common cold, or stomach flu. In treating these diseases, there will be nothing left to treat when the patient is scheduled to receive the second or later treatments. Thus, the crossover design should generally be reserved for non-curable chronic diseases for which the symptoms can be relieved only for a short time period after treatments and will reoccur shortly after the applied treatment is removed. These chronic diseases may commonly include asthma, epilepsy, angina pectoris, migraine, hypertension, and so forth (Fleiss, 1986a; Senn, 2002). The crossover design is also popular in studying the effects of antianxiety drugs on human performance (McNair, 1971).

1.2   Inappropriateness for treatments with long-lasting effects

The crossover design is appropriate for treatments that have a rapid, short, and reversible effect (e.g., bronchodilators in asthma) (Senn, 2002). The crossover design is not adequate for studying treatments that have a long-lasting effect, such as steroids or vaccine for rabies or rubella. The carry-over effect – that is, the persistent effect of a treatment applied in one period on patient responses in a subsequent period of treatments – is one of the major concerns for the use of a crossover trial. If there are carry-over effects in a crossover trial, the effect of a treatment observed at one time point can be confounded with the residual effects due to earlier treatments. Thus, our comparison between treatments and assessment of the relative treatment effect can be biased if we cannot appropriately adjust the carry-over effects due to earlier treatments. As noted by Hills and Armitage (1979), it can be difficult or even impossible to disentangle the treatment effect from the residual effects of earlier treatments. Although we may find intensive research in the development of models or testing strategies to account for the carry-over effect (Balaam, 1968; Kershner and Federer, 1981; Laska, Meisner, and Kushner, 1983; Ebbutt, 1984; Laska and Meisner, 1985; Willan and Pater, 1986; Lehmacher, 1991; Jones and Donev, 1996), most of these models are assumed for mathematical interests and convenience rather than practical utility (Fleiss, 1986a, 1986b, 1989; Senn, 1992, 2002; Senn, D'Angelo, and Potvin, 2004). Senn (1992) and Fleiss (1989) contended that the best strategy to deal with the carry-over effect is to employ an adequate washout period to assure that patients are weaned off these residual effects from earlier treatments.

1.3   Loss of efficiency in the presence of carry-over effects

As mentioned, the main motivation of employing a crossover trial instead of a parallel groups design is to increase the power of test procedures or reduce the number of patients needed. Grizzle (1965) focused attention on the AB/BA design and proposed a random effects linear additive risk model. Grizzle (1965) showed that incorporating the carry-over effects into test procedures and estimators is equivalent to carrying out data analysis based on only the data at the first period as done in the parallel groups design. Thus, the gain of efficiency in use of an AB/BA crossover trial in the presence of carry-over effect under the random effects linear additive risk model will completely disappear. On the other hand, if we originally planned to carry out a parallel groups design, we would be able to take advantage of the resources that were used to take patient responses at period 2 in use of a crossover trial to recruit more patients for the parallel groups design. This implies that for a given fixed budget, we may even end up of losing the opportunity to detect what we are interested in if we employ an AB/BA crossover trial in the presence of carry-over effects. Thus, it is advisable that we put more efforts into prior consideration in the design stage of a crossover trial. If we cannot assure ourselves of elimination of the carry-over effect with an adequate washout period based on our subjective knowledge, we may not wish to consider using the crossover trial (Brown, 1980; Fleiss, 1986a, 1989; Senn and Hildebrand, 1991; Senn, 2002; Schouten and Kester, 2010).

1.4   Concerns of treatment-by-period interaction

The treatment-by-period interaction means that the effect of a treatment on patient responses varies between periods. The interaction between treatments and periods can result from (i) a treatment effect that may carry over from one period to the next period physically or psychologically; or (ii) a treatment effect that may vary according to the level of patient response (Hills and Armitage, 1979; Ebbutt, 1984; Jones and Kenward, 1989, p. 42). If there is an interaction between treatments and periods, as for studying the association between risk factors and diseases in epidemiology, a summary conclusion between treatments across periods can be misleading (Lui, 2004). Furthermore, interpretation of our findings about the treatment effect in the presence of treatment-by-period interaction can also be more difficult. Note that the carry-over effect is a special type of treatment-by-period interaction, except that for the carry-over effect, we cannot eliminate all other kinds of treatment-by-period interactions (Hills and Armitage, 1979; Jones and Kenward, 1989) by use of a washout period. When employing an AB/BA design, we often need to implicitly assume that the treatment-by-period interaction does not exist. The treatment-by-period interaction (or carry-over effect) is not really unique in a crossover trial and can exist in the parallel groups trial as well (Senn and Hildebrand, 1991; Senn, 2002).

1.5   Flaw of the commonly used two-stage test procedure

The carry-over effect and treatment-by-period interaction are not separately identifiable under an AB/BA design (Senn, 2002). Either of these effects can cause a bias in our inference of the treatment effect. Although we may employ an adequate washout period to attenuate the carry-over effects, we can never be certain that the washout period has worked. Grizzle (1965) proposed a two-stage test procedure as follows. We first test whether the carry-over effect exists. Because the test itself for the carry-over effect is subject to the response variation between patients, the power of this test is generally low and thereby a high nominal level of Type I error (10 or 15%) is usually chosen. If the test for the carry-over effect is nonsignificant, we will carry on analyses based on the difference between responses within patients as done for the crossover trial with assuming no carry-over effects. Otherwise, the test procedure using the data at the first period only is carried out as for the parallel groups design, and all data obtained at the second period are excluded from data analysis. Freeman (1989) carried out a thorough investigation of the two-stage test approach and concluded that this approach could be potentially misleading. This is because the statistic for testing the carry-over effect is highly correlated to that for testing equality based on the data at the first period. Thus, the test result based on the data at the first period is likely to be significant as well when the test result for the carry-over effect is significant. This leads to the actual Type I error for the two-stage test being higher than the nominal α-level. Due to this concern, we do not recommend use of the two-stage test procedure in practice (Senn, 1988, 1991, 1997, 2000, 2002, 2004, 2006). Other notes in use of the two-stage test in a crossover trial can be found elsewhere (Jones and Kenward, 2003, pp. 44–49; Cleophas, 1991; Freeman, 1991; Senn, 1996).

1.6   Higher risk of dropping out or being lost to follow-up

Because each patient is to receive more than one treatment, the duration of a crossover trial is expected to be longer than that of a parallel groups design. The longer the time length of a trial, the more difficult is to obtain patients' consent to participate in a trial and the higher is the risk for patients dropping out or being lost to follow-up after consent (Senn and Lee, 2004). Extra effort is also needed, as compared with a parallel groups design, to ensure that patients follow the study protocol closely for a crossover trial with a long duration. All the above concerns can be exacerbated if it is necessary for all patients to receive even more than two treatments. Thus, the crossover trial should generally be reserved for trials in which the number of treatments under comparison is not numerous to reduce the risk of dropping out in participating patients, while the acute effect of treatments can be quickly measured.

1.7   More assumptions needed in use of a crossover design

In a crossover trial, responses taken from the same patients are likely correlated and the period effect on patient responses often exists. Furthermore, in an AB/BA trial the carry-over effect, the group effect, and the treatment-by-period interaction are all aliased and not separately estimatible (Jones and Kenward, 1989, 2003; Senn, 2002). Thus, we need to make more model assumptions to account for the above factors, and statistical analyses for a crossover design are generally more complicated than those for a parallel groups design. Although many subtle and sophisticated models have been developed recently for a crossover design, the need to make more model assumptions for the crossover design than that for the parallel groups trial is undesirable. This is because our inferences can be vulnerable to more model assumptions, which are often difficult to be completely justified in practice. To alleviate this concern, it is logically appealing that we should put more effort into designing a trial to simplify the underlying assumed model structure instead of constructing complicated models and developing sophisticated analyses.

1.8   General principle and conditional approach used in the book

To avoid the possible loss of substantial efficiency in adjusting carry-over effects and the bias of our estimators derived under models unable to appropriately account for the complicated structure of carry-over effects (Senn, D'Angelo, and Potvin, 2004), we follow Fleiss (1986a, 1989), Senn (1992, 2002) and Schouten and Kester (2010) and recommend use of the study design to deal with the carry-over effect. We focus our discussions on situations in which the carry-over effect is ignorable by assuming that practitioners will use their best knowledge to cautiously apply an adequate washout period. In case we should unexpectedly encounter carry-over effects (which are found and supported by internal evidence rather than by statistical tests exclusively), however, we discuss hypothesis tests and estimation related to the carry-over effect, as well as assess the relative treatment effect in the presence of carry-over effect at the end of some chapters.

To account for the intraclass correlation between responses taken within patients, we assume that the effects due to individual patients are random rather than fixed (Gart, 1969). Except for a section (discussing the test for carry-over effects) in Chapter 2 (for continuous data), we do not assume the random effects due to patients to follow any specified parametric distribution (such as a normal distribution as commonly done in random effects models). To eliminate these random effects, we adopt the conditional approach rather than the likelihood-based approach. The former may be less efficient than the latter if the random effects of patients do follow the assumed normal distribution. However, it is difficult or impossible to justify any specified distribution for these random effects in practice. From the practical point of view, using a simple valid method that is easy to understand and calculate, as well as requires fewer assumptions, can be more useful and desirable than using a possibly more efficient approach derived under more restricted situations. Furthermore, using the conditional arguments can easily lead to deriving the exact tests and exact interval estimators. These exact methods and results will be of use for investigators who have the concerns of employing asymptotic test procedures and interval estimators when the size of their trials is actually small.

To consider a period or simple trend effect, we focus discussions on models including the period effect throughout the book. When there is a period effect, test procedures (or estimators) without accounting for the period effect can lose accuracy (or be biased). Because one of the main reasons for using more than one treatment-receipt sequence in a crossover design is to allow for a possible period effect (Jones and Kenward, 2014, p. 99), an analysis with assuming no period effect seems to internally contradict the design itself. Note that a period effect may also be called an "order effect" (Gart, 1969; Prescott, 1981).

The scope of the book is modest. We concentrate our attention under the most commonly encountered basic crossover designs on various statistical aspects, including tests of non-equality, non-inferiority and equivalence, interval estimation, sample size determination, estimation and adjustment of unexpected carry-over effects, as well as tests of the period effect and treatment-by-period interaction. We consider the AB/BA design for continuous data (Chapter 2), dichotomous data (Chapter 3), ordinal data (Chapter 4), and frequency data (Chapter 5). To reduce the number of patients receiving an inert placebo in a random clinical trial, it can sometimes be appealing to compare more than one experimental treatment with a placebo in a single trial instead of separate trials, each having its own an experimental and a placebo arms. Thus, we extend the results for the AB/BA design to accommodate a three-treatment three-period crossover design for continuous data (Chapter 6), dichotomous data (Chapter 7), ordinal data (Chapter 8), and frequency data (Chapter 9). The extension of methods and ideas presented here to accommodate the cases for more than three-treatment three-period crossover trials (Senn, 2002) is simply straightforward. To decrease the number of groups with different treatment-receipt sequences in a crossover trial, we include some discussions on the use of Latin squares in exercises when comparing three or more treatments. To reduce the lengthy duration of a crossover trial comparing more than two treatments, we also include a chapter (Chapter 10) discussing hypothesis testing and estimation under an incomplete block crossover design for both continuous and dichotomous data. Using similar ideas, we can easily extend these results to accommodate the ordinal and frequency data under the incomplete block crossover design. For other specific topics, such as high-order designs, fixed effects models, the search for optimal designs, detailed discussions of carry-over effects, and the Bayesian approach, we refer readers to excellent books (Jones and Kenward, 1989, 2003, 2014; Senn, 2002), all of which were truly inspiring during the preparation of this book.

2

AB/BA design in continuous data

In a randomized clinical trial, it is quite common to encounter the underlying patient response of interest on a continuous scale (Senn, 2002). For example, consider the data in Table 2.1 taken from a crossover trial comparing two dose preparations of aspirin for their effects on gastric bleeding measured by using a radioactive tagging method (Fleiss, 1986a). Sixteen patients were randomly paired. Within each pair, one patient was randomly chosen to receive a preparation for one week, followed by a one-week washout period before the week of receiving the other preparation, and the other patient within the pair then received the reverse order of preparations. As a second example, consider the data in Table 2.2 taken from a crossover trial comparing the effect of 12 µg formoterol with that of a single inhaled dose of 200 µg salbutamol on peak expiratory flow (PEF) (in liters per minute), a measure of lung function (National Asthma Educational Program, 1991, pp. 6–9), in 13 children aged 7–14 years old with moderate or severe asthma (Senn and Auclair, 1990, p. 1290; Senn, 2002, p. 36). Children were randomly assigned to the group with the receipt of salbutamol first and then formoterol, or the group with the receipt of formoterol first and then salbutamol. There was a washout period of at least one day between two treatments. Other examples of a crossover trial in which patient responses are continuous can be found elsewhere (Rhind *et al.*, 1985; Smith *et al.*, 1985; Jones and Kenward, 1989, 2003, 2014; Steinijans, 1989; Hauschke, Steinijans, and Diletti, 1990; Senn, 2002).

On the basis of a random effects linear additive risk model (Grizzle, 1965), we focus our attentions on the AB/BA crossover design in continuous data. We consider both parametric and nonparametric methods. We discuss testing non-equality of two treatments. We further discuss testing non-inferiority and equivalence between an experimental treatment and an active control (or a standard) treatment. We address

Crossover Designs: Testing, Estimation, and Sample Size, First Edition. Kung-Jong Lui.
© 2016 John Wiley & Sons, Ltd. Published 2016 by John Wiley & Sons, Ltd.
Companion website: www.wiley.com/go/lui/crossover

Table 2.1   The measurements of gastric bleeding obtained using a radioactive tagging method between two dose preparations A and B of aspirin.

Group	A – B		B – A	
	Periods		Periods	
	I	II	I	II
	5.1	3.8	2.9	3.9
	0.6	1.0	1.6	2.3
	4.8	3.1	4.0	5.8
	4.4	4.9	1.6	0.8
	2.3	1.3	4.1	4.7
	4.9	2.3	3.2	0.9
	6.8	4.5	2.3	4.0
	6.1	2.2	3.4	3.6

Table 2.2   PEF in l/m measured 8 h after treatments: salbutamol (treatment A) and formoterol (treatment B).

Group	Salbutamol/formoterol		Formoterol/salbutamol	
	Periods		Periods	
	I	II	I	II
	370	385	310	270
	310	400	310	260
	380	410	370	300
	290	320	410	390
	260	340	250	210
	90	220	380	350
			330	365

interval estimation of the mean difference between two treatments, and we provide sample size determination procedures for testing non-equality, non-inferiority, and equivalence. We discuss hypothesis testing and interval estimation for the period effect. When unexpectedly encountering carry-over effects (found and supported by internal evidence instead of statistical test exclusively after collecting data) due to an inadequate washout period, we discuss hypothesis testing and estimation of the carry-over effect, as well as its adjustment in estimation of the relative treatment effect. We present SAS program codes of PROC MIXED and PROC GLIMMIX (SAS Institute Inc., 2009), as well as the corresponding results, to illustrate the use of the procedures and estimators discussed here.

Consider comparing an experimental treatment B with an active control treatment A (or a placebo) under a two-period crossover design. Suppose that we randomly assign n_1 patients to group $g = 1$ with the treatment-receipt sequence A-then-B, in which patients receive treatment A at period 1 and then cross over to receive treatment B at period 2, and n_2 patients to group $g = 2$ with the treatment-receipt sequence B-then-A, in which patients receive treatment B at period 1 and then cross over to receive treatment A at period 2. We assume that there are no carry-over effects due to the treatment administered at an earlier period with an adequate washout period. If we cannot ensure with an adequate washout period this assumption of no carry-over effects to be satisfied on the basis of our subjective knowledge, as noted in Chapter 1, we may not want to consider use of the crossover design (Fleiss, 1986a, 1989; Senn, 2002). For patient i ($= 1, 2, \cdots, n_g$) assigned to group g ($= 1, 2$), let $Y_{iz}^{(g)}$ denote the patient response at period z ($= 1, 2$). We assume that $Y_{iz}^{(g)}$ can be expressed by the following random effects linear additive risk model (Grizzle, 1965):

$$Y_{iz}^{(g)} = \mu_i^{(g)} + \eta_{BA} X_{iz}^{(g)} + \gamma Z_{iz}^{(g)} + \varepsilon_{iz}^{(g)}, \tag{2.1}$$

where $\mu_i^{(g)}$ denotes the random effect due to the *ith* patient in group g and all $\mu_i^{(g)}$'s are assumed to independently follow an unspecified probability density function $f_g(\mu)$ with variance σ_μ^2; $X_{iz}^{(g)}$ denotes the treatment-received covariate for treatment B, and $X_{iz}^{(g)} = 1$ if the *ith* patient in group g at period z receives treatment B, and $= 0$ otherwise; $Z_{iz}^{(g)}$ represents the period covariate, and $Z_{iz}^{(g)} = 1$ for period $z = 2$, and $= 0$ otherwise; and random errors $\varepsilon_{iz}^{(g)}$'s are assumed to be independent and identically distributed as a continuous distribution with mean 0 and variance σ_e^2 and are assumed to be independent of all $\mu_i^{(g)}$'s. Parameters η_{BA} and γ in model (2.1) denote the difference in effects between treatments B and A, and that between periods 2 and 1, respectively. When the effects between treatments B and A on patient responses are equal, $\eta_{BA} = 0$. When the mean response of a patient receiving treatment B is larger than that of the patient receiving treatment A for given a fixed period, $\eta_{BA} > 0$. On the other hand, when the mean response of a patient receiving treatment B is smaller than that of the patient receiving treatment A for given a fixed period, $\eta_{BA} < 0$. Similar interpretations as those for η_{BA} are applicable to γ for the period effect. Under model (2.1), we can easily see that the covariance between $Y_{i1}^{(g)}$ and $Y_{i2}^{(g)}$ on a randomly selected patient i is $Cov\left(Y_{i1}^{(g)}, Y_{i2}^{(g)}\right) = Var\left(\mu_i^{(g)}\right) = \sigma_\mu^2 > 0$ (Problem 2.1), and thereby, $Y_{i1}^{(g)}$ and $Y_{i2}^{(g)}$ are positively correlated with the intraclass correlation $\rho = \sigma_\mu^2 / \sigma_t^2$, where $\sigma_t^2 = \sigma_\mu^2 + \sigma_e^2$. Thus, the larger the variation σ_μ^2 of responses between patients, the higher is the intraclass correlation between responses within patients.

For patient i ($= 1, 2, \cdots, n_g$) in group g ($= 1, 2$), we define $D_i^{(g)} = Y_{i2}^{(g)} - Y_{i1}^{(g)}$, representing the response difference between period 2 and period 1. Note that $D_i^{(g)}$ is no longer a function of random effects $\mu_i^{(g)}$'s under model (2.1). We define

$\bar{D}^{(g)} = \sum_{i=1}^{n_g} D_i^{(g)}/n_g$ as the average of response differences between two periods over patients in group g. We obtain an unbiased consistent estimator for η_{BA} under model (2.1) as (Problem 2.2):

$$\hat{\eta}_{BA} = \left(\bar{D}^{(1)} - \bar{D}^{(2)}\right)/2, \qquad (2.2)$$

and its variance:

$$Var(\hat{\eta}_{BA}) = \sigma_d^2(1/n_1 + 1/n_2)/4, \qquad (2.3)$$

where $\sigma_d^2 = Var\left(D_i^{(g)}\right) = 2\sigma_e^2$. Furthermore, we can estimate the variance σ_d^2 by the unbiased pooled-sample variance (Problem 2.3):

$$\hat{\sigma}_d^2 = \sum_{g=1}^{2}\sum_{i=1}^{n_g}\left(D_i^{(g)} - \bar{D}^{(g)}\right)^2/(n_+ - 2), \qquad (2.4)$$

where $n_+ = n_1 + n_2$ denotes the total number of patients in the trial. When substituting $\hat{\sigma}_d^2$ (2.4) for σ_d^2 in $Var(\hat{\eta}_{BA})$ (2.3), we obtain the variance estimator $\widehat{Var}(\hat{\eta}_{BA})$.

2.1   Testing non-equality of treatments

We are generally interested in finding out whether an experimental treatment is better than a placebo or a control treatment, but we may wish to do a two-sided test (rather than a one-sided test) to detect the case of whether the experimental treatment could be unexpectedly worse than the placebo for ethical and safety reason (Fleiss, 1981; Fleiss, Levin, and Paik, 2003). Thus, we consider testing the null hypothesis $H_0 : \eta_{BA} = 0$ versus the alternative hypothesis $H_a : \eta_{BA} \neq 0$. When random errors $\varepsilon_{iz}^{(g)}$'s under model (2.1) follow a normal distribution, we can use the t-test on the basis of $\hat{\eta}_{BA}$ (2.2) (Chassan, 1964; Fleiss, 1986a). We will reject H_0 at the α-level if

$$|\hat{\eta}_{BA}|/\sqrt{\widehat{var}(\hat{\eta}_{BA})} > t_{\alpha/2, n_+ - 2}, \qquad (2.5)$$

where $t_{\alpha, n_+ - 2}$ is the upper $100(\alpha)$th percentile of the student t-distribution with $n_+ - 2$ degrees of freedom.

If random errors $\varepsilon_{iz}^{(g)}$'s do not follow a normal distribution, we may still use the t-test, which is known to have some robustness properties, or we may employ the following Mann–Whitney–Wilcoxon rank sum test (Koch, 1972; Hollander and Wolfe, 1973; Cornell, 1980; Fleiss, 1986a; Jones and Kenward, 1989, 2014; Senn, 2002). We order the combined sample of $n_+ (= n_1 + n_2)$ observations $D_i^{(g)} \left(= Y_{i2}^{(g)} - Y_{i1}^{(g)}\right.$ for $g = 1, 2)$ obtained in the two groups from least to largest. Let R_i be the rank assigned to $D_i^{(1)}$ in the combined sample, and compute $W = \sum_{i=1}^{n_1} R_i$, the total of ranks assigned to group $g = 1$. We will reject $H_0 : \eta_{BA} = 0$ at the α-level if

$$|W - n_1(n_+ + 1)/2| / \sqrt{Var(W)} > Z_{\alpha/2}, \tag{2.6}$$

where $Var(W) = n_1 n_2 (n_+ + 1)/12$ and Z_α is the upper $100(\alpha)$th percentile of the standard normal distribution. When there are ties between values $D_i^{(g)}$ in the combined sample, we use the average ranks to compute $W\left(= \sum_{i=1}^{n_1} R_i\right)$ and replace $Var(W)$ in (2.6) by $Var(W) = n_1 n_2 (n_+ + 1)/12 \left\{ 1 - \sum_{i=1}^{q} t_i(t_i + 1)(t_i - 1) / [n_+ (n_+ - 1)(n_+ + 1)] \right\}$, where q is the number of tied groups and t_i is the size of the tied group (Hollander and Wolfe, 1973, p. 69). If n_1 and n_2 are small and the normal approximation for the test procedure (2.6) is not valid, we can do the exact test by using tables for the Mann–Whitney–Wilcoxon rank sum test statistic W (Hollander and Wolfe, 1973).

Example 2.1   Consider the data in Table 2.1 taken from a crossover trial studying two dose preparations of aspirin for their effects on gastric bleeding measured using a radioactive tagging method (Fleiss, 1986a, p. 266). When employing test statistics (2.5) and (2.6), we obtain the p-values 0.021 and 0.018, respectively. Because $\hat{\eta}_{BA} = -0.925 < 0$, there is significant evidence that the dose preparation A is associated with more gastric bleeding than the dose preparation B at the 5% level.

Example 2.2   Consider the data in Table 2.2 taken from a crossover trial comparing the effects of 12 µg formoterol (treatment B) with a single inhaled dose of 200 µg salbutamol (treatment A) on PEF (in liters per minute [l/m]) measured at 8 h after treatments on 13 children with moderate or severe asthma (Senn and Auclair, 1990, p. 1290; Senn, 2002, p. 36). When employing test statistics (2.5) and (2.6), we obtain the p-values 0.001 and 0.010. Because $\hat{\eta}_{BA} = 46.61$ (l/m) > 0, these small p-values suggest that there may be strong evidence that formoterol can increase PEF as compared with salbutamol.

2.2   Testing non-inferiority of an experimental treatment to an active control treatment

When treatment A represents an active control (or a standard) treatment, we may sometimes be satisfied if we can establish the non-inferiority of an experimental treatment B to the active control treatment A. This is true especially when the experimental treatment B has fewer side effects and less expense or is easier to administer than the control treatment A. Suppose that the higher the patient response, the better is the patient outcome. Thus, when assessing the non-inferiority of an experimental treatment B to a standard treatment A, we want to test $H_0 : \eta_{BA} \leq \eta_l$ versus $H_a : \eta_{BA} > \eta_l$, where η_l ($\eta_l < 0$) is the maximum clinically acceptable lower margin such that treatment B can be regarded as non-inferior to treatment A when $\eta_{BA} > \eta_l$ holds. The determination of the non-inferior margin is generally predetermined by clinicians based on their medical knowledge rather than by statisticians. When random errors $\varepsilon_{iz}^{(g)}$'s follow a normal distribution, we can use the t-test based on $\hat{\eta}_{BA}$ (2.2) and reject $H_0 : \eta_{BA} \leq \eta_l$ at the α-level if

$$(\hat{\eta}_{BA} - \eta_l) / \sqrt{\widehat{\mathrm{Var}}(\hat{\eta}_{BA})} > t_{\alpha, n_+ - 2}. \tag{2.7}$$

When random errors $\varepsilon_{iz}^{(g)}$'s do not follow a normal distribution but a nonskewed distribution, we may still use (2.7) due to the robustness of the t-test. In this case, we can also apply the following asymptotic distribution-free procedure to test non-inferiority with assuming n_1 and n_2 to be reasonably large (Hollander and Wolfe, 1973, pp. 75–79).

We define $U_{ij} = \left(D_i^{(1)} - D_j^{(2)} \right) / 2$ for $i = 1, 2, \ldots, n_1$ and $j = 1, 2, \ldots, n_2$. Let $U^{(1)} < U^{(2)} < \cdots < U^{(n_1 n_2)}$ be the ordered statistics of $n_1 n_2$ pairwise differences U_{ij}. We will reject the null hypothesis $H_0 : \eta_{BA} \leq \eta_l$ at the α-level if (Problem 2.4)

$$U^{(C_a)} - \eta_l > 0, \tag{2.8}$$

where $C_a \approx n_1 n_2 / 2 - Z_\alpha \sqrt{n_1 n_2 (n_+ + 1)/12}$. Note that when n_1 and n_2 are small, we can use the same idea and employ test procedure (2.8) with C_α calculated by using tables for the exact distribution of the Wilcoxon rank sum test (Hollander and Wolfe, 1973, p. 78).

2.3   Testing equivalence between an experimental treatment and an active control treatment

When an experimental treatment is much more effective than an active control treatment, the former may also be more toxic than the latter. If we have this concern, we may wish to consider testing equivalence rather than non-inferiority. That is, we want to test $H_0 : \eta_{BA} \leq \eta_l$ or $\eta_{BA} \geq \eta_u$ versus $H_a : \eta_l < \eta_{BA} < \eta_u$, where η_l ($\eta_l < 0$) and η_u ($\eta_u > 0$) are the maximum clinically acceptable lower and upper margins such that treatment B can be regarded as equivalent to treatment A when $\eta_l < \eta_{BA} < \eta_u$ holds (Hauck and Anderson, 1986). When random errors $\varepsilon_{iz}^{(g)}$'s follow the normal distribution, we employ the intersection-union test (Casella and Berger, 1990) and the t-test based on $\hat{\eta}_{BA}$ (2.2). We will reject $H_0 : \eta_{BA} \leq \eta_l$ or $\eta_{BA} \geq \eta_u$ at the α-level if

$$(\hat{\eta}_{BA} - \eta_l)/\sqrt{\widehat{Var}(\hat{\eta}_{BA})} > t_{\alpha, n_+ - 2}, \quad \text{and}$$

$$(\hat{\eta}_{BA} - \eta_u)/\sqrt{\widehat{var}(\hat{\eta}_{BA})} < -t_{\alpha, n_+ - 2}. \tag{2.9}$$

When random errors $\varepsilon_{iz}^{(g)}$'s do not follow the normal distribution, we may employ the above test procedure (2.9) as long as the underlying distribution for $\varepsilon_{iz}^{(g)}$ is not skewed. We may also use the following asymptotic distribution-free method (Hollander and Wolfe, 1973, pp. 75–79). We will reject $H_0 : \eta_{BA} \leq \eta_l$ or $\eta_{BA} \geq \eta_u$ at the α-level (Problem 2.5) if

$$U^{(C_\alpha)} - \eta_l > 0, \quad \text{and}$$

$$U^{(D_\alpha)} - \eta_u < 0, \tag{2.10}$$

where $C_\alpha \approx n_1 n_2/2 - Z_\alpha \sqrt{n_1 n_2 (n_+ + 1)/12}$ and $D_\alpha \approx n_1 n_2/2 + Z_\alpha \sqrt{n_1 n_2 (n_+ + 1)/12} + 1$.

2.4 Interval estimation of the mean difference

When assessing the magnitude of the mean difference between treatments B and A, we want to obtain an interval estimator of η_{BA}. When random errors $\varepsilon_{iz}^{(g)}$'s follow a normal distribution, we obtain a $100(1 - \alpha)\%$ confidence interval for η_{BA} on the basis of $\hat{\eta}_{BA}$ (2.2) and $\widehat{Var}(\hat{\eta}_{BA})$ as

$$\left[\hat{\eta}_{BA} - t_{\alpha/2, n_+ - 2} \sqrt{\widehat{Var}(\hat{\eta}_{BA})}, \ \hat{\eta}_{BA} + t_{\alpha/2, n_+ - 2} \sqrt{\widehat{Var}(\hat{\eta}_{BA})} \right]. \tag{2.11}$$

When $\varepsilon_{iz}^{(g)}$'s do not follow a normal distribution (but a nonskewed distribution), we may still use the interval estimator (2.11). We can also consider use of the Mann–Whitney–Wilcoxon distribution-free method (Hollander and Wolfe, 1973). The latter leads us to obtain an asymptotic $100(1 - \alpha)\%$ confidence interval as given by

$$\left[U^{(C_{\alpha/2})}, \ U^{(D_{\alpha/2})} \right], \tag{2.12}$$

where $C_{\alpha/2} \approx n_1 n_2/2 - Z_{\alpha/2} \sqrt{n_1 n_2 (n_+ + 1)/12}$ and $D_{\alpha/2} \approx n_1 n_2/2 + Z_{\alpha/2}$ $\sqrt{n_1 n_2 (n_+ + 1)/12} + 1$. Note that when n_1 and n_2 are small, we can use tables for the exact distribution of W (Hollander and Wolfe, 1973, p. 78) to calculate the exact $100(1 - \alpha)\%$ confidence interval for η_{BA} as well. Note also that procedure (2.9) for testing equivalence at the α-level is identical to what we claim as two treatments are equivalent if the resulting $100(1 - 2\alpha)\%$ confidence interval using the interval estimator (2.11) lies entirely in the acceptance interval (η_l, η_u). Similarly, use of procedure (2.10) for testing equivalence at the α-level is identical to what we claim as two treatments are equivalent if the asymptotic distribution-free $100(1 - 2\alpha)\%$ confidence interval $[U^{(C_a)}, U^{(D_a)}]$ (2.12) completely falls in (η_l, η_u).

Example 2.3   Consider the data in Table 2.2 comparing the effects of 12 μg formoterol (treatment B) with a single inhaled dose of 200 μg salbutamol (treatment A) on PEF of 13 children (Senn, 2002, p. 36). When employing the point estimator $\hat{\eta}_{BA}$ (2.2) and interval estimator (2.11), we obtain $\hat{\eta}_{BA} = 46.61$ (in l/m) and 95% confidence interval [22.89, 70.33]. Because the lower limit of this 95% confidence interval falls above 0, there is significant evidence that taking formoterol can increase, as compared with taking salbutamol, the PEF at the 5% level. This is certainly consistent with the previous finding based on hypothesis testing discussed in Example 2.2. Note that if we employ the distribution-free approach by using the Hodges–Lehmann estimator based on the median of $\left\{ U_{ij} \left(= \left(D_i^{(1)} - D_j^{(2)}\right) / 2 \right) | i = 1, 2, \cdots, n_1; \; j = 1, 2, \cdots, n_2 \right\}$ (Hollander and Wolfe, 1973, p. 75) to estimate η_{BA}, we obtain 45.0 (l/m). When employing interval estimator (2.12), we obtain the asymptotic 95% confidence interval for η_{BA} (in l/m) as [25, 75]. As shown here, these resulting point and interval estimates based on the distribution-free method are similar to those using $\hat{\eta}_{BA}$ (2.2) and interval estimator (2.11) based on the parametric approach.

When testing bioequivalence between different preparations of the same drug substance, we often compare treatments with respect to extent and rate of drug absorption (Hauschke, Steinijans, and Diletti, 1990). The area under the concentration time curve/ (AUC) generally serves as characteristic of the extent of absorption, while the time $t_{\max}$ to reach the maximum concentration $C_{\max}$ in fast-releasing formulations may serve as characteristic of the rate of absorption. In the case of controlled-release formulations, other pharmacokinetic characteristics such as plateau time may be more appropriate for the rate of absorption (Steinijans, 1989). Because the values of these characteristics are always positive and their sampling distributions are frequently skewed, we may wish to employ the logarithmic transformation. We assume that the patient response $Y_{iz}^{(g)}$ follows the following random effects exponential multiplicative risk model (Westlake, 1988):

$$Y_{iz}^{(g)} = \exp\left(\mu_i^{(g)} + \eta_{BA} X_{iz}^{(g)} + \gamma Z_{iz}^{(g)} + \varepsilon_{iz}^{(g)} \right), \tag{2.13}$$

where $\varepsilon_{iz}^{(g)}$'s are assumed to be independent and identically distributed as a normal distribution with mean 0 and variance σ_e^2 and to be independent of all random effects $\mu_i^{(g)}$'s. In this case, we may apply the above test procedures and interval estimators based on t-distribution on $\log\left(Y_{iz}^{(g)}\right)$ when studying the relative treatment effect η_{BA}. If random errors $\varepsilon_{iz}^{(g)}$'s do not follow a normal distribution, we can then employ the distribution-free method based on $\log\left(Y_{iz}^{(g)}\right)$ as done previously for hypothesis testing and interval estimation of η_{BA}. Because $\exp(x)$ is an increasing function of x, we can apply this exponential transformation to the resulting confidence limits for η_{BA} to obtain a confidence interval for $\exp(\eta_{BA})$ if the relative effect of treatment B to treatment A is of our interest.

Example 2.4   Consider the data in Table 2.3 taken from a crossover trial studying a dose equivalence of two preparations with one-week washout period between treatments (Steinijans *et al.*, 1989; Hauschke, Steinijans, and Diletti, 1990). Different capsule sizes of theophylline sustained-release pellets were compared in 18 healthy, normal male volunteers. The reference (R) treatment (corresponding to treatment A) consists of two capsules of 200 mg and two capsules of 300 mg theophylline, while the test (T) treatment (corresponding to treatment B) consists of two capsules of 500 mg theophylline. We summarize in Table 2.3 the bioavailability characteristic AUC of the 18 volunteers in the two groups with different treatment-receipt sequences (Hauschke, Steinijans, and Diletti, 1990). When applying the point estimator (2.2) and the interval estimator (2.11) to $\log\left(Y_{iz}^{(g)}\right)$ (instead of $Y_{iz}^{(g)}$) under model (2.13), we obtain $\exp(\hat{\eta}_{TR}) = 1.002$ and a 90% confidence interval for $\exp(\eta_{TR})$ as given by [0.925, 1.085]. Furthermore, when using the Hodges–Lehmann estimator based on the median of $\left\{U_{ij}|i=1,2\cdots n_1, j=1,2,\cdots n_2\right\}$ and the distribution-free interval estimator (2.12), we obtain 1.034 and a 90% confidence interval for $\exp(\eta_{TR})$ as [0.942, 1.097]. If we decide the acceptance interval to be (0.80, 1.25) for the ratio $\exp(\eta_{TR})$ of AUC between test and reference treatments, then we can claim that there is evidence at the 5% level that the test dose and reference preparations are equivalent. This is because both the above 90% confidence intervals fall entirely in the acceptance interval (0.80, 1.25).

Table 2.3   Bioavailability characteristic AUC taken from a crossover trial comparing test (T): 1,000 mg theophylline (2 × 500 mg) with reference (R): 1,000 mg theophylline (2 × 200 mg + 2 × 300 mg).

Group	Reference/test		Test/reference	
	Periods		Periods	
	I	II	I	II
	339.03	329.76	228.04	288.79
	242.64	258.19	288.21	343.37
	249.94	201.56	217.97	225.77
	184.32	249.64	133.13	235.89
	209.30	231.98	213.78	215.14
	207.40	234.19	248.98	245.48
	239.84	241.25	163.93	134.89
	211.24	255.60	245.92	223.39
	230.36	256.55	188.05	169.70

Note that we focus the above discussion on testing bioequivalence with respect to the average of patient responses between two treatments. When the variance of patient responses depends on the treatment-receipt, two treatments can be equivalent with respect to mean responses but have different variations of response distributions. This may motivate us to consider testing "individual bioequivalence" (Anderson and Hauck, 1990). For brevity, we do not discuss this topic further and refer readers to those publications with a focus on testing individual bioequivalence (Hauck and Anderson, 1991, 1992; Sheiner, 1992; Schall and Luus, 1993; Chow and Liu, 2009).

2.5   Sample size determination

To assure that we have a good opportunity to achieve the goal of our study, we need to recruit an adequate number of patients into a trial. Thus, it is of essential importance to determine the minimum required number of patients in the planning stage of a study design. For simplicity, we consider equal sample allocation (i.e., $n_1 = n_2$) and let n denote this common number of patients per group in the following discussion.

2.5.1   Sample size for testing non-equality

When the resulting estimate of the minimum required sample size n is large, we may approximate t-test (2.5) by z-test. This leads us to obtain an approximate minimum required number n of patients per group for a desired power $1-\beta$ of detecting non-equality with a given specified value $\eta_{BA} \neq 0$ of clinical interest at a nominal α-level as (Problem 2.6):

$$
\begin{aligned}
n &= Ceil\left\{ \left(Z_{\alpha/2} + Z_\beta\right)^2 \sigma_e^2 / \eta_{BA}^2 \right\}, \\
&= Ceil\left\{ \left(Z_{\alpha/2} + Z_\beta\right)^2 \sigma_t^2 (1-\rho) / \eta_{BA}^2 \right\},
\end{aligned}
\tag{2.14}
$$

where $Ceil\{x\}$ is the smallest integer $\geq x$ and $\sigma_t^2 = \sigma_\mu^2 + \sigma_e^2$. By contrast, an approximate minimum required number of patients per group for a desired power $1-\beta$ of detecting non-equality with a given specified value $\eta_{BA} \neq 0$ at a nominal α-level under the parallel groups design is given by

$$
n_{PAR} = Ceil\left\{ \left(Z_{\alpha/2} + Z_\beta\right)^2 2\sigma_t^2 / \eta_{BA}^2 \right\}.
\tag{2.15}
$$

Except for rounding errors, the proportional reduction of minimum required number of patients (PRMRS) using a crossover trial versus the parallel groups design on the basis of n (2.14) and n_{PAR} (2.15) is then (Problem 2.7)

$$
(n_{PAR} - n)/n_{PAR} = (1+\rho)/2,
\tag{2.16}
$$

which is an increasing function of the intraclass correlation ρ between responses within patients. In other words, the higher the intraclass correlation (or equivalently, the larger the variation of responses between patients), the larger is the proportional reduction of patients needed for a crossover trial versus a parallel groups design. Based on a report regarding an empirical comparison of the efficiency for the AB/BA design versus the corresponding parallel groups design (Garcia *et al.*, 2004) in real life, the estimate of the intraclass correlation ranged from approximately 13 to 85%. This would translate to the PRMRS being approximately from 57 to 93% by use of (2.16). When applying n (2.14) to calculate the minimum required sample size per group, we need to know the value for σ_e^2. Because $\sigma_d^2 = 2\sigma_e^2$, we can estimate σ_e^2 by $\hat{\sigma}_d^2/2$, where $\hat{\sigma}_d^2$ is given in (2.4) from a pilot study. On the other hand, note that $\sigma_e^2 = (1-\rho)\sigma_t^2$, where the total variance $\sigma_t^2 \left(= \sigma_\mu^2 + \sigma_e^2 \right)$ can usually be obtained from a parallel groups design. Thus, if we assign various possible values to ρ, we can obtain a range of the corresponding sample size estimates n (2.14) given a fixed σ_t^2. In practice, we can estimate the intraclass correlation ρ under the AB/BA crossover trial (Lui, 2015a). Note that because we use the t-test rather than the z-test in practice, the estimated n (2.14) may underestimate the minimum required sample size based on t-test. To alleviate this concern, we may apply an ad hoc arbitrary adjustment procedure by finding the appropriate percentiles $t_{\alpha/2,2(n-1)}$ and $t_{\beta,2(n-1)}$ with the resulting sample size estimate n (2.14) and recalculate n by substituting $(t_{\alpha/2,2(n-1)} + t_{\beta,2(n-1)})^2$ for $\left(Z_{\alpha/2} + Z_\beta\right)^2$ in (2.14).

2.5.2   Sample size for testing non-inferiority

Assuming that the resulting minimum required sample size n per group is so large that we can approximate the test procedure (2.7) by z-test, we may obtain an approximate minimum required number n of patients per group for a desired power $1-\beta$ of detecting non-inferiority with a specified value $\eta_{BA}(>\eta_l)$ at a nominal α-level as given by (Problem 2.8)

$$n = Ceil\left\{ \left(Z_\alpha + Z_\beta\right)^2 \sigma_e^2 / \left(\eta_{BA} - \eta_l\right)^2 \right\}$$
$$= Ceil\left\{ \left(Z_\alpha + Z_\beta\right)^2 \sigma_t^2 (1-\rho) / \left(\eta_{BA} - \eta_l\right)^2 \right\}. \tag{2.17}$$

In application of n (2.17), we may apply the same procedure as described in Section 2.5.1 for testing non-equality to determine values for σ_e^2. Furthermore, we may also apply the ad hoc arbitrary procedure, as noted previously, to adjust n (2.17), if we have the concern that n (2.17) may underestimate the minimum required sample size because we use the t-test rather than the z-test. We can also simply add one to the resulting n (2.17) by employing the adjustment procedure as suggested by Bristol (1993).

2.5.3   Sample size for testing equivalence

When the resulting minimum required sample size n per group is large, we may obtain the power function for testing equivalence based on the normal approximation of the test procedure (2.9) as (Problem 2.9)

$$
\begin{aligned}
\psi(\eta_{BA}) &= \Phi\left(\frac{\eta_u - \eta_{BA}}{\sqrt{\sigma_e^2/n}} - Z_\alpha\right) - \Phi\left(\frac{\eta_l - \eta_{BA}}{\sqrt{\sigma_e^2/n}} + Z_\alpha\right) \\
&= \Phi\left(\frac{\eta_u - \eta_{BA}}{\sqrt{\sigma_t^2(1-\rho)/n}} - Z_\alpha\right) - \Phi\left(\frac{\eta_l - \eta_{BA}}{\sqrt{\sigma_t^2(1-\rho)/n}} + Z_\alpha\right),
\end{aligned}
\tag{2.18}
$$

where $\eta_l < \eta_{BA} < \eta_u$ and $\Phi(X)$ is the cumulative standard normal distribution. On the basis of the power function $\psi(\eta_{BA})$ (2.18), we cannot find the closed-form formula in calculation of the approximate minimum required number n of patients per group such that $\psi(\eta_{BA}) \geq 1 - \beta$ unless we can make a good approximation of $\psi(\eta_{BA})$ (2.18) under certain assumptions and conditions. However, we can easily use the trial-and-error procedure to find the minimum required sample size by searching for the smallest positive integer n satisfying $\psi(\eta_{BA}) \geq 1 - \beta$.

If the resulting minimum required number of patients n per group is large, we can approximate the power function $\psi(\eta_{BA})$ (2.18) for $\eta_l < \eta_{BA} < 0$ by (Liu and Chow, 1992; Tu, 1998; Wang, Chow and Li, 2002)

$$
1 - \Phi\left(\frac{\eta_l - \eta_{BA}}{\sqrt{\sigma_e^2/n}} + Z_\alpha\right).
\tag{2.19}
$$

On the basis of (2.19), we may obtain an approximate minimum required number n of patients per group for the desired power $(1 - \beta)$ of detecting equivalence with a specified value for η_{BA} (where $\eta_l < \eta_{BA} < 0$) at a nominal α-level as

$$
\begin{aligned}
n &= Ceil\left\{(Z_\alpha + Z_\beta)^2 \sigma_e^2 / (\eta_l - \eta_{BA})^2\right\} \\
&= Ceil\left\{(Z_\alpha + Z_\beta)^2 \sigma_t^2 (1-\rho) / (\eta_l - \eta_{BA})^2\right\}.
\end{aligned}
\tag{2.20}
$$

On the other hand, when the number of patients assigned to both treatments is large and $0 < \eta_{BA} < \eta_u$, we can approximate the power function $\psi(\eta_{BA})$ (2.18) by

$$
\Phi\left(\frac{\eta_u - \eta_{BA}}{\sqrt{\sigma_e^2/n}} - Z_\alpha\right).
\tag{2.21}
$$

On the basis of (2.21) we may obtain an approximate minimum required number n of patients per group for a desired power $(1 - \beta)$ of detecting equivalence with a specified η_{BA} (where $0 < \eta_{BA} < \eta_u$) at a nominal α-level as

$$n = Ceil\left\{ (Z_\alpha + Z_\beta)^2 \sigma_e^2 / (\eta_u - \eta_{BA})^2 \right\}$$

$$= Ceil\left\{ (Z_\alpha + Z_\beta)^2 \sigma_t^2 (1-\rho) / (\eta_u - \eta_{BA})^2 \right\}.$$

(2.22)

When $\eta_{BA} = 0$, the power function $\psi(\eta_{BA})$ (2.18) simply reduces to

$$\psi(\eta_{BA} = 0) = \Phi\left(\frac{\eta_u}{\sqrt{\sigma_e^2/n}} - Z_\alpha \right) - \Phi\left(\frac{\eta_l}{\sqrt{\sigma_e^2/n}} + Z_\alpha \right).$$

(2.23)

When $\eta_l = -\eta_u$ (i.e., the acceptable range of equivalence is symmetric with respect to 0), we may obtain an approximate minimum required number n of patients per group for the desired power $(1 - \beta)$ of detecting equivalence with a specified value $\eta_{BA} = 0$ at a nominal α-level based on (2.23) as

$$n = Ceil\left\{ (Z_\alpha + Z_{\beta/2})^2 \sigma_e^2 / (\eta_u)^2 \right\}$$

$$= Ceil\left\{ (Z_\alpha + Z_{\beta/2})^2 \sigma_t^2 (1-\rho) / (\eta_u)^2 \right\}.$$

(2.24)

Note that when deriving n (2.20) or n (2.22), we need to assume that the approximations of the power function $\psi(\eta_{BA})$ (2.18) by (2.19) and (2.21) are accurate. When the predetermined equivalence margins η_l and η_u are far away from 0, or the underlying η_{BA} of interest is chosen to be in the neighborhood of 0, the resulting minimum required number of patients n may not be large enough to assure these approximations to be good. Because the power function (2.19) (or the power function (2.21)) is larger than $\psi(\eta_{BA})$ (2.18), using n (2.20) (or n (2.22)) tends to underestimate the minimum required number of patients per group. Thus, we may use n (2.20) (or n (2.22)) as the initial estimate and apply a trial-and-error procedure to find the minimum positive integer n such that $\psi(\eta_{BA}) \geq 1 - \beta$. The same ad hoc arbitrary adjustment procedure as described previously or the adjustment procedure suggested by Bristol (1993) can be used if we also have the concern about using the t-test (rather than the z-test) for testing equivalence in practice.

2.6 Hypothesis testing and estimation for the period effect

The period effect γ can sometimes be of interest in a crossover trial. If we wish to investigate the period effect γ, we can easily modify the above test procedures and estimators for studying the treatment effect to investigate the period effect. When estimating the period effect γ, we may consider use of the following unbiased estimator for γ (Problem 2.10):

$$\hat{\gamma} = \left(\bar{D}^{(1)} + \bar{D}^{(2)} \right)/2. \tag{2.25}$$

An estimated variance for $\hat{\gamma}$ is $\widehat{Var}(\hat{\gamma}) = \hat{\sigma}_d^2(1/n_1 + 1/n_2)/4$, which is actually the same as $\widehat{Var}(\hat{\eta}_{BA})$. For testing $H_0 : \gamma = 0$ versus $H_a : \gamma \neq 0$, we reject $H_0 : \gamma = 0$ at the α-level if

$$|\hat{\gamma}|/\sqrt{\widehat{var}(\hat{\gamma})} > t_{\alpha/2, n_+ - 2}. \tag{2.26}$$

If random errors $\varepsilon_{iz}^{(g)}$'s do not follow a normal distribution, we can still use the Mann–Whitney–Wilcoxon rank sum test as follows. We first order the combined sample of $n_+ (= n_1 + n_2)$ observations $\{D_i^{(1)}$ and $-D_j^{(2)} \mid i = 1, 2, \cdots, n_1, j = 1, 2, \cdots, n_2\}$ from least to largest. We let R_i^* be the rank assigned to $D_i^{(1)}$ in the combined sample and compute $W^* = \sum_{i=1}^{n_1} R_i^*$, the total of ranks assigned to group $g = 1$. We will reject $H_0 :$ $\gamma = 0$ at the α-level if

$$|W^* - n_1(n_+ + 1)/2|/\sqrt{Var(W^*)} > Z_{\alpha/2}, \tag{2.27}$$

where $Var(W^*) = n_1 n_2(n_+ + 1)/12$. When there are ties between observations, we use the average ranks of tied observations in the combined sample to compute $W^* = \sum_{i=1}^{n_1} R_i^*$ and replace $Var(W^*)$ in (2.27) by

$$Var(W^*) = n_1 n_2(n_+ + 1)/12 \left\{ 1 - \sum_{i=1}^{q^*} t_i^* \left(t_i^* + 1 \right) \left(t_i^* - 1 \right) / [n_+ (n_+ - 1)(n_+ + 1)] \right\},$$

where q^* is the number of tied groups and t_i^* is the size of the tied group (Hollander and Wolfe, 1973, p. 69). Using similar ideas as those for studying the treatment effect, we can derive interval estimators for γ on the basis of t-distribution and the Mann–Whitney–Wilcoxon rank sum statistic.

Example 2.5   Consider the data in Table 2.2 comparing the effects of 12 μg formo-terol with a single inhaled dose of 200 μg salbutamol on PEF in 13 children consid-ered in Examples 2.2 and 2.3. When employing the test procedure (2.26), we obtain the p-value 0.168; there is no significant evidence that the period effect is different from 0 at the 5% level. When using the point estimator $\hat{\gamma}$ (2.25) and $\widehat{Var}(\hat{\gamma}) \left(= \hat{\sigma}_d^2(1/n_1 + 1/n_2)/4 \right)$, we obtain $\hat{\gamma} = 15.893$ (l/m) and the 95% confidence interval [−7.826 l/m, 39.612 l/m]. Thus, there is a tendency that the PEF tends to be larger at the second period than at the first period, but this increase is not significant at the 5% level. As noted by Senn (2002, pp. 51, 89), however, no statistical signif-icance does not constitute a reason for determining that we should not adjust the period effect in a crossover trial.

2.7 Estimation of the relative treatment effect in the presence of differential carry-over effects

We shall not employ, as noted previously, a crossover trial if we cannot assure that there are no carry-over effects with an adequate washout period. We include this section only for readers' information if readers should unexpectedly encounter carry-over effects suggested by internal evidence post–data collection. To avoid the concern of inflating Type I error in application of the commonly used two-stage test procedure (Freeman, 1989), we should not apply the two-stage test procedure (Grizzle, 1965) to determine whether we should adjust these carry-over effects in data analysis.

For patient i ($= 1, 2, \ldots, n_g$) assigned to group g ($= 1, 2$), we extend model (2.1) to include carry-over effects by assuming the patient response $Y_{iz}^{(g)}$ as given by (Grizzle, 1965)

$$Y_{iz}^{(g)} = \mu_i^{(g)} + \eta_{BA} X_{iz}^{(g)} + \gamma Z_{iz}^{(g)} + \lambda_A I_{\{g=1\}} Z_{iz}^{(g)} + \lambda_B \left(1 - I_{\{g=1\}}\right) Z_{iz}^{(g)} + \varepsilon_{iz}^{(g)}, \qquad (2.28)$$

where $I_{\{g=1\}} = 1$ for group $g = 1$, and $= 0$ otherwise; λ_A and λ_B are the carry-over effects due to treatments A and B, respectively; $E\left(\mu_i^{(1)}\right) = E\left(\mu_i^{(2)}\right)$ due to randomization; and other parameters and covariates are defined exactly as those in model (2.1). We can show that (Problem 2.12) the expectation of $\hat{\eta}_{BA}$ (2.2) under model (2.28) is

$$E(\hat{\eta}_{BA}) = \eta_{BA} + (\lambda_A - \lambda_B)/2. \qquad (2.29)$$

Thus, $\hat{\eta}_{BA}$ is no longer an unbiased estimator of η_{BA} unless $\lambda_A = \lambda_B$.

We define $S_i^{(g)} = Y_{i2}^{(g)} + Y_{i1}^{(g)}$, representing the sum of responses over the two periods for each patient. We further define $\bar{S}^{(g)} = \sum_{i=1}^{n_g} S_i^{(g)}/n_g$ for $g = 1, 2$. Under model (2.28), we can show that the expectation of $\bar{S}^{(1)} - \bar{S}^{(2)}$ is (Problem 2.13)

$$E\left(\bar{S}^{(1)} - \bar{S}^{(2)}\right) = \lambda_A - \lambda_B. \qquad (2.30)$$

The variance of $\bar{S}^{(1)} - \bar{S}^{(2)}$ is given by

$$Var\left(\bar{S}^{(1)} - \bar{S}^{(2)}\right) = \sigma_s^2(1/n_1 + 1/n_2), \qquad (2.31)$$

where $\sigma_s^2 = \left(4\sigma_\mu^2 + 2\sigma_e^2\right)$. We can estimate the variance σ_s^2 by the unbiased pooled-sample variance:

$$\hat{\sigma}_s^2 = \sum_{g=1}^{2} \sum_{i=1}^{n_g} \left(S_i^{(g)} - \bar{S}^{(g)}\right)^2/(n_+ - 2). \qquad (2.32)$$

Therefore, when substituting $\hat{\sigma}_s^2$ (2.32) for σ_s^2 in $Var\left(\bar{S}^{(1)} - \bar{S}^{(2)}\right)$ (2.31), we obtain the variance estimator $\widehat{Var}\left(\bar{S}^{(1)} - \bar{S}^{(2)}\right)$. When testing $H_0 : \lambda_A = \lambda_B$ versus $H_a : \lambda_A \neq \lambda_B$ on the basis of (2.30)–(2.32), we will reject $H_0 : \lambda_A = \lambda_B$ at the α-level if

$$|\bar{S}^{(1)} - \bar{S}^{(2)}| / \sqrt{\widehat{Var}\left(\bar{S}^{(1)} - \bar{S}^{(2)}\right)} > t_{\alpha/2, n_+ - 2}. \tag{2.33}$$

Note that we need to assume the random effects $\mu_i^{(g)}$'s to follow a normal distribution here in order to assure the above test procedure (2.33) to be exact. Note also that the test procedure (2.33) is expected to lack power, because $Var\left(\bar{S}^{(1)} - \bar{S}^{(2)}\right)$ $\left(= \sigma_s^2(1/n_1 + 1/n_2), \text{ where } \sigma_s^2 = \left(4\sigma_\mu^2 + 2\sigma_e^2\right)\right)$ can be quite large when the variation σ_μ^2 of responses between patients is large. Note further that since $\bar{S}^{(1)} - \bar{S}^{(2)}$ is an unbiased estimator for $\lambda_A - \lambda_B$, we may consider adjusting the bias of $\hat{\eta}_{BA}$ given in (2.29) by using the following unbiased estimator for η_{BA} under model (2.28) as

$$\hat{\eta}_{BA}^* = \hat{\eta}_{BA} - \left(\bar{S}^{(1)} - \bar{S}^{(2)}\right)/2, \tag{2.34}$$

which can be shown to actually equal $\bar{Y}_{+1}^{(2)} - \bar{Y}_{+1}^{(1)}$ (Problem 2.14). In other words, if there are differential carry-over effects, we will do data analysis using only the data at period 1 and ignore all data at period 2. Using the crossover design in this case will not help us gain any efficiency as compared with the parallel groups design. Conversely, as noted in Chapter 1, the power of the crossover design can be even less than that of the corresponding parallel groups design for a given fixed budget. This is because we could employ the resources for getting the information on patient responses at period 2 in a crossover design to recruit more patients if we originally employed the parallel groups design in the beginning of a trial.

2.8   Examples of SAS programs and results

Note that all procedures and formulas presented in this chapter are in simple closed forms. Thus, we can easily use a hand pocket calculator or write our own programs when using these formulas to do hypothesis testing and obtain parameter estimates. We can also apply the SAS packages to carry out the task of calculations. Under model (2.1), we assume that patient effects $\mu_i^{(g)}$'s are random rather than fixed. When estimating the relative treatment effect η_{BA}, we use the difference $D_i^{(g)}$, which does not depend on $\mu_i^{(g)}$. Thus, it does not usually matter whether $\mu_i^{(g)}$ is regarded as random or fixed if our focus is to estimate the relative treatment effect under model (2.1) with no missing data.

When the patient effect $\mu_i^{(g)}$ is regarded as fixed, we may use the following SAS codes to obtain estimates for the relative treatment effect of two dose preparations of aspirin on gastric bleeding and the relative effect between periods, as well as test results regarding whether these effects are different from 0 based on the data in Table 2.1. Note that the two dose preparations A and B are coded as treatments 1 and 2, respectively.

```
data step1;
input patient treatment period resp;
cards;
   1   1   1 5.1
   1   2   2 3.8
   2   1   1 0.6
   2   2   2 1.0
...
;;;
proc mixed data = step1;
   class patient period treatment;
   model resp = patient period treatment/solution;
run;
```

We present, for example, the outputs for testing non-equality of the two periods and of the two treatments in the following box. We see that p-values for testing these effect differences are 0.1368 and 0.0212, respectively.

Effect	DF	DF	F Value	Pr > F
patient	15	14	3.94	0.0071
period	1	14	2.49	0.1368
treatment	1	14	6.74	0.0212

When the patient effect $\mu_i^{(g)}$ is regarded as random, we can use the following SAS codes to obtain estimates for the relative treatment and period effects, as well as the p-value for testing differential carry-over effects using the data in Table 2.1.

```
data step1;
input patient treatment period resp group;
cards;
   1   1   1 5.1   1
   1   2   2 3.8   1
   2   1   1 0.6   1
   2   2   2 1.0   1
```

```
. . .
;;;
proc mixed data = step1;
  class group patient period treatment;
  model resp = group period treatment/solution;
    random patient (group);
run;
```

For brevity, we present only a partial output of the results in the following box.

Solution for Fixed Effects

Effect	group	period	treatment	Estimate	Standard Error	DF	t Value	Pr > |t|
Intercept				2.3250	0.5657	14	4.11	0.0011
group	1			0.5625	0.7163	14	0.79	0.4454
group	2			0	.	.	.	.
period		1		0.5625	0.3564	14	1.58	0.1368
period		2		0	.	.	.	.
treatment			1	0.9250	0.3564	14	2.60	0.0212
treatment			2	0	.	.	.	.

Type 3 Tests of Fixed Effects

Effect	Num DF	Den DF	F Value	Pr > F
group	1	14	0.62	0.4454
period	1	14	2.49	0.1368
treatment	1	14	6.74	0.0212

Note that SAS treats period 2 and treatment B as references (coded 0 as shown in the above output). Thus, the estimates of the mean response differences for period 2 versus period 1 and for treatment B versus treatment A are $\hat{\gamma} = -0.5625 \ (= 0 - 0.5625)$ and $\hat{\eta}_{BA} = -0.9250 \ (= 0 - 0.925)$, respectively. However, these different coding schemes do not affect the p-values for testing non-equality of two-period or testing non-equality of two treatments, because we consider a two-sided test here. We note that p-values 0.1368 and 0.0212 obtained under the random effects model are identical to those obtained under the fixed effects model. We also note that the p-value for testing whether there are differential carry-over effects is 0.4454. Thus, we have no significant evidence that there are differential carry-over effects, although this test should not be used to justify the assumption that there are no differential carry-over effects (Senn, 2002).

Similarly, we can apply the following SAS codes to the data in Table 2.2 regarding the PEF between salbutamol (coded as treatment 1) and formoterol (coded as treatment 2) when the patient effects are regarded as random.

```
data step1;
input patient treatment period resp group;
cards;
   1   1   1 370   1
   1   2   2 385   1
   2   1   1 310   1
   2   2   2 400   1

   . . .
  15   2   1 330   2
  15   1   2 365   2
;;;
proc mixed data = step1;
   class patient period treatment group;
   model resp = group period treatment/solution;
   random patient(group);
run;
```

Again, for brevity we present only a partial output in the following box.

Effect	period	treatment	group	Estimate	Standard Error	DF	t Value	Pr > |t|
Intercept				353.04	28.4341	11	12.42	<.0001
group			1	-7.2024	40.2026	11	-0.18	0.8611
group			2	0	.	.	.	.
period	1			-15.8929	10.7766	11	-1.47	0.1683
period	2			0	.	.	.	.
treatment		1		-46.6071	10.7766	11	-4.32	0.0012
treatment		2		0				

```
                  Type 3  Tests of Fixed Effects

                       Num  Den
           Effect       DF   DF   F Value    Pr > F

           group        1    11    0.03      0.8611
           period       1    11    2.17      0.1683
           treatment    1    11   18.70      0.0012
      ~

      ~    .      .       .       .
```

For example, the p-value for testing non-equality between salbutamol and formoterol under the assumption of no carry-over effects is 0.0012. Thus, there is significant evidence that formoterol can increase the PEF as compared with salbutamol. On the other hand, the p-value for testing non-equality of two periods under the assumption of no carry-over effects is, as found in Example 2.5, 0.168. This suggests that the difference in period effects is not significant at the 0.05 level, though the patient response at period 2 is likely larger than that at period 1. Note that one can also apply PROC GLIMMIX in the SAS software (SAS Institute, 2009) to analyze the data for a crossover design when patient effects are treated as random. To illustrate the use of this program, we present under the assumption of no carry-over effects the following SAS codes of PROC GLIMMIX to analyze, for example, the data in Table 2.2.

```
data step1;
ls = 80;
input patient treatment period resp group;
cards;
   1   1   1 370   1
   1   2   2 385   1
   2   1   1 310   1
   2   2   2 400   1
 . . .
  15   2   1 330   2
  15   1   2 365   2
;;;;
proc glimmix data = step1;
   class patient period treatment group;
   model resp = period treatment/solution
                    dist = normal link = id;
   random intercept/subject = patient;
```

```
    estimate "treatment effect" treatment -1 1;
    estimate "period effect" period -1 1;
run;
```

Because the outputs for using PROC GLIMMIX are essentially identical to those for using PROC MIXED, we do not include these results. Note that a discussion on how to use PROC GLIMMIX to adjust for differential carry-over effects can be found elsewhere (Jones and Kenward, 2014, p. 192).

Exercises

Problem 2.1.   Show that the covariance between $Y_{i1}^{(g)}$ and $Y_{i2}^{(g)}$ under model (2.1) is $Cov\left(Y_{i1}^{(g)}, Y_{i2}^{(g)}\right) = Var\left(\mu_i^{(g)}\right) = \sigma_\mu^2 > 0$ and hence the correlation between $Y_{i1}^{(g)}$ and $Y_{i2}^{(g)}$ is $\rho = \sigma_\mu^2 / \left(\sigma_e^2 + \sigma_\mu^2\right)$.

Problem 2.2.   Show that $\hat\eta_{BA} = \left(\bar{D}^{(1)} - \bar{D}^{(2)}\right)/2$ is an unbiased estimator for η_{BA} under model (2.1) and has variance $Var(\hat\eta_{BA}) = \sigma_d^2(1/n_1 + 1/n_2)/4$, where $\sigma_d^2 = 2\sigma_e^2$.

Problem 2.3.   Show   that   the   pooled-sample   variance $\hat\sigma_d^2 = \sum_{g=1}^{2}\sum_{i=1}^{n_g}\left(D_i^{(g)} - \bar{D}^{(g)}\right)^2/(n_+ - 2)$ is   an   unbiased   estimator   for σ_d^2,   where $n_+ = n_1 + n_2$.

Problem 2.4.   Show that Type I error for the test procedure in which we reject $H_0 : \eta_{BA} \le \eta_l$ if $U^{(C_\alpha)} - \eta_l > 0$, where $C_\alpha \approx n_1 n_2/2 - Z_\alpha\sqrt{n_1 n_2(n_+ + 1)/12}$, is approximately equal to α-level.

Problem 2.5.   Show that Type I error for the test procedure in which we reject $H_0 : \eta_{BA} \le \eta_l$ or $\eta_{BA} \ge \eta_u$ if $U^{(C_\alpha)} - \eta_l > 0$ and $U^{(D_\alpha)} - \eta_u < 0$,   where $C_\alpha \approx n_1 n_2/2 - Z_\alpha\sqrt{n_1 n_2(n_+ + 1)/12}$ and $D_\alpha \approx n_1 n_2/2 + Z_\alpha\sqrt{n_1 n_2(n_+ + 1)/12} + 1$,   is approximately equal to α-level.

Problem 2.6.   Assume that the resulting sample size n is so large that we can approximate t-test by z-test using the test procedure (2.5). Show that the approximate minimum required number of patients per group for a desired power $1 - \beta$ of detecting non-equality with a specified value $\eta_{BA} \ne 0$ at a nominal α-level is given by $n = Ceil\left\{\left(Z_{\alpha/2} + Z_\beta\right)^2 \sigma_e^2/\eta_{BA}^2\right\}$, where $Ceil\{x\}$ is the smallest integer $\ge x$.

Problem 2.7.   Except rounding errors, show that the proportional reduction of the minimum required sample size n (2.14) for a crossover trial versus that of n_{PAR} (2.15) for a parallel groups design is $(n_{PAR} - n)/n_{PAR} = (1 + \rho)/2$, where $\rho = \sigma_\mu^2/\sigma_t^2$.

Problem 2.8. Show that the approximate minimum required number n of patients per group for a desired power $1-\beta$ of detecting non-inferiority with a specified value $\eta_{BA}(>\eta_l)$ at a nominal α-level is given by $n = Ceil\left\{ (Z_\alpha + Z_\beta)^2 \sigma_e^2 / (\eta_{BA} - \eta_l)^2 \right\}$.

Problem 2.9. When the estimate of the minimum required sample size n per group is large, show that the power function for testing equivalence based on the test procedure (2.9) and the normal approximation is given by

$$\psi(\eta_{BA}) = \Phi\left(\frac{\eta_u - \eta_{BA}}{\sqrt{\sigma_e^2/n}} - Z_\alpha \right) - \Phi\left(\frac{\eta_l - \eta_{BA}}{\sqrt{\sigma_e^2/n}} + Z_\alpha \right),$$

where $\eta_l < \eta_{BA} < \eta_u$ and $\Phi(X)$ is the cumulative standard normal distribution.

Problem 2.10. Show that an unbiased estimator for γ is given by $\hat{\gamma} = \left(\bar{D}^{(1)} + \bar{D}^{(2)} \right)/2$ with an estimated variance $\widehat{Var}(\hat{\gamma}) = \hat{\sigma}_d^2(1/n_1 + 1/n_2)/4$.

Problem 2.11. Suppose that we employ a simple linear regression $Y_i = a + bx_i + \varepsilon_i$, where ε_i is independent and identically distributed as a normal distribution with mean 0 and variance σ^2 on the data $\{(x_i, Y_i) = (1, D_1^{(1)}/2), (1, D_2^{(1)}/2), \ldots, (1, D_{n_1}^{(1)}/2),$ $(0, D_1^{(2)}/2), (0, D_2^{(2)}/2), \ldots, (0, D_{n_2}^{(2)}/2)\}$. Show that the least-squared estimator for the slope b is $\hat{b} = \left(\bar{D}^{(1)} - \bar{D}^{(2)} \right)/2$, the uniformly minimum variance unbiased estimator (UMVUE) for σ^2 is $\hat{\sigma}^2 = \hat{\sigma}_d^2/4$, as well as $\widehat{Var}(\hat{b}) = \hat{\sigma}^2 / \sum_i (x_i - \bar{x})^2 = \hat{\sigma}_d^2(1/n_1 + 1/n_2)/4$. Thus, we can apply a linear regression analysis to test whether the slope equals 0 when testing non-equality of two treatments (Senn, 2002, p. 47).

Problem 2.12. Show that the expectation of $\hat{\eta}_{BA}$ (2.2) under model (2.28) is

$$E(\hat{\eta}_{BA}) = \eta_{BA} + (\lambda_A - \lambda_B)/2.$$

Problem 2.13. Show that the expectation of $\bar{S}^{(1)} - \bar{S}^{(2)}$ under model (2.28) is

$$E\left(\bar{S}^{(1)} - \bar{S}^{(2)} \right) = \lambda_A - \lambda_B.$$

Problem 2.14. Show that the estimator $\hat{\eta}_{BA}^* = \hat{\eta}_{BA} - (\bar{S}^{(1)} - \bar{S}^{(2)})/2$ is identical to the estimator $\bar{Y}_{+1}^{(2)} - \bar{Y}_{+1}^{(1)}$.

Problem 2.15. Show that we can estimate the total variance $\sigma_t^2 \left(= \sigma_\mu^2 + \sigma_e^2 \right)$ by the unbiased estimator $\hat{\sigma}_t^2 = \left(\hat{\sigma}_s^2 + \hat{\sigma}_d^2 \right)/4$, where $\hat{\sigma}_s^2$ is given by (2.32).

Problem 2.16.   Under the assumption that $\mu_i^{(g)}$'s and $\varepsilon_{iz}^{(g)}$'s are all mutually independent and normally distributed, show that (a) $D_i^{(g)} \left(= Y_{i2}^{(g)} - Y_{i1}^{(g)} \right)$ and $S_i^{(g)}$ $\left(= Y_{i2}^{(g)} + Y_{i1}^{(g)} \right)$ are mutually independent and have the variances $\sigma_d^2 = 2\sigma_e^2$ and $\sigma_s^2 = 4\sigma_\mu^2 + 2\sigma_e^2$, respectively. (b) Show that the intraclass correlation between responses $Y_{i1}^{(g)}$ and $Y_{i2}^{(g)}$ can be re-expressed as $\rho = 1 - 2\sigma_d^2 / \left(\sigma_s^2 + \sigma_d^2 \right)$. Thus, we can estimate the intraclass correlation by $\hat{\rho} = 1 - 2\hat{\sigma}_d^2 / \left(\hat{\sigma}_s^2 + \hat{\sigma}_d^2 \right)$, where $\hat{\sigma}_d^2$ and $\hat{\sigma}_s^2$ are given by (2.4) and (2.32), respectively. (c) Show that we can obtain an exact $100(1 - \alpha)\%$ confidence interval for the ratio $R = \sigma_d^2 / \sigma_s^2$ (< 1) as given by $[R_l, R_u]$, where $R_l = \left(\hat{\sigma}_d^2 / \hat{\sigma}_s^2 \right) \left(1 / F_{\alpha/2, n_+ - 2, n_+ - 2} \right)$, $R_u = \min \{ \left(\hat{\sigma}_d^2 / \hat{\sigma}_s^2 \right) \left(1 / F_{1 - \alpha/2, n_+ - 2, n_+ - 2} \right), 1 \}$, $\min\{a, b\}$ denotes the smaller number of a and b; and F_{α, df_1, df_2} is the upper $100(\alpha)$th percentile of the central F-distribution with df_1 and df_2 degrees of freedom. (d) Note that $f(R) = \rho$, where $f(x) = 1 - 2x / (1 + x)$ is a decreasing function of x. Thus, we may obtain the exact $100(1 - \alpha)\%$ confidence interval for ρ as given by $[1 - 2R_u / (1 + R_u), 1 - 2R_l / (1 + R_l)]$ (Lui, 2015a).

Problem 2.17.   The following random effects linear additive risk model is assumed elsewhere (Jones and Kenward, 1989; Senn, 2002) for the AB/BA crossover trial:

$$Y_{i1}^{(1)} = \alpha_i^{(1)} + \pi_1 + \tau_1 + \varepsilon_{i1}^{(1)},$$

$$Y_{i2}^{(1)} = \alpha_i^{(1)} + \pi_2 + \tau_2 + \varepsilon_{i2}^{(1)},$$

$$Y_{i1}^{(2)} = \alpha_i^{(2)} + \pi_1 + \tau_2 + \varepsilon_{i1}^{(2)}, \quad \text{and}$$

$$Y_{i2}^{(2)} = \alpha_i^{(2)} + \pi_2 + \tau_1 + \varepsilon_{i2}^{(2)},$$

where $\alpha_i^{(g)}$'s denote the random effects due to the underlying characteristics of patient i assigned to group g; π_z ($z = 1, 2$) denotes the period effect z; and τ_i (for $i = 1, 2$) denotes the effect (for treatments A and B) and where $\pi_1 + \pi_2 = 0$ and $\tau_1 + \tau_2 = 0$. Show that the above model is equivalent to model (2.1) (Lui, 2015a).

3

AB/BA design in dichotomous data

In a randomized clinical trial (RCT), we frequently encounter the patient outcome or clinical endpoint of interest on a dichotomous scale – positive/negative or improvement/no improvement. For example, when we compared treatments for the relief of primary dysmenorrhea, each patient rated the treatment as giving relief or no relief (Jones and Kenward, 1989). The common assumption of normal distribution for continuous data is obviously not satisfied when the underlying patient response is binary (= 1 or 0). Although one can apply the linear additive risk model (Grizzle, 1965) to the marginal probabilities of dichotomous responses (Zimmermann and Rahlfs, 1978), because a probability must fall between 0 and 1, we need to implicitly put parameter constraints in use for the linear additive risk model. Furthermore, it is unlikely that the treatment and period effects are additive on the probability of patient responses in most situations in practice. To alleviate these concerns, the logistic regression is probably the most commonly used model (Gart, 1969, 1970; Cox and Snell, 1989; Agresti, 1990; Hosmer and Lemeshow, 2000) for dichotomous data.

In this chapter, we assume a random effects logistic regression model but do not require random effects to follow any specified parametric distribution (Lui and Chang, 2011), such as the normal distribution, as frequently done elsewhere (Ezzet and Whitehead, 1992). Based on the conditional approach, we provide asymptotic and exact procedures for testing non-equality of two treatments. We give procedures for testing non-inferiority and equivalence with respect to the odds ratio (OR) recommended by Garrett (2003). We address interval estimation of the OR and sample size determination for testing non-equality, non-inferiority, and equivalence. We discuss hypothesis testing and estimation for the period effect. In the

Crossover Designs: Testing, Estimation, and Sample Size, First Edition. Kung-Jong Lui.
© 2016 John Wiley & Sons, Ltd. Published 2016 by John Wiley & Sons, Ltd.
Companion website: www.wiley.com/go/lui/crossover

Table 3.1   The observed frequencies of patients with dichotomous response (success, failure) taken from a simple crossover trial comparing the treatment of 200 μg salbutamol solution aerosol (drug A) with the treatment of 12 μg formoterol solution aerosol (drug B).

		Group I (A-then-B drug sequence)		
			Period II	
		Success	Failure	Total
Period I	Success	5	1	6
	Failure	6	0	6
	Total	11	1	`12

		Group II (B-then-A drug sequence)		
			Period II	
		Success	Failure	Total
Period I	Success	2	9	11
	Failure	0	1	1
	Total	2	10	`12

presence of unexpected carry-over effects, we discuss in exercises estimation of the relative treatment effect with adjustment of the bias due to carry-over effects. We include SAS codes by applying PROC NLMIXED and PROC GLIMMIX to analyze the data in Table 3.1 when assuming normal random effects (Ezzet and Whitehead, 1992), and we compare the test results with those obtained by use of the conditional approach focused on here.

Consider comparing an experimental treatment B with an active control treatment (or a placebo) A. Suppose that we randomly assign n_1 patients to group ($g =$) 1 with A-then-B sequence, in which patients receive treatment A at period 1 and then cross over to receive treatment B at period 2, and n_2 patients to group ($g =$) 2 with B-then-A sequence, in which patients receive treatment B at period 1 and then cross over to receive treatment A at period 2. With an adequate washout period, we assume that there are no carry-over effects due to treatments administered at period 1. If the assumption of no carry-over effects cannot be ensured on the basis of our subjective knowledge, we will not recommend use of the crossover design (Fleiss, 1986a, p. 270; Senn, 2002; Schouten and Kester, 2010). For patient i (= 1, 2, $\cdots$, n_g) assigned to group g (= 1, 2), let $Y_{iz}^{(g)}$ denote the response of the patient at period z (= 1, 2), and $Y_{iz}^{(g)} = 1$ if the patient has the positive response of interest, and = 0 otherwise. Let $X_{iz}^{(g)}$ denote the treatment-received covariate for the corresponding patient at period z, and $X_{iz}^{(g)} = 1$ if the patient receives treatment B, and = 0 otherwise. Further-more, let $Z_{iz}^{(g)}$ denote the period covariate, and $Z_{iz}^{(g)} = 1$ for period (z =) 2, and = 0 otherwise. Following Ezzet and Whitehead (1992), we assume that the probability of a positive response for patient i ($= 1, 2, \cdots, n_g$) assigned to group g ($= 1, 2$) at period z ($= 1, 2$) is given by the following random effects logistic regression model (Cox and Snell, 1989):

$$P\left(Y_{iz}^{(g)} = 1\right) = \frac{\exp\left(\mu_i^{(g)} + \eta_{BA}X_{iz}^{(g)} + \gamma Z_{iz}^{(g)}\right)}{1 + \exp\left(\mu_i^{(g)} + \eta_{BA}X_{iz}^{(g)} + \gamma Z_{iz}^{(g)}\right)}, \qquad (3.1)$$

where $\mu_i^{(g)}$ denotes the random effect due to the ith patient in group g and $\mu_i^{(g)}$'s are assumed to independently follow an unspecified probability density function $f_g(\mu)$, η_{BA} denotes the effect of treatment B relative to treatment A (or placebo), and γ denotes the effect of period 2 relative to period 1. On the basis of model (3.1), the OR of a positive response for a fixed period on a given patient between treatment B and treatment A is simply equal to $\varphi_{BA} = \exp(\eta_{BA})$. When the effects between treatments B and A are equal, $\varphi_{BA} = 1$ (or $\eta_{BA} = 0$). When treatment B increases the probability of a positive response as compared with treatment A, $\varphi_{BA} > 1$ (or $\eta_{BA} > 0$). On the other hand, when treatment B decreases the probability of a positive response as compared with treatment A, $\varphi_{BA} < 1$ (or $\eta_{BA} < 0$). Let $n_{rc}^{(g)}$ denote the number of patients among n_g patients in group g ($= 1, 2$) with the response vector ($Y_{i1}^{(g)} = r$, $Y_{i2}^{(g)} = c$), where $r = 1, 0$ and $c = 1, 0$. The random frequencies $\{n_{rc}^{(g)} | r = 1, 0, c = 1, 0\}$ then follow the quadrinomial distribution with parameters n_g and $\{\pi_{rc}^{(g)} | r = 1, 0, c = 1, 0\}$, where $\pi_{rc}^{(g)}$ denotes the cell probability that a randomly selected patient from group g has the bivariate response vector ($Y_{i1}^{(g)} = r$, $Y_{i2}^{(g)} = c$). For example, the parameter $\pi_{10}^{(g)}$ denotes the cell probability that a randomly selected patient from group g ($= 1, 2$) has a positive response at period 1 and a negative response at period 2. Similarly, the parameter $\pi_{01}^{(g)}$ denotes the cell probability that a randomly selected patient from group g has a negative response at period 1 and a positive response at period 2. The OR of a positive response φ_{BA} between treatments B and A under model (3.1) can be expressed in terms of $\pi_{rc}^{(g)}$'s as (Problem 3.1)

$$\varphi_{BA} = \left[\left(\pi_{01}^{(1)}\pi_{10}^{(2)}\right) / \left(\pi_{10}^{(1)}\pi_{01}^{(2)}\right)\right]^{1/2}, \qquad (3.2)$$

regardless of any given probability density function $f_g(\mu)$. Note that labels "A" and "B" for treatments can sometimes be arbitrary. If the OR of a positive response φ_{AB} for treatment A versus treatment B (rather than treatment B versus treatment A) is our interest, then we have $\varphi_{AB} = 1/\varphi_{BA}$. Note also that we can estimate $\pi_{rc}^{(g)}$ by using the unbiased consistent sample proportion estimator $\hat{\pi}_{rc}^{(g)} = n_{rc}^{(g)}/n_g$. Thus, when substituting $\hat{\pi}_{rc}^{(g)}$ for $\pi_{rc}^{(g)}$ in (3.2), we obtain a consistent estimator for φ_{BA} as given by

$$\hat{\varphi}_{BA} = \left[\left(\hat{\pi}_{01}^{(1)} \hat{\pi}_{10}^{(2)} \right) / \left(\hat{\pi}_{10}^{(1)} \hat{\pi}_{01}^{(2)} \right) \right]^{1/2},$$

$$= \left[\left(n_{01}^{(1)} n_{10}^{(2)} \right) / \left(n_{10}^{(1)} n_{01}^{(2)} \right) \right]^{1/2}. \tag{3.3}$$

Similarly, we may obtain a consistent estimator for φ_{AB} as $\hat{\varphi}_{AB} = 1/\hat{\varphi}_{BA}$. Using the delta method (Agresti, 1990; Lui, 2004), we can show that an estimated asymptotic variance for $\hat{\varphi}_{BA}$ (3.3) with the logarithmic transformation is (Problem 3.2)

$$\widehat{Var}(\log(\hat{\varphi}_{BA})) = \frac{1}{4} \left[\frac{1}{n_{01}^{(1)}} + \frac{1}{n_{10}^{(1)}} + \frac{1}{n_{01}^{(2)}} + \frac{1}{n_{10}^{(2)}} \right]. \tag{3.4}$$

We can easily see that an estimated asymptotic variance $\widehat{Var}(\log(\hat{\varphi}_{AB}))$ for the estimator $\hat{\varphi}_{AB}$ with the logarithmic transformation is the same as $\widehat{Var}(\log(\hat{\varphi}_{BA}))$ (3.4).

Define $n_{dis}^{(g)} = n_{10}^{(g)} + n_{01}^{(g)}$ as the total number of patients with discordant responses between two periods in group g (= 1, 2). The conditional distribution of $n_{01}^{(g)}$, given $n_{dis}^{(g)}$ fixed, follows the binomial distribution with parameters $n_{dis}^{(g)}$ and $p^{(g)} = \pi_{01}^{(g)} / \left(\pi_{01}^{(g)} + \pi_{10}^{(g)} \right)$ (Problem 3.3). We can show that the conditional distribution of $n_{01}^{(1)} = x_1$, given the total number $n_{01}^{(+)} = n_{01}^{(1)} + n_{01}^{(2)}$ of patients whose response is negative at period 1 and is positive at period 2 over the two groups fixed, follows the noncentral hypergeometric distribution (Problem 3.4) (Gart, 1970; Gart and Thomas, 1972) as

$$P\left(n_{01}^{(1)} = x_1 \big| n_{01}^{(+)}, n_{dis}^{(1)}, n_{dis}^{(2)}, Q_{BA} \right)$$

$$= \binom{n_{dis}^{(1)}}{x_1} \binom{n_{dis}^{(2)}}{n_{01}^{(+)} - x_1} Q_{BA}^{x_1} / \sum_x \binom{n_{dis}^{(1)}}{x} \binom{n_{dis}^{(2)}}{n_{01}^{(+)} - x} Q_{BA}^{x}, \tag{3.5}$$

where $Q_{BA} = \left(\pi_{01}^{(1)} \pi_{10}^{(2)} \right) / \left(\pi_{10}^{(1)} \pi_{01}^{(2)} \right) = \varphi_{BA}^2$ and the summation for x in the denominator is over the range $\max\{0, n_{01}^{(+)} - n_{dis}^{(2)}\} \le x \le \min\left\{ n_{dis}^{(1)}, n_{01}^{(+)} \right\}$. Note that the probability mass function (3.5) is a function of the parameter φ_{BA} only and does not depend on any other nuisance parameter. Note also that when $\varphi_{BA} = 1$ (or equivalently, $Q_{BA} = 1$), the conditional distribution (3.5) reduces to the central hypergeometric distribution given by

$$P\left(n_{01}^{(1)} = x_1 \big| n_{01}^{(+)}, n_{dis}^{(1)}, n_{dis}^{(2)}, Q_{BA} = 1 \right) = \binom{n_{dis}^{(1)}}{x_1} \binom{n_{dis}^{(2)}}{n_{01}^{(+)} - x_1} \bigg/ \binom{n_{dis}^{(1)} + n_{dis}^{(2)}}{n_{01}^{(+)}}, \tag{3.6}$$

where $\max\{0, n_{01}^{(+)} - n_{dis}^{(2)}\} \le x_1 \le \min\left\{ n_{dis}^{(1)}, n_{01}^{(+)} \right\}$.

3.1   Testing non-equality of treatments

Suppose that we wish to study whether the effects between treatments A and B are equal to each other. We want to test the null hypothesis $H_0 : \varphi_{BA} = 1$ (or $\eta_{BA} = 0$) versus the alternative hypothesis $H_a : \varphi_{BA} \neq 1$ (or $\eta_{BA} \neq 0$). On the basis of (3.3) and (3.4), we will reject $H_0 : \varphi_{BA} = 1$ at the α-level if

$$|\log(\hat{\varphi}_{BA})| / \sqrt{\widehat{Var}(\log(\hat{\varphi}_{BA}))} > Z_{\alpha/2}, \qquad (3.7)$$

where $\log(\hat{\varphi}_{BA}) = (1/2)\log\left(\left(n_{01}^{(1)} n_{10}^{(2)}\right) / \left(n_{10}^{(1)} n_{01}^{(2)}\right)\right)$ and Z_α is the upper $100(\alpha \text{th})$ percentile of the standard normal distribution. Note that if any of $n_{10}^{(g)}$ and $n_{01}^{(g)}$ (for $g = 1$, 2) equaled 0, the test procedure (3.7) would be inapplicable. To alleviate this concern, we may employ the commonly used ad hoc adjustment procedure for sparse data by adding 0.5 to each observed cell frequency when calculating (3.7) (Gart and Thomas, 1972; Lui and Lin, 2003). This leads us to reject the null hypothesis $H_0 : \varphi_{BA} = 1$ at the α-level if the test statistic is

$$\left|\log\left(\hat{\varphi}_{BA}^{adj}\right)\right| / \sqrt{\widehat{Var}\left(\log\left(\hat{\varphi}_{BA}^{adj}\right)\right)} > Z_{\alpha/2}, \qquad (3.8)$$

where

$$\hat{\varphi}_{BA}^{adj} = \left\{ \left[\left(n_{01}^{(1)} + 0.50\right)\left(n_{10}^{(2)} + 0.5\right) \right] / \left[\left(n_{10}^{(1)} + 0.5\right)\left(n_{01}^{(2)} + 0.5\right) \right] \right\}^{1/2}, \quad \text{and}$$

$$\widehat{Var}\left(\log\left(\hat{\varphi}_{BA}^{adj}\right)\right) = \frac{1}{4}\left[\frac{1}{n_{01}^{(1)} + 0.5} + \frac{1}{n_{10}^{(1)} + 0.5} + \frac{1}{n_{01}^{(2)} + 0.5} + \frac{1}{n_{10}^{(2)} + 0.5} \right].$$

Note that $p^{(1)} = p^{(2)}$, where $p^{(g)} = \pi_{01}^{(g)} / \left(\pi_{01}^{(g)} + \pi_{10}^{(g)}\right)$ for g = 1, 2, if and only if $\varphi_{BA} = 1$ (Problem 3.5). Thus, when testing $H_0 : \varphi_{BA} = 1$, we can also apply the two-independent-sample proportion test. We will reject $H_0 : \varphi_{BA} = 1$ at the α-level if

$$|\hat{p}^{(1)} - \hat{p}^{(2)}| / \sqrt{\hat{\bar{p}}(1 - \hat{\bar{p}})\left(1/n_{dis}^{(1)} + 1/n_{dis}^{(2)}\right)} > Z_{\alpha/2}, \qquad (3.9)$$

where $\hat{p}^{(g)} = n_{01}^{(g)} / n_{dis}^{(g)}$ for g = 1, 2, and $\hat{\bar{p}} = \left(n_{dis}^{(1)} \hat{p}^{(1)} + n_{dis}^{(2)} \hat{p}^{(2)}\right) / \left(n_{dis}^{(1)} + n_{dis}^{(2)}\right)$. Note that the test procedure (3.9) has been suggested by Fleiss (1986a) as well. Note further that all test procedures (3.7)–(3.9) are derived on the basis of large sample theory. If the observed frequency, $n_{10}^{(g)}$ or $n_{01}^{(g)}$ (for g = 1, 2), is small, these asymptotic test procedures can be inappropriate for use. In this case, we can consider the following exact test procedure based on the conditional distribution (3.6). When testing $H_0 : \varphi_{BA} = 1$ versus $H_a : \varphi_{BA} \neq 1$, we will reject H_0 at the α-level if we obtain $n_{01}^{(1)} = x_1$ such that (Gart, 1969; Fleiss, 1981; Fleiss, Levin, and Paik, 2003)

$$\min\left\{P\left(x \geq x_1 | n_{01}^{(+)}, n_{dis}^{(1)}, n_{dis}^{(2)}, Q_{BA} = 1\right), \ P\left(x \leq x_1 | n_{01}^{(+)}, n_{dis}^{(1)}, n_{dis}^{(2)}, Q_{BA} = 1\right)\right\} \leq \alpha/2,$$

$$(3.10)$$

where

$$P\left(x \geq x_1 | n_{01}^{(+)}, n_{dis}^{(1)}, n_{dis}^{(2)}, Q_{BA} = 1\right) = \sum_{x \geq x_1} P\left(n_{01}^{(1)} = x | n_{01}^{(+)}, n_{dis}^{(1)}, n_{dis}^{(2)}, Q_{BA} = 1\right),$$

$$P\left(x \leq x_1 | n_{01}^{(+)}, n_{dis}^{(1)}, n_{dis}^{(2)}, Q_{BA} = 1\right) = \sum_{x \leq x_1} P\left(n_{01}^{(1)} = x | n_{01}^{(+)}, n_{dis}^{(1)}, n_{dis}^{(2)}, Q_{BA} = 1\right), \text{ and}$$

$\min\{a, b\}$ denotes the smaller of a and b.

Note that the assumed model (3.1) with distribution-free random effects and the conditional arguments used here are different from those given by Gart (1969), who considered a fixed effects logistic regression model and derived test procedures by conditioning on the sufficient statistics for fixed patient effects. However, the asymptotic test procedures (3.7)–(3.9) and the exact test procedure (3.10) are asymptotically equivalent and identical to those asymptotic and exact test procedures suggested elsewhere, respectively (Mainland, 1963; Gart, 1969). Note also that there are other procedures for testing non-equality of two treatments. These include Prescott's test (Prescott, 1981) accounting for patients with concordant responses between two periods (Problem 3.6) to improve power, test procedures (Zimmermann and Rahlfs, 1978; Schouten and Kester, 2010) based on a similar linear additive risk model proposed by Grizzle (1965), test procedures based on a log-linear model (Kenward and Jones, 1987), and test procedures based on a random effects exponential multiplicative risk model (Lui and Chang, 2012a).

Example 3.1 Consider the data regarding 24 children suffering from exercise-induced asthma (Senn, 2002; Schouten and Kester, 2010). Children were randomly assigned to receive one of the two treatment-receipt sequences. In terms of the context as described here, we define 200 μg salbutamol solution aerosol as treatment A and 12 μg formoterol solution aerosol as treatment B. A success (or a positive response) represents a "good" response, and a failure (or a negative response) represents "poor," "fair," or "moderate" responses on a subjective four-point scale (Senn, 2002). We summarize these data in Table 3.1. Note that there is a ($n_{01}^{(2)} = $) zero frequency in the cell, and we cannot employ estimator $\hat{\varphi}_{BA}$ (3.3) to estimate the OR of a success. When using $\hat{\varphi}_{BA}^{adj}$, we obtain the estimate of the OR to be 9.074. Because both $n_{dis}^{(1)}$ and $n_{dis}^{(2)}$ are small, we do not recommend using asymptotic test procedures (3.7)–(3.9). For the purpose of illustration only, however, if we employ test procedure (3.8), we will obtain the p-value as 0.010. When using the exact test procedure (3.10), we obtain the p-value as 0.002. Both of these small p-values suggest that there may be strong evidence that the effects between 12 μg formoterol solution aerosol and 200 μg salbutamol solution aerosol on the patient response are not equal to each other. The former seems to be more effective than the latter, because $\hat{\varphi}_{BA}^{adj} > 1$.

Table 3.2   The observed frequencies of patients with dichotomous response (yes, no) taken from a simple crossover trial comparing two new inhalation devices delivering salbutamol.

		Group I (A-then-B device sequence)		
			Period II	
		Yes	No	Total
Period I	Yes	26	41	67
	No	15	57	72
	Total	41	98	139
		Group II (B-then-A device sequence)		
			Period II	
		Yes	No	Total
Period I	Yes	38	16	54
	No	32	54	86
	Total	70	70	140

Example 3.2   Consider the AB/BA crossover trial (conducted by 3M-Riker) comparing the suitability of two new inhalation devices (A and B) in patients who were using a standard inhaler device delivering salbutamol (Ezzet and Whitehead, 1992). Group 1 used device A for one week followed by device B for another week, while Group 2 used the devices in reverse order. No washout period was felt necessary. Patients reported whether there were particular features that they liked about each device, and their responses were either "yes" or "no." There were very few ($\approx 3\%$) patients with missing outcomes. We assume that these missing outcomes occur completely at random and summarize the frequencies of patients with known responses in Table 3.2. Suppose that we want to study whether there is a difference in the patient favor rates between devices B and A. Given these data, we obtain the estimates $\hat{\varphi}_{BA} = 0.428$ and $\hat{\varphi}_{BA}^{adj} = 0.435$ for the OR of favor responses. When applying asymptotic test procedures (3.7) and (3.8), as well as the exact test procedure (3.10), we obtain p-values to be all < 0.001. All these small p-values strongly suggest that the patient favor response rate of device A is higher than that of device B, because $\hat{\varphi}_{BA}$ (or $\hat{\varphi}_{BA}^{adj}$) < 1.

3.2   Testing non-inferiority of an experimental treatment to an active control treatment

In an RCT, it can sometimes be nonethical to use a placebo control instead of an active control treatment (or a standard treatment). Because it is more difficult to show that an experimental treatment beats an active control treatment than that an experimental treatment beats a placebo, we may be satisfied if one demonstrates that the experimental treatment is non-inferior to the active control treatment with respect to efficacy (Rousson and Seifert, 2008). This is true especially when the experimental treatment has fewer side effects and less expense and is easier to administer than the active control treatment.

For certain treatments, such as drugs designed not to produce an appreciable absorption into the systemic circulation, the pharmacokinetics parameters are no longer adequate for the assessment of non-inferiority (Liu and Chow, 1993; Tu, 1998, 2001, 2003; Chen, Tsong, and Kang, 2000; Tsong, Zhang, and Wang, 2004; Chow and Liu, 2009). These may include, for example, metered dose inhalers (MDI) for the relief of bronchospasm in patients with reversible obstructive airway disease, antiulcer agents, and topical antifungal agents (Liu and Chow, 1993; Tu, 1998). In these cases, we may wish to assess whether the experimental treatment is non-inferior to the active control treatment with respect to clinical endpoints (Dunnett and Gent, 1977; Liu and Chow, 1993; Tu, 1998, 2003; Chen, Tsong, and Kang, 2000; Chow and Liu, 2009).

When we assess non-inferiority of an experimental treatment, the choice of the maximum clinically acceptable non-inferior margin for the risk difference (RD) can depend heavily on the underlying patient response rate in the active control treatment (Lui and Cumberland, 2001). This is because the range of the RD is between -1 and 1. If the underlying patient response rate in the active control treatment equaled 0.1, for example, it would be senseless to choose the non-inferior margin to be larger than 0.1. Furthermore, a fixed value for the non-inferior margin of the RD can possess different clinical meanings and implications depending on the underlying response rate in the active control treatment. Thus, the choice of a fixed constant clinically non-inferior margin for the RD is likely difficult. Though the risk ratio (RR) has been often used in both RCTs and etiological studies, it is well known that the RR lacks symmetry when "success" and "failure" are interchanged. Thus, we may come across the situation in which an experimental treatment is non-inferior to an active control treatment with respect to the positive outcome, but the former is not non-inferior to the latter with respect to the negative outcome, and vice versa. Furthermore, for a given fixed non-inferior margin of the RR, one can easily show that the larger the underlying patient response rate in the active control treatment, the larger is the corresponding non-inferior margin on the RD scale (Garrett, 2003; Rousson and Seifert, 2008). This may contradict, for example, in establishing the effectiveness of a new *Helicobacter Pylori* regimen that a general Food and Drug Administration (FDA) (1997) desirable guideline for the non-inferior margin on the RD scale should shrink as the underlying patient response rate increases from 0.50 to 1.0. Thus, Garrett (2003) contended that the OR should be the most rational measure for assessing the therapeutic non-inferiority or equivalence in binary data. One clinically desirable property of using the OR is that given a fixed non-inferior margin for the OR, the corresponding non-inferior margin on the RD scale is getting small when the underlying patient response rate in the standard treatment becomes large and close to 1 (Tu, 1998; Garrett, 2003). In fact, we may find numerous publications based on the OR in testing non-inferiority or equivalence (Weng and Liu, 1994; Tu, 1998, 2003; Chen,

Tsong, and Kang, 2000; Senn, 2000; Wang, Chow, and Li, 2002; Garrett, 2003; Liu, Fan, and Ma, 2005; Rousson and Seifert, 2008).

Suppose that the higher the positive response rate to a treatment, the better is the treatment. When assessing non-inferiority of an experimental treatment B to an active control treatment A with respect to the OR, we want to test the null hypothesis H_0 : $\varphi_{BA} \leq \varphi_l$ (where $0 < \varphi_l < 1$) versus the alternative hypothesis $H_a : \varphi_{BA} > \varphi_l$, where φ_l is the maximum clinically acceptable low margin such that treatment B can be regarded as non-inferior to treatment A when $\varphi_{BA} > \varphi_l$ holds. Note that the determination of the non-inferior margin is generally predetermined by clinicians based on their subjective clinical knowledge rather than by statisticians. A discussion on various possible choices of φ_l in practice can be found elsewhere (Garrett, 2003).

When the expected frequencies $n_g \pi_{rc}^{(g)}$ (for $(r, c) = (0, 1), (1, 0)$) are all reasonably large (say ≥ 5), we may apply estimator $\hat{\varphi}_{BA}$ (3.3) with the logarithmic transformation and $\widehat{Var}(\log(\hat{\varphi}_{BA}))$ (3.4) to test the null hypothesis $H_0 : \varphi_{BA} \leq \varphi_l$ versus $H_a : \varphi_{BA} > \varphi_l$. We will reject $H_0 : \varphi_{BA} \leq \varphi_l$ at the α-level and claim that treatment B is non-inferior to treatment A for the following test statistic (Lui and Chang, 2011):

$$(\log(\hat{\varphi}_{BA}) - \log(\varphi_l)) / \sqrt{\widehat{Var}(\log(\hat{\varphi}_{BA}))} > Z_\alpha, \qquad (3.11)$$

where $\log(\hat{\varphi}_{BA}) = (1/2)\log\left(\left(n_{01}^{(1)} n_{10}^{(2)}\right) / \left(n_{10}^{(1)} n_{01}^{(2)}\right)\right)$. If any of $n_{10}^{(g)}$ and $n_{01}^{(g)}$ ($g = 1, 2$) equaled 0, the test procedure (3.11) would be inapplicable. When this occurs, we may use the ad hoc adjustment procedure for sparse data by adding 0.5 to each observed cell frequency in calculation of (3.11). Thus, we will reject $H_0 : \varphi_{BA} \leq \varphi_l$ at the α-level for the test statistic

$$\left(\log\left(\hat{\varphi}_{BA}^{adj}\right) - \log(\varphi_l)\right) / \sqrt{\widehat{Var}\left(\log\left(\hat{\varphi}_{BA}^{adj}\right)\right)} > Z_\alpha, \qquad (3.12)$$

where

$$\hat{\varphi}_{BA}^{adj} = \left\{\left[\left(n_{01}^{(1)} + 0.50\right)\left(n_{10}^{(2)} + 0.5\right)\right] / \left[\left(n_{10}^{(1)} + 0.5\right)\left(n_{01}^{(2)} + 0.5\right)\right]\right\}^{1/2}, \text{ and}$$

$$\widehat{Var}\left(\log\left(\hat{\varphi}_{BA}^{adj}\right)\right) = \frac{1}{4}\left[\frac{1}{n_{01}^{(1)} + 0.5} + \frac{1}{n_{10}^{(1)} + 0.5} + \frac{1}{n_{01}^{(2)} + 0.5} + \frac{1}{n_{10}^{(2)} + 0.5}\right].$$

When $n_{10}^{(g)}$ or $n_{01}^{(g)}$ (for $g = 1, 2$) is small, we can consider the following exact test procedure based on the conditional distribution (3.5). When testing $H_0 : \varphi_{BA} \leq \varphi_l$ versus $H_a : \varphi_{BA} > \varphi_l$, we calculate the exact p-value for an observed value $n_{01}^{(1)} = x_1$ as given by (Lui and Chang, 2011)

$$P\left(x \geq x_1 | n_{01}^{(+)}, n_{dis}^{(1)}, n_{dis}^{(2)}, \varphi_l^2\right) = \sum\nolimits_{x \geq x_1} \binom{n_{dis}^{(1)}}{x} \binom{n_{dis}^{(2)}}{n_{01}^{(+)} - x} \varphi_l^{2x} / \sum\nolimits_x \binom{n_{dis}^{(1)}}{x} \binom{n_{dis}^{(2)}}{n_{01}^{(+)} - x} \varphi_l^{2x}.$$

(3.13)

If the resulting p-value (3.13) is less than the α-level, we will reject $H_0 : \varphi_{BA} \leq \varphi_l$ and claim that treatment B is non-inferior to treatment A. Note that if our interest is to test non-inferiority (or equivalence) of treatment A to treatment B, we can simply employ the above test procedures with obvious modifications. For example, for testing non-inferiority of treatment A to treatment B, we may replace $\log(\hat{\varphi}_{BA})$ by $\log(\hat{\varphi}_{AB})$ in use of test procedure (3.11).

Example 3.3   Consider again the simple crossover trial (conducted by 3M-Riker) comparing the suitability of two new inhalation devices (A and B) in Table 3.2. Note that the labels for devices "A" and "B" here are arbitrary. To illustrate the use of test procedures (3.11)–(3.13) and how to modify the estimators and test procedures presented here to accommodate the case of studying device A versus device B (instead of device B versus A), for example, we are interested in estimation of φ_{AB} and testing the non-inferiority of device A to device B with respect to the OR of patient favor responses. Given these data, we obtain the estimates $\hat{\varphi}_{AB}(= 1/\hat{\varphi}_{BA}) = 2.338$ and $\hat{\varphi}_{AB}^*(= 1/\hat{\varphi}_{BA}^*) = 2.296$. Suppose that we arbitrarily choose the maximum clinically acceptable non-inferior margin $\varphi_l = 0.80$. When employing test procedures (3.11)–(3.13), we obtain p-values to be all < 0.001. These small p-values strongly suggest that the patient favor response rate of device A is non-inferior to that of device B.

3.3   Testing equivalence between an experimental treatment and an active control treatment

When an experimental treatment B is much more effective than an active control treatment A, the former can be more toxic than the latter. Thus, we may wish to test equivalence rather than non-inferiority in this case. When assessing equivalence between treatments B and A, we want to test $H_0 : \varphi_{BA} \leq \varphi_l$ or $\varphi_{BA} \geq \varphi_u$ versus $H_a : \varphi_l < \varphi_{BA} < \varphi_u$, where φ_l and φ_u are the maximum clinically acceptable margins such that the efficacy of treatment B can be regarded as equivalent to that of treatment A when $\varphi_l < \varphi_{BA} < \varphi_u$ holds. If the expected frequencies $n_g \pi_{rc}^{(g)}$ [for $(r, c) = (0, 1)$, $(1, 0)$] are all reasonably large, we may apply the intersection-union test (Casella and Berger, 1990) to modify the asymptotic test procedures for testing non-inferiority to accommodate testing equivalence. For example, on the basis of $\log\left(\hat{\varphi}_{BA}^{adj}\right)$, we will reject $H_0 : \varphi_{BA} \leq \varphi_l$ or $\varphi_{BA} \geq \varphi_u$ at the α-level and claim that treatment B is equivalent to treatment A if

$$\left(\log\left(\hat{\varphi}_{BA}^{adj}\right)-\log(\varphi_l)\right)\Big/\sqrt{\widehat{Var}\left(\log\left(\hat{\varphi}_{BA}^{adj}\right)\right)}>Z_\alpha,\ \text{ and}$$

$$\left(\log\left(\hat{\varphi}_{BA}^{adj}\right)-\log(\varphi_u)\right)\Big/\sqrt{\widehat{Var}\left(\log\left(\hat{\varphi}_{BA}^{adj}\right)\right)}<-Z_\alpha. \tag{3.14}$$

When either $n_{10}^{(g)}$ or $n_{01}^{(g)}$ is small, we may again consider using the exact test procedure based on the conditional distribution (3.5). Given an observed value $n_{01}^{(1)}=x_1$, we will reject $H_0: \varphi_{BA}\le\varphi_l$ or $\varphi_{BA}\ge\varphi_u$ at the α-level and claim that the two treatments are equivalent if the following two inequalities simultaneously hold (Lui and Chang, 2011):

$$P\left(x\ge x_1|n_{01}^{(+)},n_{dis}^{(1)},n_{dis}^{(2)},\varphi_l^2\right)<\alpha,\ \text{ and}$$

$$P\left(x\le x_1|n_{01}^{(+)},n_{dis}^{(1)},n_{dis}^{(2)},\varphi_u^2\right)<\alpha. \tag{3.15}$$

Note that the inequality $\varphi_l<\varphi_{BA}<\varphi_u$ holds if and only if $1/\varphi_u<\varphi_{AB}<1/\varphi_l$. Because labels "A" and "B" can be arbitrary, it is desirable to choose $\varphi_u=1/\varphi_l$ (i.e., the equivalence limits are symmetric with respect to 0 on the logarithmic scale). This is because it is not intuitively appealing to define an equivalence interval for the OR of a patient response between two treatments as a function of which treatment is called "A" or which treatment is called "B."

3.4 Interval estimation of the odds ratio

It is well known that one can find statistical significance even for a tiny difference of no clinical importance between treatments as long as the number of patients in a trial is large. Thus, it is always desirable to obtain an interval estimator of the relative treatment effect especially when we obtain significant test results.

On the basis of $\hat{\varphi}_{BA}$ (3.3) and $\widehat{Var}(\log(\hat{\varphi}_{BA}))$ (3.4), we obtain an asymptotic $100(1-\alpha)\%$ confidence interval for $\varphi_{BA}(=\exp(\eta_{BA}))$ as

$$\left[\hat{\varphi}_{BA}\exp\left(-Z_{\alpha/2}\sqrt{\widehat{Var}(\log(\hat{\varphi}_{BA}))}\right),\ \hat{\varphi}_{BA}\exp\left(Z_{\alpha/2}\sqrt{\widehat{Var}(\log(\hat{\varphi}_{BA}))}\right)\right]. \tag{3.16}$$

Similarly, when either $n_{10}^{(g)}$ or $n_{01}^{(g)}$ is zero, we may use the ad hoc adjustment procedure of adding 0.50 for sparse data and obtain an asymptotic $100(1-\alpha)\%$ confidence interval for φ_{BA} as

$$\left[\hat{\varphi}_{BA}^{adj}\exp\left(-Z_{\alpha/2}\sqrt{\widehat{Var}\left(\log\left(\hat{\varphi}_{BA}^{adj}\right)\right)}\right),\ \hat{\varphi}_{BA}^{adj}\exp\left(Z_{\alpha/2}\sqrt{\widehat{Var}\left(\log\left(\hat{\varphi}_{BA}^{adj}\right)\right)}\right)\right].$$

$$\tag{3.17}$$

When the number of $n_{10}^{(g)}$ or $n_{01}^{(g)}$ is small, we can use of the interval estimator based on the exact conditional distribution (3.5). Given an observed value $n_{01}^{(1)} = x_1$, we obtain an exact $100(1 - \alpha)\%$ confidence interval for φ_{BA} as

$$\left[Q_{BAL}^{1/2}, \; Q_{BAU}^{1/2} \right], \tag{3.18}$$

where

$$P\left(x \geq x_1 \big| n_{01}^{(+)}, n_{dis}^{(1)}, n_{dis}^{(2)}, Q_{BAL} \right) = \alpha/2, \quad \text{and}$$

$$P\left(x \leq x_1 \big| n_{01}^{(+)}, n_{dis}^{(1)}, n_{dis}^{(2)}, Q_{BAU} \right) = \alpha/2.$$

Example 3.4 Consider the simple crossover trial (conducted by 3M-Riker) comparing the suitability of two new inhalation devices (A and B) in Table 3.2 (Ezzet and Whitehead, 1992). Suppose that we want to assess the magnitude of the relative device effect by providing an interval estimator for the OR of patient favor responses between devices B and A. When employing interval estimators (3.16) and (3.17), we obtain 95% confidence intervals for φ_{BA} between devices B and A as [0.281, 0.652] and [0.287, 0.660]. When using the exact interval estimator (3.18), we obtain the 95% confidence interval for φ_{BA} as [0.268, 0.677]. Because observed values for $n_{10}^{(g)}$ and $n_{01}^{(g)}$ in the example are not small, all these resulting interval estimates are similar to one another. Furthermore, since all the above resulting upper confidence limits fall below 1, there is significant evidence that the patient favor response rate of device B is less than that of device A. This is consistent with the test result found in Example 3.2. Note that PROC FREQ in the SAS software (SAS Institute, 2009) can be used to obtain both asymptotic and exact 95% confidence intervals for $Q_{BA} \left(= \varphi_{BA}^2 \right)$. To obtain the corresponding 95% confidence interval for φ_{BA}, we can simply take the square root of these confidence limits for Q_{BA}.

Note that an asymptotic one-sided $100(1 - \alpha)\%$ confidence lower bound for the underlying OR of a positive response φ_{BA} for treatment B versus treatment A based on statistic $\hat{\varphi}_{BA}$ with the logarithmic transformation can be shown to be given by

$$\left[\hat{\varphi}_{BA} \exp\left(-Z_\alpha \sqrt{\widehat{Var}(\log(\hat{\varphi}_{BA}))} \right), \; \infty \right). \tag{3.19}$$

Using procedure (3.11) for testing non-inferiority is actually identical to rejecting the null hypothesis $H_0 : \varphi_{BA} \leq \varphi_l$ whenever the lower confidence limit (3.19) falls above the maximum clinically acceptable low margin φ_l. Similarly, given an observed value $n_{01}^{(1)} = x_1$, we can obtain the one-sided exact $100(1 - \alpha)\%$ lower confidence limit by finding the solution φ_{BAL} satisfying $P\left(x \geq x_1 \big| n_{01}^{(+)}, n_{dis}^{(1)}, n_{dis}^{(2)}, \varphi_{BAL}^2 \right) = \alpha$. Using the exact tail probability (3.13) for testing non-inferiority is identical to rejecting H_0: $\varphi_{BA} \leq \varphi_l$ whenever the one-sided exact $100(1-\alpha)\%$ confidence lower limit φ_{BAL} falls above the acceptable non-inferior margin φ_l (Problem 3.7). We can also show an analogous relationship as noted in the above between the test procedure (3.14) (or (3.15)) at the α-level and the corresponding $100(1-2\alpha)\%$ (two-sided) confidence interval (3.17) (or (3.18)) for φ_{BA} when testing equivalence. For example, we can show that the test procedure (3.14) is equivalent to rejecting the null hypothesis H_0: $\varphi_{BA} \leq \varphi_l$ or $\varphi_{BA} \geq \varphi_u$ at the α-level whenever the asymptotic $100(1-2\alpha)\%$ confidence interval (3.17) lies entirely in the equivalence interval (φ_l, φ_u) (Problem 3.8).

3.5   Sample size determination

It is essentially important that we obtain an adequate number of patients for detecting the primary goal of a trial. Thus, calculation of the minimum required sample size becomes one of the most important steps for designing a good RCT. For simplicity, we consider equal sample allocation (i.e., $n_1 = n_2 = n$) between two groups in the following discussion.

3.5.1   Sample size for testing non-equality

Note that we can re-express the statistic $\log(\hat{\varphi}_{BA})$, where $\hat{\varphi}_{BA}$ is given in (3.3), as

$$(1/2)\left[\log\left(\hat{\pi}_{01}^{(1)}/\hat{\pi}_{10}^{(1)}\right) - \log\left(\hat{\pi}_{01}^{(2)}/\hat{\pi}_{10}^{(2)}\right)\right]. \tag{3.20}$$

We can further show that an asymptotic variance for $\log(\hat{\varphi}_{BA})$ is given by

$$V(\log(\hat{\varphi}_{BA}))/n, \tag{3.21}$$

where $V(\log(\hat{\varphi}_{BA})) = \dfrac{1}{4}\left[\dfrac{1}{\pi_{01}^{(1)}} + \dfrac{1}{\pi_{10}^{(1)}} + \dfrac{1}{\pi_{01}^{(2)}} + \dfrac{1}{\pi_{10}^{(2)}}\right]$. On the basis of the test procedure (3.7) (two-sided test), an approximate minimum required number n of patients per group for a desired power $1-\beta$ of detecting non-equality with a specified value $\varphi_{BA}^* \neq 1$ at a nominal α-level is approximately given by (Problem 3.9)

$$n = Ceil\left\{\left(Z_{\alpha/2} + Z_\beta\right)^2 V(\log(\hat{\varphi}_{BA}))/\left(\log(\varphi_{BA}^*)\right)^2\right\}, \tag{3.22}$$

where $Ceil\{x\}$ is the smallest integer $\geq x$ and $V(\log(\hat{\varphi}_{BA}))$ is defined in (3.21).

3.5.2   Sample size for testing non-inferiority

On the basis of test procedure (3.11), we can show that an approximate minimum required number n of patients per group for a desired power $1-\beta$ of detecting non-inferiority with a specified value $\varphi^*_{BA}(>\varphi_l)$ at a nominal α-level is given by (Problem 3.10)

$$n = Ceil\left\{ (Z_\alpha + Z_\beta)^2 V(\log(\hat{\varphi}_{BA})) / \left(\log(\varphi_l) - \log\left(\varphi^*_{BA}\right)\right)^2 \right\}. \qquad (3.23)$$

Note that if the resulting estimate n (3.23) is not large, then the sample size calculation formula (3.23) derived from the asymptotic test procedure (3.11) based on the normal approximation can lose accuracy. In this case, we may employ the exact sample size calculation procedure (Lui and Chang, 2012b) for testing non-inferiority under the AB/BA crossover trial. Note that the above sample size calculation procedure can be easily modified for testing non-inferiority of treatment A to treatment B rather than testing non-inferiority of treatment B to treatment A.

Example 3.5   To illustrate the use of sample size formula (3.23) for testing non-inferiority, we consider the situation with the configurations determined by the parameter estimates from data in Table 3.2: $\hat{\pi}^{(1)}_{01} = 0.11$, $\hat{\pi}^{(1)}_{10} = 0.29$, $\hat{\pi}^{(2)}_{01} = 0.23$, and $\hat{\pi}^{(2)}_{10} = 0.11$. Given these parameter values, suppose that we want to find out how large the approximate minimum required number of patients per group needed is to achieve 80% power of detecting non-inferiority when the underlying OR of favor responses for device A versus device B (rather than device B versus A) is equal to 2.0 when $\varphi_l = 0.80$ at the 5% level. When employing sample size calculation formula (3.23) replacing $\log\left(\varphi^*_{BA}\right)$ by $\log\left(\varphi^*_{AB}\right)$ $(= \log(2))$, we obtain an approximate minimum required number n of patients per group of 48 patients.

3.5.3 Sample size for testing equivalence

When the number n of patients is reasonably large, we may obtain the power function for testing equivalence based on the test procedure (3.14) and normal approximation as given by (Problem 3.11)

$$\psi\left(\varphi^*_{BA}\right) = \Phi\left(\frac{\log(\varphi_u) - \log\left(\varphi^*_{BA}\right)}{\sqrt{V(\log(\hat{\varphi}_{BA}))/n}} - Z_\alpha \right) - \Phi\left(\frac{\log(\varphi_l) - \log\left(\varphi^*_{BA}\right)}{\sqrt{V(\log(\hat{\varphi}_{BA}))/n}} + Z_\alpha \right), \qquad (3.24)$$

where $\varphi_l < \varphi^*_{BA} < \varphi_u$ and $\Phi(X)$ is the cumulative standard normal distribution. On the basis of the power function $\psi\left(\varphi^*_{BA}\right)$ (3.24), we cannot find the closed-form formula in calculation of the approximate minimum required number n of patients per group such that $\psi\left(\varphi^*_{BA}\right) \geq 1 - \beta$ unless we can make a good approximation of $\psi\left(\varphi^*_{BA}\right)$ (3.24) under certain assumptions. However, we can use the trial-and-error procedure to find an approximate minimum required sample size by searching for the smallest positive integer n such that $\psi\left(\varphi^*_{BA}\right) \geq 1 - \beta$.

   If the resulting estimate for the minimum required number of patients is large, we can approximate the power function $\psi\left(\varphi^*_{BA}\right)$ (3.24) for $\varphi_l < \varphi^*_{BA} < 1$ by (Tu, 1998; Wang, Chow, and Li, 2002)

$$1 - \Phi\left(\frac{\log(\varphi_l) - \log\left(\varphi_{BA}^*\right)}{\sqrt{V(\log(\hat{\varphi}_{BA}))/n}} + Z_\alpha\right). \tag{3.25}$$

On the basis of (3.25), we obtain an approximate minimum required number n of patients per group for the desired power $(1 - \beta)$ of detecting equivalence with a specified $\varphi_l < \varphi_{BA}^* < 1$ at a nominal α-level as

$$n = Ceil\left\{ (Z_\alpha + Z_\beta)^2 V(\log(\hat{\varphi}_{BA})) / \left(\log(\varphi_l) - \log\left(\varphi_{BA}^*\right)\right)^2 \right\}. \tag{3.26}$$

On the other hand, if the resulting estimate for the minimum required number of patients per group is large and $1 < \varphi_{BA}^* < \varphi_u$, we can approximate the power function $\psi\left(\varphi_{BA}^*\right)$ (3.24) by

$$\Phi\left(\frac{\log(\varphi_u) - \log\left(\varphi_{BA}^*\right)}{\sqrt{V(\log(\hat{\varphi}_{BA}))/n}} - Z_\alpha\right). \tag{3.27}$$

On the basis of (3.27) we obtain an approximate minimum required number n of patients per group for a desired power $(1 - \beta)$ of detecting equivalence with a specified $1 < \varphi_{BA}^* < \varphi_u$ at a nominal α-level as

$$n = Ceil\left\{ (Z_\alpha + Z_\beta)^2 V(\log(\hat{\varphi}_{BA})) / \left(\log(\varphi_u) - \log\left(\varphi_{BA}^*\right)\right)^2 \right\}. \tag{3.28}$$

When $\varphi_{BA}^* = 1$, the power function $\psi\left(\varphi_{BA}^*\right)$ (3.24) simply reduces to

$$\psi\left(\varphi_{BA}^* = 1\right) = \Phi\left(\frac{\log(\varphi_u)}{\sqrt{V(\log(\hat{\varphi}_{BA}))/n}} - Z_\alpha\right) - \Phi\left(\frac{\log(\varphi_l)}{\sqrt{V(\log(\hat{\varphi}_{BA}))/n}} + Z_\alpha\right). \tag{3.29}$$

When $\log(\varphi_l) = -\log(\varphi_u)$ (i.e., the acceptable range is symmetric with respect to 0 on the logarithmic scale), we obtain an approximate minimum required number n of patients per group for the desired power $(1 - \beta)$ of detecting equivalence with a specified value $\varphi_{BA}^* = 1$ at a nominal α-level based on (3.29) as

$$n = Ceil\left\{ \left((Z_\alpha + Z_{\beta/2})^2 V(\log(\hat{\varphi}_{BA})) / (\log(\varphi_u))^2 \right) \right\}. \tag{3.30}$$

Note that when deriving n (3.26) and n (3.28), we need to assume that the approximations of the power function $\psi\left(\varphi_{BA}^*\right)$ (3.24) by (3.25) and (3.27) are accurate. When the predetermined equivalence margins φ_l (e.g., 0.55 suggested by Senn (2000) and hence $\varphi_u = 1.82$ such that $\log(\varphi_l) = -\log(\varphi_u)$) are away from 1, or the underlying $\varphi_{BA}^*(\neq 1)$ of interest is chosen to be in the neighborhood of 1, the resulting approximate minimum required number n of patients may not be large enough to assure these approximations to be good. In these cases, because the power function (3.25) (or the power function (3.27)) is larger than $\psi\left(\varphi_{BA}^*\right)$ (3.24), using n (3.26) (or n (3.28)) tends to underestimate the minimum required number of patients per group. Thus, we may use n (3.26) (or n (3.28)) as the initial estimate and apply a trial-and-error procedure to find the approximate minimum positive integer n such that $\psi\left(\varphi_{BA}^{*}\right)$ (3.24) is $\geq 1-\beta$.

3.6   Hypothesis testing and estimation for the period effect

Under model (3.1), we can easily show that the OR of a positive response between periods 2 and 1 for a fixed treatment on a given patient is equal to $\phi = \exp(\gamma)$. From Problem 3.1, we can easily see that

$$\phi = \left[\left(\pi_{01}^{(1)}\pi_{01}^{(2)}\right)/\left(\pi_{10}^{(1)}\pi_{10}^{(2)}\right)\right]^{1/2}. \tag{3.31}$$

Thus, we can estimate the OR of a positive response for period 2 versus period 1 by

$$\begin{aligned}
\hat{\phi} &= \left[\left(\hat{\pi}_{01}^{(1)}\hat{\pi}_{01}^{(2)}\right)/\left(\hat{\pi}_{10}^{(1)}\hat{\pi}_{10}^{(2)}\right)\right]^{1/2}, \\
&= \left[\left(n_{01}^{(1)}n_{01}^{(2)}\right)/\left(n_{10}^{(1)}n_{10}^{(2)}\right)\right]^{1/2}.
\end{aligned} \tag{3.32}$$

We can easily show that an estimated asymptotic variance $\widehat{Var}\left(\log(\hat{\phi})\right)$ for $\log(\hat{\phi})$ is identical to $\widehat{Var}\left(\log(\hat{\varphi}_{BA})\right)$ (3.4). Similarly, when $n_{10}^{(g)}$ or $n_{01}^{(g)}$ is zero, we may employ the ad hoc adjustment procedure for sparse data and obtain

$$\hat{\phi}^{adj} = \left\{\left[\left(n_{01}^{(1)}+0.50\right)\left(n_{01}^{(2)}+0.50\right)\right]/\left[\left(n_{10}^{(1)}+0.50\right)\left(n_{10}^{(2)}+0.50\right)\right]\right\}^{1/2}. \tag{3.33}$$

Using the delta method (Agresti, 1990), we may obtain an estimated asymptotic variance for $\widehat{Var}\left(\log\left(\hat{\phi}^{adj}\right)\right)$ to be the same as $\widehat{Var}\left(\log\left(\hat{\varphi}_{BA}^{adj}\right)\right)$. Based on either $\hat{\phi}$ (3.32) or $\hat{\phi}^{adj}$ (3.33), we can do testing non-equality of two-period effects. For example, we will reject $H_0 : \phi = 1$ at the α-level if

$$\left|\log\left(\hat{\phi}^{adj}\right)\right|/\sqrt{\widehat{Var}\left(\log\left(\hat{\phi}^{adj}\right)\right)} > Z_{\alpha/2}. \tag{3.34}$$

Also, using $\hat{\phi}^{adj}$ (3.33) and $\widehat{Var}\left(\log\left(\hat{\phi}^{adj}\right)\right)$, we may obtain an asymptotic $100(1-\alpha)\%$ confidence interval for ϕ as

$$\left[\hat{\phi}^{adj}\exp\left(-Z_{\alpha/2}\sqrt{\widehat{Var}\left(\log\left(\hat{\phi}^{adj}\right)\right)}\right), \hat{\phi}^{adj}\exp\left(Z_{\alpha/2}\sqrt{\widehat{Var}\left(\log\left(\hat{\phi}^{adj}\right)\right)}\right)\right]. \tag{3.35}$$

When observed frequencies $n_{rc}^{(g)}$ [for $(r, c) = (0, 1), (1, 0)$] are not large, we may consider using an exact $100(1 - \alpha)\%$ confidence interval for ϕ based on the following conditional distribution. Given the total number $n_{01}^{(1)} + n_{10}^{(2)} = x_+$ of patients whose responses are negative when they receive treatment A and are positive when they receive treatment B, over the two groups fixed, the random number $n_{01}^{(1)} = x_1$ then follows the probability mass function:

$$
\begin{aligned}
& P\left(n_{01}^{(1)} = x_1 | n_{01}^{(1)} + n_{10}^{(2)} = x_+, n_{dis}^{(1)}, n_{dis}^{(2)}, \Theta\right) \\
& = \binom{n_{dis}^{(1)}}{x_1} \binom{n_{dis}^{(2)}}{x_+ - x_1} \Theta^{x_1} / \sum_x \binom{n_{dis}^{(1)}}{x} \binom{n_{dis}^{(2)}}{x_+ - x} \Theta^x,
\end{aligned}
\tag{3.36}
$$

where $\Theta = \left(\pi_{01}^{(1)} \pi_{01}^{(2)}\right) / \left(\pi_{10}^{(1)} \pi_{10}^{(2)}\right) = (\phi)^2$ and the summation for x is over the range $\max\{0, x_+ - n_{dis}^{(2)}\} \leq x \leq \min\left\{n_{dis}^{(1)}, x_+\right\}$. On the basis of the probability mass function (3.36), we obtain an exact $100(1 - \alpha)\%$ confidence interval for ϕ given an observed value $\left(n_{01}^{(1)} = \right) x_1^*$ as given by

$$
\left[\Theta_{PL}^{1/2}, \Theta_{PU}^{1/2}\right],
\tag{3.37}
$$

where

$$
P\left(n_{01}^{(1)} \geq x_1^* | n_{01}^{(1)} + n_{10}^{(2)} = x_+, n_{dis}^{(1)}, n_{dis}^{(2)}, \Theta_{PL}\right) = \alpha/2, \quad \text{and}
$$

$$
P\left(n_{01}^{(1)} \leq x_1^* | n_{01}^{(1)} + n_{10}^{(2)} = x_+, n_{dis}^{(1)}, n_{dis}^{(2)}, \Theta_{PU}\right) = \alpha/2.
$$

Example 3.6   Consider the simple crossover trial comparing the suitability of two new inhalation devices (A and B) in Table 3.2. When assessing the magnitude of the relative period effect, we obtain the OR of patient favor response rates $\hat{\phi} = 0.855$ with the 95% confidence interval [0.561, 1.304], and $\hat{\phi}^{adj} = 0.858$ with 95% confidence interval [0.566, 1.308]. Using the exact interval estimator (3.37), we obtain the exact 95% confidence interval as [0.537, 1.361]. Note that all these resulting interval estimates cover 1. Thus, we may conclude that there seems to be a decrease in patient favor response rates at period 2 versus period 1, but this decrease is not significant at the 0.05 level.

Finally, if we wish to find out whether both the treatment and period effects are 0, then we can test $H_0 : \eta_{BA} = \gamma = 0$ versus $H_a : \eta_{BA} \neq 0$ or $\gamma \neq 0$. Recall that the conditional distribution of $n_{01}^{(g)}$, given $n_{dis}^{(g)}$ fixed, follows the binomial distribution with parameters $n_{dis}^{(g)}$ and $p^{(g)} = \pi_{01}^{(g)} / \left(\pi_{01}^{(g)} + \pi_{10}^{(g)} \right)$ (see Problem 3.3). Note that when $\eta_{BA} = \gamma = 0$, $p_2^{(g)} = 1/2$ for both g. Thus, if $n_{10}^{(g)}$ and $n_{01}^{(g)}$ are reasonably large, we can apply the following test procedure (Problem 3.12). We will reject $H_0 : \eta_{BA} = \gamma = 0$ at the α-level if

$$\left(n_{01}^{(1)} - n_{10}^{(1)} \right)^2 / n_{dis}^{(1)} + \left(n_{01}^{(2)} - n_{10}^{(2)} \right)^2 / n_{dis}^{(2)} > \chi_\alpha^2(2). \tag{3.38}$$

Note the above test statistic is actually the sum of two McNemar's tests. On the other hand, if $n_{10}^{(g)}$ or $n_{01}^{(g)}$ is small for either group g, we may apply the following exact test procedure. We will reject $H_0 : \eta_{BA} = \gamma = 0$ at the α-level if we obtain an observed bivariate response vector $(n_{01}^{(1)}, n_{01}^{(2)}) = \left(x_1^*, x_2^* \right)$ such that

$$\sum_{\{(x_1,x_2) \in C\}} \binom{n_{dis}^{(1)}}{x_1} \binom{n_{dis}^{(2)}}{x_2} \left(\frac{1}{2} \right)^{n_{dis}^{(1)} + n_{dis}^{(2)}} < \alpha, \tag{3.39}$$

where $C = \left\{ (x_1, x_2) | \binom{n_{dis}^{(1)}}{x_1} \binom{n_{dis}^{(2)}}{x_1} \left(\frac{1}{2} \right)^{n_{dis}^{(1)} + n_{dis}^{(2)}} \le \binom{n_{dis}^{(1)}}{x_1^*} \binom{n_{dis}^{(2)}}{x_2^*} \left(\frac{1}{2} \right)^{n_{dis}^{(1)} + n_{dis}^{(2)}} \right\}.$

3.7   Testing and estimation for carry-over effects

We shall not employ, as noted previously, a crossover trial unless one can assure that there will be no carry-over effects with an adequate washout period. The purpose of this section is included only for readers' information (if they should unexpectedly encounter differential carry-over effects) and is not to advocate the use of a crossover design in the presence of carry-over effects.

To account for the possible differential carry-over effects due to treatments A and B, we assume that the probability of a positive response for patient i ($= 1, 2, \ldots, n_g$) assigned to group g ($= 1, 2$) at period z ($= 1, 2$) is given by

$$P\left(Y_{iz}^{(g)} = 1 \right) = \frac{\exp\left(\mu_i^{(g)} + \eta_{BA} X_{iz}^{(g)} + \gamma Z_{iz}^{(g)} + \lambda_A I_{\{g=1\}} Z_{iz}^{(g)} + \lambda_B \left(1 - I_{\{g=1\}} \right) Z_{iz}^{(g)} \right)}{1 + \exp\left(\mu_i^{(g)} + \eta_{BA} X_{iz}^{(g)} + \gamma Z_{iz}^{(g)} + \lambda_A I_{\{g=1\}} Z_{iz}^{(g)} + \lambda_B \left(1 - I_{\{g=1\}} \right) Z_{iz}^{(g)} \right)}, \tag{3.40}$$

where $I_{\{g=1\}} = 1$ for group $g = 1$, and $= 0$ otherwise; λ_A and λ_B are the carry-over effects due to treatments A and B, respectively, and the other parameters and covariates are defined as those in model (3.1). We can show that (Problem 3.15)

$$\left[\left(\pi_{01}^{(1)} \pi_{10}^{(2)} \right) / \left(\pi_{10}^{(1)} \pi_{01}^{(2)} \right) \right]^{1/2} = \varphi_{BA} \exp((\lambda_A - \lambda_B)/2). \tag{3.41}$$

Thus, the estimator $\hat{\varphi}_{BA} \left(= \left[\left(\hat{\pi}_{01}^{(1)} \hat{\pi}_{10}^{(2)} \right) / \left(\hat{\pi}_{10}^{(1)} \hat{\pi}_{01}^{(2)} \right) \right]^{1/2} \right)$ (3.2) is no longer a consist-

ent estimator of φ_{BA} unless $\lambda_A = \lambda_B$. On the basis of (3.41), we can see that $\hat{\varphi}_{BA}$ tends to overestimate (or underestimate) φ_{BA} when $\lambda_A > \lambda_B$ (or $\lambda_A < \lambda_B$). Note that Hills and Armitage (1979) suggested that we test whether there is a treatment-by-period interaction by testing if there is an association for the 2×2 tables with cell probabilities $(\pi_{00}^{(1)}, \pi_{00}^{(2)})$ in the first row and $(\pi_{11}^{(1)}, \pi_{11}^{(2)})$ in the second row. However, we can show that this test procedure may not work adequately under model (3.40) (Problem 3.16). To assess and adjust differential carry-over effects, we may want to extend the design AB/BA to ABB/BAA (Lucas, 1957; Kershner and Federer, 1981; Ebbutt, 1984; Laska and Meisner, 1985) under the simple carry-over model (Senn, 1992). To avoid diverting the attentions of readers from the situations covered in the book, we include the discussion in detail on the carry-over effects in Problem 3.17. Some other discussions on estimations of the proportion ratio in the presence of differential carry-over effects under an AB/BA design can be found elsewhere (Lui, 2015d).

3.8   SAS Program codes and likelihood-based approach

Ezzet and Whitehead (1992) assumed that random effects $\mu_i^{(g)}$'s under model (3.1) followed a normal distribution with mean $E\left(\mu_i^{(g)}\right) = m$ and variance $Var\left(\mu_i^{(g)}\right) = \sigma_\mu^2$ and suggested use of the likelihood-based approach on the basis of $\pi_{rc}^{(g)}$'s, which are in non-closed form integrals as given in Problem 3.1. The likelihood is proportional to

$$L = \prod_{g=1}^{2} \prod_{r=0}^{1} \prod_{c=0}^{1} \left(\pi_{rc}^{(g)} \right)^{n_{rc}^{(g)}}, \tag{3.42}$$

which is a function of η_{BA}, γ, m, and σ_μ^2. We can apply PROC NLMIXED to obtain the maximum likelihood estimators (MLEs) of these parameters based on the likelihood (3.42). Following Senn (2002), we present the SAS codes of applying PROC NLMIXED to the data in Table 3.1 in the following box, in which salbutamol is coded as "treat = 1" and formoterol is coded as "treat = 2."

```
Data step1;
input patient period treat bineff;
  if period eq 1 then period = 0;
  if period eq 2 then period = 1;
  if treat eq 1 then treat = 0;
```

```
    if treat eq 2 then treat = 1;
cards;
    1  1  1  0
    1  2  2  1
    2  1  1  0
    2  2  2  1
.  .  .  .
;;;;
proc sort;
by patient;
run;
proc nlmixed;
parms m = 0 eta = 0.0 gamma = 0.0 s2u = 1;
bounds s2u > 0;
pred = m + eta*treat + gamma*period + u;
p = exp(pred)/(1 + exp(pred));
model bineff ~ binomial(1,p);
random u ~ normal(0,s2u) subject = patient;
run;
```

Some explanations of these SAS codes for PROC NLMIXED can be found elsewhere (Senn, 2002, p. 133). The parameter s2u in the above SAS codes represents the random effects variance σ_μ^2. We obtain the following computer output:

Parameter	Estimate	Standard Error	DF	t Value	Pr > |t|	Alpha	Lower	Upper
m	-0.1651	0.5522	23	-0.30	0.7677	0.05	-1.3074	0.9772
eta	3.2884	0.9114	23	3.61	0.0015	0.05	1.4029	5.1738
gamma	-1.1729	0.8054	23	-1.46	0.1588	0.05	-2.8390	0.4932
s2u	1E-8	.	23	.	.	0.05	.	.

Note that since the codes used here to represent salbutamol and formoterol happen to be in the reverse order of those used by Senn (2002), our estimate of the relative treatment effect is different from that obtained elsewhere (Senn, 2002, p. 133) by switching the sign. This also accounts for the reason why there is a difference in the resulting estimates of the intercept. We can see that the p-value for testing non-equality of treatment effects is 0.0015. Thus, there is strong evidence that the effects on patient responses are not equal between 12 µg formoterol solution aerosol and 200 µg salbutamol solution aerosol. This is similar to the p-value 0.00175, as obtained by use of the exact test (Example 3.1). As noted by Senn (2002), however, the variance estimate σ_u^2 for random effects in the above computer output is on the low bound of zero. Thus, it is probably not completely suitable to employ the assumed model with normal random effects to fit the data in Table 3.1. Note that one may also apply the following SAS codes of PROC GLIMMIX (SAS Institute, 2009) to obtain the MLEs of the above parameters.

```
Data step1;
input patient period treat bineff;
  if period eq 1 then period = 0;
  if period eq 2 then period = 1;
  if treat eq 1 then treat = 0;
  if treat eq 2 then treat = 1;
   n = 1;
cards;
    1  1  1  0
    1  2  2  1
    2  1  1  0
    2  2  2  1
;;;;
proc print;
proc glimmix;
  class patient;
    model bineff/n = period treat /solution;
    random intercept / subject = patient;
run;
```

Because we obtain the same results as those using PROC NLMIXED, we do not present the outputs in use of PROC GLIMMIX for brevity. Jones and Kenward (2014, p. 295) recommended that we use "method = quad" rather than "default method" when employing PROC GLIMMIX in binary data. Thus, we have rerun PROC GLIMMIX with specifying "method = quad". We have gotten essentially identical estimates when using the data in Table 3.1 as well.

Using Monte Carlo simulation, McCulloch and Neuhaus (2011) noted that misspecifying the shape of distribution for random effects might not matter much in estimation of parameters for "within-cluster" covariates under random effects models. However, we prefer to use methods derived from conditional arguments because we make fewer assumptions and our test procedures and estimators are applicable and remain unchanged regardless of the assumed distribution for random effects. Furthermore, using the conditional arguments, we can derive the exact test procedure, which is of use especially when the number of patients in a crossover trial is small and asymptotic test procedures are theoretically invalid (Lui, 2015e). On the other hand, if the random effects do follow the assumed normal distribution, the likelihood-based approach is expected to be more efficient than the conditional approach focused on here. Also, using the likelihood-based approach, we can easily extend the model to include a parameter representing carry-over effects and employ the likelihood ratio or Wald's test to test whether there is a difference in carry-over effects. As noted by Senn (2002, p. 134), however, we do not recommend use of these tests to verify the assumption of no differential carry-over effects based on significance of a test because there can be the same concern as that for use of the two-stage test in continuous data (Freeman, 1989).

Exercises

Problem 3.1. Show that the OR of a positive response between an experimental treatment B and an active control treatment (or a placebo) A under model (3.1) is $\varphi_{BA} = \left[\left(\pi_{01}^{(1)} \pi_{10}^{(2)} \right) / \left(\pi_{10}^{(1)} \pi_{01}^{(2)} \right) \right]^{1/2}$ despite the form for the probability density function $f_g(\alpha)$. (Hint: The cell probabilities $\pi_{rc}^{(g)}$ in group (g =) 1 for $r = 1, 0$, and $c = 1, 0$ are equal to

$$\pi_{11}^{(1)} = \int \left(\frac{\exp(\mu)}{1 + \exp(\mu)} \right) \left(\frac{\exp(\mu + \eta_{BA} + \gamma)}{1 + \exp(\mu + \eta_{BA} + \gamma)} \right) f_1(\mu) d\mu;$$

$$\pi_{10}^{(1)} = \int \left(\frac{\exp(\mu)}{1 + \exp(\mu)} \right) \left(\frac{1}{1 + \exp(\mu + \eta_{BA} + \gamma)} \right) f_1(\mu) d\mu;$$

$$\pi_{01}^{(1)} = \int \left(\frac{1}{1 + \exp(\mu)} \right) \left(\frac{\exp(\mu + \eta_{BA} + \gamma)}{1 + \exp(\mu + \eta_{BA} + \gamma)} \right) f_1(\mu) d\mu;$$

$$\pi_{00}^{(1)} = \int \left(\frac{1}{1 + \exp(\mu)} \right) \left(\frac{1}{1 + \exp(\mu + \eta_{BA} + \gamma)} \right) f_1(\mu) d\mu;$$

$$\pi_{11}^{(2)} = \int \left(\frac{\exp(\mu + \eta_{BA})}{1 + \exp(\mu + \eta_{BA})} \right) \left(\frac{\exp(\mu + \gamma)}{1 + \exp(\mu + \gamma)} \right) f_2(\mu) d\mu;$$

$$\pi_{10}^{(2)} = \int \left(\frac{\exp(\mu + \eta_{BA})}{1 + \exp(\mu + \eta_{BA})} \right) \left(\frac{1}{1 + \exp(\mu + \gamma)} \right) f_2(\mu) d\mu;$$

$$\pi_{01}^{(2)} = \int \left(\frac{1}{1 + \exp(\mu + \eta_{BA})} \right) \left(\frac{\exp(\mu + \gamma)}{1 + \exp(\mu + \gamma)} \right) f_2(\mu) d\mu; \text{ and}$$

$$\pi_{00}^{(2)} = \int \left(\frac{1}{1 + \exp(\mu + \eta_{BA})} \right) \left(\frac{1}{1 + \exp(\mu + \gamma)} \right) f_2(\mu) d\mu.$$

Thus, we obtain

$$\pi_{01}^{(1)} / \pi_{10}^{(1)} = \exp(\eta_{BA} + \gamma) \text{ and } \pi_{01}^{(2)} / \pi_{10}^{(2)} = \exp(-\eta_{BA} + \gamma).$$

Problem 3.2. Show that an estimated asymptotic variance for $\hat{\varphi}_{BA}$ (3.3) with the logarithmic transformation is given by $\widehat{Var}(\log(\hat{\varphi}_{BA})) = \frac{1}{4}\left[\frac{1}{n_{01}^{(1)}} + \frac{1}{n_{10}^{(1)}} + \frac{1}{n_{01}^{(2)}} + \frac{1}{n_{10}^{(2)}}\right]$.

Problem 3.3. Show that the conditional distribution of $n_{01}^{(g)}$, given $n_{dis}^{(g)}$ fixed, follows the binomial distribution with parameters $n_{dis}^{(g)}$ and $p^{(g)} = \pi_{01}^{(g)} / \left(\pi_{01}^{(g)} + \pi_{10}^{(g)}\right)$.

Problem 3.4. Show that the conditional distribution of $n_{01}^{(1)} = x_1$, given the total number $n_{01}^{(+)} = n_{01}^{(1)} + n_{01}^{(2)}$ of patients whose response is negative at period 1 and positive at period 2 over the two groups fixed, follows the noncentral hypergeometric distribution:

$$P\left(n_{01}^{(1)} = x_1 | n_{01}^{(+)}, n_{dis}^{(1)}, n_{dis}^{(2)}, Q_{BA}\right) = \binom{n_{dis}^{(1)}}{x_1}\binom{n_{dis}^{(2)}}{n_{01}^{(+)} - x_1} Q_{BA}^{x_1} / \sum_x \binom{n_{dis}^{(1)}}{x}\binom{n_{dis}^{(2)}}{n_{01}^{(+)} - x} Q_{BA}^x.$$

where $Q_{BA} = \left(\pi_{01}^{(1)} \pi_{10}^{(2)}\right) / \left(\pi_{10}^{(1)} \pi_{01}^{(2)}\right) = \varphi_{BA}^2$ and the summation for x is over the range $\max\{0, n_{01}^{(+)} - n_{dis}^{(2)}\} \leq x \leq \min\{n_{dis}^{(1)}, n_{01}^{(+)}\}$.

Problem 3.5. Show that $p^{(1)} = p^{(2)}$, where $p^{(g)} = \pi_{01}^{(g)} / \left(\pi_{01}^{(g)} + \pi_{10}^{(g)}\right)$ for g = 1, 2, if and only if $\varphi_{BA} = 1$.

Problem 3.6. Define the response score for a success as 1 and failure as 0. Prescott (1981) considered the difference in response scores between the first and second periods. In other words, we assign patients with response vector (1, 0) at the two periods the score $X = 1$, patients with response vector (1, 1) and (0, 0) the score $X = 0$, and patients with response vector (0, 1) the score $X = -1$. Thus, we may summarize our data in the following table:

Response vector		(1, 0)	(1, 1) or (0, 0)	(0, 1)	Total
g	Score	X = 1	X = 0	X = -1	
1		$n_{10}^{(1)}$	$n_{11}^{(1)} + n_{00}^{(1)}$	$n_{01}^{(1)}$	n_1
2		$n_{10}^{(2)}$	$n_{11}^{(2)} + n_{00}^{(2)}$	$n_{01}^{(2)}$	n_2
Total		$n_{10}^{(+)}$	$n_{11}^{(+)} + n_{00}^{(+)}$	$n_{01}^{(+)}$	n_+

When there is no difference in treatment effects, we may regard group $g = 1$ as a random sample of size n_1 taken from a population of size n_+. Show that the expectation $E(n_{10}^{(1)} - n_{01}^{(1)}) = n_1(n_{10}^{(+)} - n_{01}^{(+)})/n_+$ and variance given by $Var(n_{10}^{(1)} - n_{01}^{(1)}) = n_1 n_2\{(n_{10}^{(+)} + n_{01}^{(+)}) - (n_{10}^{(+)} - n_{01}^{(+)})^2/n_+\}/\{n_+(n_+ - 1)\}$. (Hint: Use Theorems 2.1 and

2.2 in Cochran (1977, pp. 22–23).) We can use test statistic $z = [|(n_{10}^{(1)} - n_{01}^{(1)}) - E(n_{10}^{(1)} - n_{01}^{(1)})| - 1/2]/[Var(n_{10}^{(1)} - n_{01}^{(1)})]^{1/2}$ based on normal approximation to test $H_0 : \eta = 0$. Note that Prescott (1981) has also provided an exact test procedure on the basis of the distribution of random permutations. Note also that a discussion on the use of PROC FREQ to implement Prescott's test procedures can be found elsewhere (Jones and Kenward, 2014, pp. 102–104).

Problem 3.7.   Show that using procedure (3.13) based on the exact conditional distribution for testing non-inferiority is identical to rejecting $H_0 : \varphi_{BA} \leq \varphi_l$ whenever the one-sided exact $100(1 - \alpha)\%$ confidence lower limit φ_{BAL} falls above the acceptable non-inferior margin φ_l.

Problem 3.8.   Show that the test procedure (3.14) is equivalent to rejecting $H_0 : \varphi_{BA} \leq \varphi_l$ or $\varphi_{BA} \geq \varphi_u$ at the α-level whenever the asymptotic $100(1 - 2\alpha)\%$ confidence interval (3.17) lies entirely in the equivalence interval (φ_l, φ_u).

Problem 3.9.   On the basis of the test procedure (3.7) (two-sided test), show that an approximate minimum required number of patients n per group for a desired power $1 - \beta$ of detecting non-equality with a specified value $\varphi_{BA}^* \neq 0$ at a nominal α-level is given by (3.22).

Problem 3.10.   Show that an approximate minimum required number of patients n per group for a desired power $1 - \beta$ of detecting non-inferiority with a specified value $\varphi_{BA}^* (> \varphi_l)$ at a nominal α-level based on the test procedure (3.11) is given by (3.23).

Problem 3.11.   As the number n of patients is reasonably large, show that the power function for testing equivalence based on the test procedure (3.14) is approximately given by (3.24).

Problem 3.12.   When $n_{10}^{(g)}$ and $n_{01}^{(g)}$ are reasonably large, show that one can use the test procedure (3.38) to test $H_0 : \eta_{BA} = \gamma = 0$. (Hint: The conditional probability mass function $n_{01}^{(g)}$, given $n_{dis}^{(g)}$ fixed, follows the binomial distribution with parameters $n_{dis}^{(g)}$ and $p_g = 1/2$ under $H_0 : \eta_{BA} = \gamma = 0$.)

Problem 3.13.   Suppose that in an AB/BA design we obtain the following data:

Response vector	(1, 0)	(1, 1) or (0, 0)	(0, 1)	Total
g Score	X = 1	X = 0	X = -1	
1 (AB sequence)	3	20	7	30
2 (BA sequence)	8	18	4	30
Total	11	38	11	60

(a) What are the p-values for using test procedures (3.7)–(3.9) to test non-equality?

(b) What is the p-value for using the exact test procedure (3.10)?

(c) What is the p-value for using Prescott's test procedure?

Problem 3.14.   The following data are taken from a simple crossover trial comparing a placebo (A) with an active drug (B) in cerebrovascular deficiency from one of the two centers (Jones and Kenward, 1989, p. 90). The response was defined according to whether an electrocardiogram was considered as normal (coded as 1) or abnormal (coded as 0).

Response vector at two periods		(1, 0)	(1, 1) or (0, 0)	(0, 1)	Total
g	Score	$X = 1$	$X = 0$	$X = -1$	
1 (AB sequence)		6	28	0	34
2 (BA sequence)		2	27	4	33
Total		8	55	4	67

(a) What is the p-value for using the exact test procedure (3.10)?

(b) What is the p-value for using Prescott's asymptotic test procedure?

Problem 3.15.   Show that under model (3.40), we have $\left[\left(\pi_{01}^{(1)}\pi_{10}^{(2)}\right)\Big/\right.$ $\left.\left(\pi_{10}^{(1)}\pi_{01}^{(2)}\right)\right]^{1/2} = \varphi_{BA}\exp((\lambda_A - \lambda_B)/2).$

Problem 3.16.   Show why the procedure for testing whether there is an association for the 2×2 tables with the vector of cell probabilities $(\pi_{11}^{(1)}, \pi_{11}^{(2)})$ in the first row and $(\pi_{00}^{(1)}, \pi_{00}^{(2)})$ in the second row under model (3.40) does not work exactly for testing treatment-by-period interaction.

Problem 3.17.   Consider use of ABB/BAA design (Lucas, 1957; Patterson and Lucas, 1959; Kershner and Federer, 1981; Ebbutt, 1984; Senn, D'Angelo, and Potvin, 2004) in the simple carry-over model, in which the carry-over effect of a treatment depends exclusively on the treatment received at the previous period and is not modified by the treatment received at the current period. Patients are randomly assigned to the group ($g = 1$) with the treatment-receipt sequence A-B-B, in which patients receive treatments A at period 1, treatment B at periods 2 and 3, or the group ($g = 2$) with the treatment-receipt sequence B-A-A, in which patients receive treatment B at period 1, treatment A at periods 2 and 3. We assume that the patient response

$$P\left(Y_{iz}^{(g)} = 1\right)$$
$$= \frac{\exp\left(\mu_i^{(g)} + \eta_{BA}X_{iz}^{(g)} + \gamma_1 Z_{iz1}^{(g)} + \gamma_2 Z_{iz2}^{(g)} + \lambda_A I_{\{g=1\}}Z_{iz1}^{(g)} + \lambda_B I_{\{g=1\}}Z_{iz2}^{(g)} + \lambda_B\left(1 - I_{\{g=1\}}\right)Z_{iz1}^{(g)} + \lambda_A\left(1 - I_{\{g=1\}}\right)Z_{iz2}^{(g)}\right)}{1 + \exp\left(\mu_i^{(g)} + \eta_{BA}X_{iz}^{(g)} + \gamma_1 Z_{iz1}^{(g)} + \gamma_2 Z_{iz2}^{(g)} + \lambda_A I_{\{g=1\}}Z_{iz1}^{(g)} + \lambda_B I_{\{g=1\}}Z_{iz2}^{(g)} + \lambda_B\left(1 - I_{\{g=1\}}\right)Z_{iz1}^{(g)} + \lambda_A\left(1 - I_{\{g=1\}}\right)Z_{iz2}^{(g)}\right)},$$

where $\mu_i^{(g)}$ denotes the random effect due to the ith patient in group g and all $\mu_i^{(g)}$'s are assumed to independently follow an unspecified probability density function $f_g(\mu)$,

η_{BA} denotes the effect of treatment B relative to treatment A; $I_{\{g=1\}} = 1$ for group $g = 1$, and $= 0$ otherwise; $Z_{i1}^{(g)}$ and $Z_{i2}^{(g)}$ represent the indicator functions of period covariates, defining $Z_{i1}^{(g)} = 1$ for period $z = 2$, and $= 0$ otherwise; as well as $Z_{i2}^{(g)} = 1$ for period $z = 3$, and $= 0$ otherwise; γ_1 and γ_2 represent the respective effect of periods 2 and 3 versus period 1; and λ_A and λ_B are the carry-over effects due to treatments A and B, respectively. For brevity in notation, let "+" denote the summation over that subscript for notation in the following discussion. Under the above model, (a) show that the following equalities:

$$\pi_{+11}^{(1)} = \int \left(\frac{\exp(\mu + \eta_{BA} + \gamma_1 + \lambda_A)}{1 + \exp(\mu + \eta_{BA} + \gamma_1 + \lambda_A)} \right) \left(\frac{\exp(\mu + \eta_{BA} + \gamma_2 + \lambda_B)}{1 + \exp(\mu + \eta_{BA} + \gamma_2 + \lambda_B)} \right) f_1(\mu) d\mu;$$

$$\pi_{+01}^{(1)} = \int \left(\frac{1}{1 + \exp(\mu + \eta_{BA} + \gamma_1 + \lambda_A)} \right) \left(\frac{\exp(\mu + \eta_{BA} + \gamma_2 + \lambda_B)}{1 + \exp(\mu + \eta_{BA} + \gamma_2 + \lambda_B)} \right) f_1(\mu) d\mu;$$

$$\pi_{+10}^{(1)} = \int \left(\frac{\exp(\mu + \eta_{BA} + \gamma_1 + \lambda_A)}{1 + \exp(\mu + \eta_{BA} + \gamma_1 + \lambda_A)} \right) \left(\frac{1}{1 + \exp(\mu + \eta_{BA} + \gamma_2 + \lambda_B)} \right) f_1(\mu) d\mu;$$

$$\pi_{+00}^{(1)} = \int \left(\frac{1}{1 + \exp(\mu + \eta_{BA} + \gamma_1 + \lambda_A)} \right) \left(\frac{1}{1 + \exp(\mu + \eta_{BA} + \gamma_2 + \lambda_B)} \right) f_1(\mu) d\mu;$$

$$\pi_{+11}^{(2)} = \int \left(\frac{\exp(\mu + \gamma_1 + \lambda_B)}{1 + \exp(\mu + \gamma_1 + \lambda_B)} \right) \left(\frac{\exp(\mu + \gamma_2 + \lambda_A)}{1 + \exp(\mu + \gamma_2 + \lambda_A)} \right) f_2(\mu) d\mu;$$

$$\pi_{+01}^{(2)} = \int \left(\frac{1}{1 + \exp(\mu + \gamma_1 + \lambda_B)} \right) \left(\frac{\exp(\mu + \gamma_2 + \lambda_A)}{1 + \exp(\mu + \gamma_2 + \lambda_A)} \right) f_2(\mu) d\mu;$$

$$\pi_{+10}^{(2)} = \int \left(\frac{\exp(\mu + \gamma_1 + \lambda_B)}{1 + \exp(\mu + \gamma_1 + \lambda_B)} \right) \left(\frac{1}{1 + \exp(\mu + \gamma_2 + \lambda_A)} \right) f_2(\mu) d\mu;$$

$$\pi_{+00}^{(2)} = \int \left(\frac{1}{1 + \exp(\mu + \gamma_1 + \lambda_B)} \right) \left(\frac{1}{1 + \exp(\mu + \gamma_2 + \lambda_A)} \right) f_2(\mu) d\mu.$$

(b) Show that $\left[\left(\pi_{+01}^{(1)} \pi_{+10}^{(2)} \right) / \left(\pi_{+10}^{(1)} \pi_{+01}^{(2)} \right) \right]^{1/2} = \exp(\lambda_B - \lambda_A)$. Let $n_{rst}^{(g)}$ denote in group g (= 1, 2) the number of patients among n_g patients with response vector ($Y_{i1}^{(g)} = r$, $Y_{i2}^{(g)} = s$, $Y_{i3}^{(g)} = t$), where $r = 1, 0$, $s = 1, 0$, $t = 1, 0$. The random frequencies $\{n_{rst}^{(g)} | r = 1, 0, s = 1, 0, t = 1, 0\}$ then follow the multinomial distribution with parameters n_g and $\{\pi_{rst}^{(g)} | r = 1, 0, s = 1, 0, t = 1, 0\}$, where $\pi_{rst}^{(g)}$ denotes the cell probability that a randomly selected patient i from group g has the response vector ($Y_{i1}^{(g)} = r$, $Y_{i2}^{(g)} = s$, $Y_{i3}^{(g)} = t$) at three periods. We can estimate $\pi_{+st}^{(g)}$ by $\hat{\pi}_{+st}^{(g)} = n_{+st}^{(g)} / n_g$ and hence we can estimate $\lambda_B - \lambda_A$ by $(1/2) \log \left(\left(\hat{\pi}_{+01}^{(1)} \hat{\pi}_{+10}^{(2)} \right) / \left(\hat{\pi}_{+10}^{(1)} \hat{\pi}_{+01}^{(2)} \right) \right)$ with its estimated asymptotic variance $(1/4) \left(1/n_{+01}^{(1)} + 1/n_{+10}^{(2)} + 1/n_{+10}^{(1)} + 1/n_{+01}^{(2)} \right)$. (c) Show how to use the above result based on equation (3.41) to adjust the bias caused by the differential carry-over effect in assessing the relative treatment effect. We can also employ the above results to do hypothesis testing and interval estimation of $\lambda_B - \lambda_A$ if we wish. Note that when using the simple carry-over model, we assume that the carry-over effect depends on only the treatment at the immediately preceding period, and the carry-over effect is not affected by the treatment received at the current period. As noted by Fleiss (1986b, 1989) and Senn (1992, 2002), this strong assumption is unlikely to hold under most situations in practice. To alleviate the above strong assumption in use of the simple carry-over model, Lui (2016) has recently suggested an alternative three-period crossover design in which the carry-over effect can depend on both the preceding and current treatments for comparing two treatments in dichotomous data.

4

AB/BA design in ordinal data

It is not uncommon that we may encounter in a randomized clinical trial the patient response on an ordinal scale – worse, same, or better. In contrast to the quantitative data, one subtle point in the analysis of ordinal data is that ordinal responses are not truly appropriate for arithmetic operations. For example, consider the data (Table 4.1) taken from an AB/BA crossover trial (Ezzet and Whitehead, 1991) conducted by 3M-Riker to compare the suitability of two inhalation devices (A and B) among asthma patients who were using a standard inhaler device delivering salbutamol. Patients were randomly assigned to either group 1 with use of device A for one week followed by device B for another week, or group 2 with use of device B for one week followed by device A for another week. Patients were then asked to assess the clarity of leaflet instructions accompanying the devices on a four-point ordinal scale: "easy," "only clear after rereading," "not very clear," and "confusing." Since these categorical levels of response are not on an interval scale, the relative distance between "easy" and "only clear after rereading" is not, for example, identical to the relative distance between "not every clear" and "confusing." Thus, the mean of differences between arbitrary scores (such as 0, 1, 2, 3) assigned to these ordinal categories generally possesses no practical meaning or easy interpretation. To alleviate this concern, Ezzet and Whitehead (1991) proposed a random effects proportional odds model (Clayton and Cuzick, 1985). However, this model-based approach requires not only the data between different ordinal categories to satisfy a very specific model structural relationship but also unobservable patient random effects to follow a normal distribution. Furthermore, we need to use a sophisticated iterative numerical procedure (which is now no longer an issue with the availability of PROC GLIMMIX (SAS Institute, 2009)) to obtain parameter estimates based on a likelihood involving non-closed form integrals. Other approaches, such as converting the difference between two periods from the ordinal data to a change score scale and using a trend test (Senn, 1993),

Crossover Designs: Testing, Estimation, and Sample Size, First Edition. Kung-Jong Lui.
© 2016 John Wiley & Sons, Ltd. Published 2016 by John Wiley & Sons, Ltd.
Companion website: www.wiley.com/go/lui/crossover

Table 4.1   The frequency of patients taken from a crossover study conducted by 3M-Riker to compare the assessment on the clarity of leaflet instructions for two inhalation devices in patients currently using a standard inhaler device delivering salbutamol between period 1 (row) versus period 2 (column).

	Group 1: A-then-B sequence				
	Easy	Only clear after rereading	Not very clear	Confusing	Total
Easy	59	35	3	2	99
Only clear after rereading	11	27	2	1	41
Not very clear	0	0	0	0	0
Confusing	1	1	0	0	2
Total	71	63	5	3	142

	Group 2: B-then-A sequence				
	Easy	Only clear after rereading	Not very clear	Confusing	Total
Easy	63	13	0	0	76
Only clear after rereading	40	15	0	0	55
Not very clear	7	2	1	0	10
Confusing	2	0	1	0	3
Total	112	30	2	0	144

or treating these artificial scores as quantitative data and using a t-test, have been suggested elsewhere (Hills and Armitage, 1979; Senn, 2002, pp. 135–139). However, using these approaches may group patients with response changes that are not truly comparable into the same category (Ezzet and Whitehead, 1993). This concern can even exacerbate when the number of ordinal categories is not few. Furthermore, besides testing whether there is a difference between treatments, we may often wish to assess the magnitude of the relative treatment effect. How to assign artificial scores to reflect the relative distance between different ordinal levels and provide a meaningful and easily understood summary measure of the relative treatment effect based on these artificial scores can be challenging.

Using the generalized odds ratio (GOR) for paired samples or Agresti's α' (Agresti, 1980; Lui, 2002a, 2002b, 2004; Lui and Chang, 2013a, 2013b) to measure the relative treatment effect, we discuss hypothesis testing and interval estimation in ordinal data under an AB/BA crossover trial (Lui and Chang, 2012c). We provide asymptotic and exact test procedures for testing non-equality of two treatments. We further provide asymptotic and exact procedures for testing non-inferiority and equivalence. We address interval estimation of the relative treatment effect and sample size determination based on the GOR. We discuss hypothesis testing and estimation for the period effect. We present SAS codes (SAS Institute, 2009) for the likelihood-based approach assuming a normal random effects proportional odds model (Ezzet and Whitehead, 1991), and compare the test results with those obtained by using the conditional arguments focused on here. An alternative model-free test procedure based on the GOR for two independent samples (or Agresti's α) (Agresti, 1980) to improve power when the number of patients is adequately large relative to the number of ordinal categories can be found elsewhere (Lui and Chang, 2012c).

Suppose we compare an experimental treatment B with an active control treatment (or a placebo) A. We randomly assign n_1 patients to group $(g =)$ 1 with A-then-B sequence, in which patients receive treatment A at period 1 and then cross over to receive treatment B at period 2, and n_2 patients to group $(g =)$ 2 with B-then-A sequence, in which patients receive treatment B at period 1 and then cross over to receive treatment A at period 2. We consider the situations in which the underlying patient response is on an ordinal scale with L possible categories: $C_1 < C_2 < C_3 < \cdots < C_L$. For patient i $(= 1, 2, \ldots, n_g)$ from group g $(= 1, 2)$ at period z $(= 1, 2)$, we let $X_{iz}^{(g)}$ $(= 1$ for the experimental treatment B, and $= 0$ otherwise) and $Z_{iz}^{(g)}$ $(= 1$ for period $z = 2$, and $= 0$ otherwise) denote the treatment and period covariates of this patient, respectively. We further let $Y_{iz}^{(g)}$ denote in group g $(= 1, 2)$ the response of the *ith* patient at period z. We assume that the joint probability of $\left(Y_{i1}^{(g)}, Y_{i2}^{(g)}\right)$ for patient i $(= 1, 2, \cdots, n_g)$ in group g satisfies

$$P\left(Y_{i1}^{(g)} < Y_{i2}^{(g)}\right) = \left[1 / \left(1 + \exp\left(\mu_i^{(g)} + \eta_{BA} X_{i1}^{(g)} + \gamma Z_{i1}^{(g)}\right)\right)\right]$$
$$\times \left[\exp\left(\mu_i^{(g)} + \eta_{BA} X_{i2}^{(g)} + \gamma Z_{i2}^{(g)}\right) / \left(1 + \exp\left(\mu_i^{(g)} + \eta_{BA} X_{i2}^{(g)} + \gamma Z_{i2}^{(g)}\right)\right)\right],$$

$$P\left(Y_{i1}^{(g)} > Y_{i2}^{(g)}\right) = \left[1 / \left(1 + \exp\left(\mu_i^{(g)} + \eta_{BA} X_{i2}^{(g)} + \gamma Z_{i2}^{(g)}\right)\right)\right]$$
$$\times \left[\exp\left(\mu_i^{(g)} + \eta_{BA} X_{i1}^{(g)} + \gamma Z_{i1}^{(g)}\right) / \left(1 + \exp\left(\mu_i^{(g)} + \eta_{BA} X_{i1}^{(g)} + \gamma Z_{i1}^{(g)}\right)\right)\right], \text{ and}$$

$$P\left(Y_{i1}^{(g)} = Y_{i2}^{(g)}\right) = 1 - P\left(Y_{i1}^{(g)} > Y_{i2}^{(g)}\right) - P\left(Y_{i1}^{(g)} < Y_{i2}^{(g)}\right), \tag{4.1}$$

where $\mu_i^{(g)}$ denotes the random effect due to the *ith* subject in group g, and $\mu_i^{(g)}$'s are assumed to independently follow an unspecified probability density $f_g(\mu)$, η_{BA} denotes the relative effect of treatment B to treatment A, and γ denotes the effect of period 2 versus period 1. Based on model (4.1), the GOR for paired samples or Agresti's α' (Agresti, 1980; Lui, 2002a, 2004) of responses on a given patient i in group g $(= 1, 2)$ when he/she has covariates $\left(X_{i2}^{(g)}, Z_{i2}^{(g)}\right)$ at period 2 versus when he/she has covariates $\left(X_{i1}^{(g)}, Z_{i1}^{(g)}\right)$ at period 1 is, by definition, equal to (Problem 4.1)

$$P\left(Y_{i1}^{(g)} < Y_{i2}^{(g)}\right) / P\left(Y_{i1}^{(g)} > Y_{i2}^{(g)}\right) = \exp\left(\eta_{BA}\left(X_{i2}^{(g)} - X_{i1}^{(g)}\right) + \gamma\left(Z_{i2}^{(g)} - Z_{i1}^{(g)}\right)\right). \tag{4.2}$$

When $\eta_{BA} = 0$, the GOR (4.2) remains, for given a fixed period, unchanged and equals 1 despite the patient receiving treatment B or treatment A. When $\eta_{BA} > 0$, the response of the patient receiving treatment B tends to fall, for given a fixed period, in a category with level C_k higher than that of the patient receiving treatment A. On the other hand, when $\eta_{BA} < 0$, the response of the patient receiving treatment B tends to fall, for given a fixed period, in a category with level C_k lower than that of the patient receiving treatment A. Similar interpretations can be applied to the parameter γ representing the period effect. On the basis of model (4.1), for a randomly selected patient from group g (= 1, 2) the probability that the patient response $Y_1^{(g)}$ (the noninformative subscript i has been deleted for simplicity in notation) at period 1 is less than his/her response $Y_2^{(g)}$ at period 2 is

$$P\left(Y_1^{(g)} < Y_2^{(g)}\right) = \int \left[1/\left(1 + \exp\left(\mu + \eta_{BA}X_1^{(g)} + \gamma Z_1^{(g)}\right)\right)\right]$$
$$\times \left[\exp\left(\mu + \eta_{BA}X_2^{(g)} + \gamma Z_2^{(g)}\right)/\left(1 + \exp\left(\mu + \eta_{BA}X_2^{(g)} + \gamma Z_2^{(g)}\right)\right)\right] f_g(\mu) d\mu.$$
(4.3)

Similarly, for a randomly selected patient from group g (= 1, 2), the probability that the patient response $Y_1^{(g)}$ at period 1 is larger than his/her response $Y_2^{(g)}$ at period 2 is

$$P\left(Y_1^{(g)} > Y_2^{(g)}\right) = \int \left[1/\left(1 + \exp\left(\mu + \eta_{BA}X_2^{(g)} + \gamma Z_2^{(g)}\right)\right)\right]$$
$$\times \left[\exp\left(\mu + \eta_{BA}X_1^{(g)} + \gamma Z_1^{(g)}\right)/\left(1 + \exp\left(\mu + \eta_{BA}X_1^{(g)} + \gamma Z_1^{(g)}\right)\right)\right] f_g(\mu) d\mu.$$
(4.4)

For brevity, we let $\Pi_C^{(g)}$ and $\Pi_D^{(g)}$ denote these probabilities $P\left(Y_1^{(g)} < Y_2^{(g)}\right)$ and $P\left(Y_1^{(g)} > Y_2^{(g)}\right)$, respectively. From (4.3) and (4.4), we can see that the GOR of patient responses between periods 2 and 1 for a randomly selected patient from group g is (Problem 4.2)

$$GOR^{(g)} = \Pi_C^{(g)}/\Pi_D^{(g)}$$
$$= \exp\left(\eta_{BA}\left(X_2^{(g)} - X_1^{(g)}\right) + \gamma\left(Z_2^{(g)} - Z_1^{(g)}\right)\right).$$
(4.5)

Under the AB/BA design as described above, we have

$$GOR^{(1)} = \Pi_C^{(1)}/\Pi_D^{(1)} = \exp(\eta_{BA} + \gamma), \quad \text{and}$$
(4.6)

$$GOR^{(2)} = \Pi_C^{(2)}/\Pi_D^{(2)} = \exp(-\eta_{BA} + \gamma).$$
(4.7)

From formulas (4.6) and (4.7), we can express the GOR of patient responses for treatment B versus treatment A (for a fixed period on a randomly selected patient), as well as that for period 2 versus period 1 (for a fixed treatment on a randomly selected patient) as given by (Problem 4.3)

$$GOR_{BA} = \exp(\eta_{BA}) = \left(GOR^{(1)}/GOR^{(2)}\right)^{1/2}, \quad \text{and} \tag{4.8}$$

$$GOR_P = \exp(\gamma) = \left(GOR^{(1)}GOR^{(2)}\right)^{1/2}, \quad \text{respectively.} \tag{4.9}$$

Note that $\Pi_C^{(g)}$ and $\Pi_D^{(g)}$ are, by definition, equal to $\sum_{r=1}^{L-1}\sum_{s=r+1}^{L}\pi_{rs}^{(g)}$ and $\sum_{r=2}^{L}\sum_{s=1}^{r-1}\pi_{rs}^{(g)}$, where $\pi_{rs}^{(g)} = P\left(Y_1^{(g)} = C_r, Y_2^{(g)} = C_s\right)$, for $r = 1, 2, \cdots, L$, and $s = 1, 2, \cdots, L$. When $L = 2$, $GOR^{(1)}$ (4.6) and $GOR^{(2)}$ (4.7) reduce to the ORs $\pi_{12}^{(1)}/\pi_{21}^{(1)}$ and $\pi_{12}^{(2)}/\pi_{21}^{(2)}$ for paired samples, respectively. Thus, we can see that formulas (4.8) and (4.9) reduce to formulas (3.2) and (3.31) when we have only two categories with C_1 and C_2 representing the negative and positive responses, respectively.

Let $n_{rs}^{(g)}$ denote the number of patients in group g ($= 1, 2$) falling in the cell with the response vector $\left(Y_1^{(g)} = C_r, Y_2^{(g)} = C_s\right)$ among n_g patients. The random frequencies $\{n_{rs}^{(g)} \mid r = 1, 2, 3, \cdots, L, s = 1, 2, 3, \cdots, L\}$ then follow the multinomial distribution with parameters n_g and $\{\pi_{rs}^{(g)} \mid r = 1, 2, 3, \cdots, L, s = 1, 2, 3, \cdots, L\}$. Note that we can estimate $\pi_{rs}^{(g)}$ by the unbiased consistent sample proportion estimator $\hat{\pi}_{rs}^{(g)} = n_{rs}^{(g)}/n_g$ based on the multinomial distribution. Thus, we obtain a consistent estimator for $GOR^{(g)}$ in group g ($= 1, 2$) as given by

$$\widehat{GOR}^{(g)} = \hat{\Pi}_C^{(g)}/\hat{\Pi}_D^{(g)}, \tag{4.10}$$

where $\hat{\Pi}_C^{(g)} = \sum_{r=1}^{L-1}\sum_{s=r+1}^{L}\hat{\pi}_{rs}^{(g)}$ and $\hat{\Pi}_D^{(g)} = \sum_{r=2}^{L}\sum_{s=1}^{r-1}\hat{\pi}_{rs}^{(g)}$. Therefore, we obtain consistent estimators for GOR_{BA} (4.8) and GOR_P (4.9) as given by

$$\widehat{GOR}_{BA} = \left(\widehat{GOR}^{(1)}/\widehat{GOR}^{(2)}\right)^{1/2}, \quad \text{and} \tag{4.11}$$

$$\widehat{GOR}_P = \left(\widehat{GOR}^{(1)}\widehat{GOR}^{(2)}\right)^{1/2}. \tag{4.12}$$

Furthermore, using the delta method (Agresti, 1990; Lui, 2004), we obtain an estimated asymptotic variance of $\log(\widehat{GOR}_{BA})$ as given by (Lui, 2002a; Lui and Chang, 2012c) (Problem 4.4)

$$\widehat{Var}\left(\log\left(\widehat{GOR}_{BA}\right)\right) = \widehat{Var}\left(\log\left(\widehat{GOR}_P\right)\right)$$
$$= \left[\sum_{g=1}^{2}\left(\hat{\Pi}_C^{(g)} + \hat{\Pi}_D^{(g)}\right)/\left(n_g\hat{\Pi}_C^{(g)}\hat{\Pi}_D^{(g)}\right)\right]/4. \tag{4.13}$$

Define $n_{dis}^{(g)} = n_C^{(g)} + n_D^{(g)}$, where $n_C^{(g)} = \sum_{r=1}^{L-1} \sum_{s=r+1}^{L} n_{rs}^{(g)}$ and $n_D^{(g)} = \sum_{r=2}^{L} \sum_{s=1}^{r-1} n_{rs}^{(g)}$ for $g = 1, 2$. Note that the number $n_{dis}^{(g)}$ simply denotes the total number of patients with responses falling into different categories between two periods in group g. We can show that the conditional distribution of $n_C^{(g)}$, given $n_{dis}^{(g)}$ fixed, follows the binomial distribution with parameters $n_{dis}^{(g)}$ and $p^{(g)} = \Pi_C^{(g)} / \left(\Pi_C^{(g)} + \Pi_D^{(g)} \right)$ for $g = 1, 2$ (Problem 4.5). We can further show that the conditional probability mass function of $n_C^{(1)} = x_1$ (where $\max\{0, n_C^{(+)} - n_{dis}^{(2)}\} \le x_1 \le \min\left\{ n_{dis}^{(1)}, n_C^{(+)} \right\}$), given $n_C^{(+)} = n_C^{(1)} + n_C^{(2)}$ fixed, is given by the noncentral hypergeometric distribution (Gart and Thomas, 1972; Agresti, 1990; Lui, 2004):

$$P\left(n_C^{(1)} = x_1 | n_C^{(+)}, n_{dis}^{(1)}, n_{dis}^{(2)}, Q_{BA} \right) = \binom{n_{dis}^{(1)}}{x_1} \binom{n_{dis}^{(2)}}{n_C^{(+)} - x_1} Q_{BA}^{x_1} / \sum_x \binom{n_{dis}^{(1)}}{x} \binom{n_{dis}^{(2)}}{n_C^{(+)} - x} Q_{BA}^x,$$

(4.14)

where $Q_{BA} = \left(\Pi_C^{(1)} \Pi_D^{(2)} \right) / \left(\Pi_D^{(1)} \Pi_C^{(2)} \right) = GOR_{BA}^2$, and the summation for x is over the range $\max\left\{0, n_C^{(+)} - n_{dis}^{(2)} \right\} \le x \le \min\left\{ n_{dis}^{(1)}, n_C^{(+)} \right\}$.

Note that when $\eta_{BA} = 0$ (i.e., $Q_{BA} = 1$), the noncentral hypergeometric distribution (4.14) reduces to the central hypergeometric distribution:

$$P\left(n_C^{(1)} = x_1 | n_C^{(+)}, n_{dis}^{(1)}, n_{dis}^{(2)}, Q_{BA} = 1 \right) = \binom{n_{dis}^{(1)}}{x_1} \binom{n_{dis}^{(2)}}{n_C^{(+)} - x_1} / \binom{n_{dis}^{(1)} + n_{dis}^{(2)}}{n_C^{(+)}}, \quad (4.15)$$

where $\max\left\{ 0, n_C^{(+)} - n_{dis}^{(2)} \right\} \le x_1 \le \min\left\{ n_{dis}^{(1)}, n_C^{(+)} \right\}$.

4.1   Testing non-equality of treatments

Suppose that we wish to find out whether there is a difference between treatments A and B. This leads us to consider testing the null hypothesis $H_0 : GOR_{BA} = 1$ (i.e., $\eta_{BA} = 0$) versus $H_a : GOR_{BA} \neq 1$ (i.e., $\eta_{BA} \neq 0$). On the basis of $\widehat{GOR}_{BA}$ (4.11) with the logarithmic transformation and the estimated asymptotic variance $\widehat{Var}\left(\log\left(\widehat{GOR}_{BA} \right) \right)$ (4.13), we will reject $H_0 : GOR_{BA} = 1$ at the α-level if the test statistic

$$|\log\left(\widehat{GOR}_{BA} \right)| / \sqrt{\widehat{Var}\left(\log\left(\widehat{GOR}_{BA} \right) \right)} > Z_{\alpha/2}, \quad (4.16)$$

where Z_α is the upper $100(\alpha)$th percentile of the standard normal distribution.

Recall that given $n_{dis}^{(g)}\left(=n_C^{(g)}+n_D^{(g)}\right)$ fixed, the conditional distribution of $n_C^{(g)}$ follows the binomial distribution with parameters $n_{dis}^{(g)}$ and $p^{(g)}=\Pi_C^{(g)}/\left(\Pi_C^{(g)}+\Pi_D^{(g)}\right)=GOR^{(g)}/\left(1+GOR^{(g)}\right)$. Note that $p^{(1)}=p^{(2)}$ if and only if $GOR_{BA}=1$ (Problem 4.6). Thus, we can employ the commonly used procedure for testing non-equality of two proportions in two independent samples. We will reject $H_0:GOR_{BA}=1$ at the α-level if the test statistic

$$\left(\hat{p}^{(1)}-\hat{p}^{(2)}\right)/\sqrt{\hat{\bar{p}}\left(1-\hat{\bar{p}}\right)\left(1/n_{dis}^{(1)}+1/n_{dis}^{(2)}\right)}>Z_{\alpha/2}, \qquad (4.17)$$

where $\hat{p}^{(g)}=n_C^{(g)}/n_{dis}^{(g)}$ for $g=1,2$, and $\hat{\bar{p}}=\left(n_C^{(1)}+n_C^{(2)}\right)/\left(n_{dis}^{(1)}+n_{dis}^{(2)}\right)$. When $n_C^{(g)}$ or $n_D^{(g)}$ is small, test procedures (4.16) and (4.17) are not appropriate for use. In this case, we may consider use of Fisher's exact test on the basis of the exact conditional distribution (4.15). We will reject $H_0:GOR_{BA}=1$ at the α-level if we observe $n_C^{(1)}=x_1$ such that

$$\min\left\{P\left(x\ge x_1|n_C^{(+)},n_{dis}^{(1)},n_{dis}^{(2)},Q_{BA}=1\right),\ P\left(x\le x_1|n_C^{(+)},n_{dis}^{(1)},n_{dis}^{(2)},Q_{BA}=1\right)\right\}\le\alpha/2, \qquad (4.18)$$

where

$$P\left(x\ge x_1|n_C^{(+)},n_{dis}^{(1)},n_{dis}^{(2)},Q_{BA}=1\right)=\sum_{x\ge x_1}P\left(n_C^{(1)}=x|n_C^{(+)},n_{dis}^{(1)},n_{dis}^{(2)},Q_{BA}=1\right),\ \text{and}$$

$$P\left(x\le x_1|n_C^{(+)},n_{dis}^{(1)},n_{dis}^{(2)},Q_{BA}=1\right)=\sum_{x\le x_1}P\left(n_C^{(1)}=x|n_C^{(+)},n_{dis}^{(1)},n_{dis}^{(2)},Q_{BA}=1\right).$$

Example 4.1   Consider the data in Table 4.1 taken from a crossover trial conducted by 3M-Riker to compare the suitability of two new inhalation devices (A and B) in asthma patients who were using a standard inhaler device delivering salbutamol (Ezzet and Whitehead, 1991). Group 1 used device A for one week followed by device B for another week, while group 2 used the devices in reverse order. No wash-out period was felt necessary. Besides the information on various outcome measures related to the use of devices, patients gave their assessment on the clarity of leaflet instructions accompanying the device, and reported on an ordinal scale: "easy," "only clear after reading," "not very clear," and "confusing." When employing test procedures (4.16)–(4.18) to test $H_0:GOR_{BA}=1$ (i.e., the clarity of leaflet instructions between devices A and B is the same), we obtain all the p-values to be less than 0.001. These results strongly suggest that the clarity of leaflet instructions are different between devices A and B.

4.2   Testing non-inferiority of an experimental treatment to an active control treatment

When an experimental treatment has fewer side effects and is easier to administer than an active control treatment, the former can be a useful alternative to the latter if we can show that the experimental treatment is non-inferior to the active control treatment with respect to treatment efficacy. For certain treatments, such as antiulcer agents and topical antifungal agents (Liu and Chow, 1993; Tu, 1998, 2001), which do not produce an appreciable absorption into the systemic circulation, we may want to assess whether the experimental treatment is non-inferior to the active control treatment with respect to clinical outcomes.

Suppose that the higher the ordinal response level C_j, the better is the outcome. When assessing the non-inferiority of an experimental treatment B to an active control treatment A, we want to test the null hypothesis $H_0 : GOR_{BA} \leq GOR_l$ versus the alternative hypothesis $H_a : GOR_{BA} > GOR_l$, where $0 < GOR_l < 1$ is the maximum clinically acceptable low margin such that treatment B can be regarded as non-inferior to treatment A when $GOR_{BA} > GOR_l$ holds. The determination of the non-inferior margin GOR_l should be, just like other statistical indices, prespecified by the experts in the fields of biopharmaceutics and medicine based on their medical judgment, instead of by statisticians (Schuirmann, 1987). Some comprehensive discussions on issues relevant to the determination of the non-inferiority margin applicable to all statistical indices appear elsewhere (Wiens, 2002; D'Agostino, Massaro, and Sullivan, 2003; Hung et al., 2003; Lui and Chang, 2012c). In general, if the endpoints were irreversible serious outcomes, presumably only the slightest decline in efficacy as compared with the active control treatment would be acceptable (Brittain and Hu, 2009). On the other hand, if the endpoints related to outcomes could be easily alleviated or reversed by further treatment or the experimental treatment has other significant benefits (e.g., less toxic, less costly, fewer side effects), a larger non-inferior margin GOR_l could be used. Also, we may follow some common practices by specifying the margin to preserve a certain fraction, for example, 50% of the benefit of an active control treatment over placebo (Hung et al., 2003). To illustrate this point, suppose that we use the GOR to measure the benefit and we have $P(Y_3 > Y_1)/P(Y_1 > Y_3) = 1/4$, where Y_1 and Y_3 represent the patient response for a randomly selected patient from the active control treatment (g = 1) and placebo (g = 3), respectively. These will lead us to set the non-inferior limit for the GOR $(=P(Y_2 > Y_1)/P(Y_1 > Y_2))$ between the experimental (g = 2) and active control (g = 1) treatments equal to 0.50 (halfway between 1 and ¼). Note that when $K = 2$, the GOR reduces to the regular OR. The above non-inferior limit 0.50 happens to coincide with the value that provides a compromise between the non-inferior margins given by the FDA and the Committee for Proprietary Medicinal Products (CPMP) in terms of the difference in proportions as well (Garrett, 2003, pp. 746–747). Because the final decision of the non-inferior margin may depend on the magnitude of the control treatment effect, safety profiles of treatments, the nature of the endpoint or disease, the type of drug, the administration factors, the cost, statistical considerations, and so forth (Hung et al., 2003), it is impossible to provide a fixed non-inferior margin GOR_l to fit all the situations in practice. Note that Munzel and Hauschke (2003) discussed testing non-inferiority with respect to the difference between $P(Y_2 > Y_1)$ and $P(Y_1 > Y_2)$ under the parallel groups design.

Given adequate numbers $n_C^{(g)}$ and $n_D^{(g)}$ (e.g., ≥ 5) of patients for both groups, we may apply the test statistic $\widehat{GOR}_{BA}$ (4.11) with the logarithmic transformation and its estimated asymptotic variance $\widehat{Var}\left(\log\left(\widehat{GOR}_{BA}\right)\right)$ (4.13) to test $H_0: GOR_{BA} \leq GOR_l$ versus $H_a: GOR_{BA} > GOR_l$. We will reject $H_0: GOR_{BA} \leq GOR_l$ at the α-level and claim that treatment B is non-inferior to treatment A if the test statistic

$$\left(\log\left(\widehat{GOR}_{BA}\right) - \log(GOR_l)\right) / \sqrt{\widehat{Var}\left(\log\left(\widehat{GOR}_{BA}\right)\right)} > Z_\alpha. \tag{4.19}$$

If $n_C^{(g)}$ or $n_D^{(g)}$ is small, then we can employ the exact test procedure based on the conditional distribution (4.14). When testing $H_0: GOR_{BA} \leq GOR_l$ versus $H_a: GOR_{BA} > GOR_l$, we can calculate the p-value for an observed number $n_C^{(1)} = x_1$ as

$$P\left(x \geq x_1 | n_C^{(+)}, n_{dis}^{(1)}, n_{dis}^{(2)}, GOR_l^2\right)$$

$$= \sum_{x \geq x_1} \binom{n_{dis}^{(1)}}{x} \binom{n_{dis}^{(2)}}{n_C^{(+)} - x} GOR_l^{2x} / \sum_x \binom{n_{dis}^{(1)}}{x} \binom{n_{dis}^{(2)}}{n_C^{(+)} - x} GOR_l^{2x}. \tag{4.20}$$

If the resulting p-value (4.20) is less than a given small α-level, we will reject the null hypothesis $H_0: GOR_{BA} \leq GOR_l$ and claim that treatment B is non-inferior to treatment A.

4.3   Testing equivalence between an experimental treatment and an active control treatment

For safety and ethical reasons, we may sometimes want to test equivalence rather than non-inferiority between an experimental treatment and an active control treatment. When assessing equivalence between treatments B and A, we want to test $H_0: GOR_{BA} \leq GOR_l$ or $GOR_{BA} \geq GOR_u$ versus $H_a: GOR_l < GOR_{BA} < GOR_u$, where GOR_l and GOR_u are the maximum clinically acceptable lower and upper margins such that treatment B can be regarded as equivalent to treatment A when $GOR_l < GOR_{BA} < GOR_u$ holds. If the frequencies $n_C^{(g)}$ and $n_D^{(g)}$ (for $g = 1, 2$) are large, we may apply the intersection-union test (Casella and Berger, 1990) to modify procedure (4.19) for testing non-inferiority to accommodate testing equivalence. On the basis of $\widehat{GOR}_{BA}$ (4.11) with the logarithmic transformation and its estimated asymptotic variance $\widehat{Var}\left(\log\left(\widehat{GOR}_{BA}\right)\right)$ (4.13), we will reject $H_0: GOR_{BA} \leq GOR_l$ or $GOR_{BA} \geq GOR_u$ at the α-level and claim that treatment B is equivalent to treatment A if

$$\left(\log\left(\widehat{GOR}_{BA}\right) - \log(GOR_l)\right) / \sqrt{\widehat{Var}\left(\log\left(\widehat{GOR}_{BA}\right)\right)} > Z_\alpha, \text{ and}$$

$$\left(\log\left(\widehat{GOR}_{BA}\right) - \log(GOR_u)\right) / \sqrt{\widehat{Var}\left(\log\left(\widehat{GOR}_{BA}\right)\right)} < -Z_\alpha. \tag{4.21}$$

If $n_C^{(g)}$ or $n_D^{(g)}$ is small, we may again consider using the test procedure based on the exact conditional distribution (4.14). For given an observed value $n_C^{(1)} = x_1$, we will reject $H_0 : GOR_{BA} \le GOR_l$ or $GOR_{BA} \ge GOR_u$ at the α-level and claim that the two treatments are equivalent if the following two inequalities simultaneously hold:

$$P\left(x \ge x_1 | n_C^{(+)}, n_{dis}^{(1)}, n_{dis}^{(2)}, GOR_l^2\right) < \alpha, \text{ and}$$

$$P\left(x \le x_1 | n_C^{(+)}, n_{dis}^{(1)}, n_{dis}^{(2)}, GOR_u^2\right) < \alpha, \tag{4.22}$$

where

$$P\left(x \ge x_1 | n_C^{(+)}, n_{dis}^{(1)}, n_{dis}^{(2)}, GOR_l^2\right)$$

$$= \sum_{x \ge x_1} \binom{n_{dis}^{(1)}}{x} \binom{n_{dis}^{(2)}}{n_C^{(+)} - x} GOR_l^{2x} / \sum_x \binom{n_{dis}^{(1)}}{x} \binom{n_{dis}^{(2)}}{n_C^{(+)} - x} GOR_l^{2x}, \text{ and}$$

$$P\left(x \le x_1 | n_C^{(+)}, n_{dis}^{(1)}, n_{dis}^{(2)}, GOR_u^2\right)$$

$$= \sum_{x \le x_1} \binom{n_{dis}^{(1)}}{x} \binom{n_{dis}^{(2)}}{n_C^{(+)} - x} GOR_u^{2x} / \sum_x \binom{n_{dis}^{(1)}}{x} \binom{n_{dis}^{(2)}}{n_C^{(+)} - x} GOR_u^{2x}.$$

4.4   Interval estimation of the generalized odds ratio

It is of importance and use to obtain an interval estimator of the GOR so that we can appreciate the magnitude of relative treatment effect and the precision of our inference drawn from our data. When $n_C^{(g)}$ and $n_D^{(g)}$ are appropriately large (≥ 5) for $g = 1, 2$, we can obtain an asymptotic $100(1 - \alpha)\%$ confidence interval for $GOR_{BA}(= \exp(\eta_{BA}))$ based on the estimator $\widehat{GOR}_{BA}$ (4.11) and $\widehat{Var}\left(\log\left(\widehat{GOR}_{BA}\right)\right)$ (4.13) as given by

$$\left[\widehat{GOR}_{BA} \exp\left(-Z_{\alpha/2}\sqrt{\widehat{Var}\left(\log\left(\widehat{GOR}_{BA}\right)\right)}\right),\right.$$

$$\left.\widehat{GOR}_{BA} \exp\left(Z_{\alpha/2}\sqrt{\widehat{Var}\left(\log\left(\widehat{GOR}_{BA}\right)\right)}\right)\right]. \tag{4.23}$$

When $n_C^{(g)}$ or $n_D^{(g)}$ is small, we can calculate the exact interval estimator on the basis of the conditional distribution (4.14). For given an observed value $n_C^{(1)} = x_1$, we obtain an exact $100(1 - \alpha)\%$ confidence interval for $GOR_{BA} (= \exp(\eta_{BA}))$ as

$$\left[GOR_{BAL}^{1/2}, \quad GOR_{BAU}^{1/2} \right], \tag{4.24}$$

where GOR_{BAL} and GOR_{BAU} are found by solving the following two equations: $P\left(x \geq x_1 | n_C^{(+)}, n_{dis}^{(1)}, n_{dis}^{(2)}, GOR_{BAL}\right) = \alpha/2$ and $P\left(x \leq x_1 | n_C^{(+)}, n_{dis}^{(1)}, n_{dis}^{(2)}, GOR_{BAU}\right) = \alpha/2$. Note that when the patient response is dichotomous ($K = 2$), interval estimators (4.23) and (4.24) reduce to interval estimators (3.16) and (3.18) for the OR in binary data.

Example 4.2   To estimate the GOR of patient opinions regarding the clarity of leaflet instructions between devices A and B based on the data in Table 4.1, we obtain $\widehat{GOR}_{BA} = 3.637$. This estimate suggests approximately 3.6 times the probability that a randomly selected patient felt more unclear of the leaflet instructions for device B than device A versus that a randomly selected patient felt more unclear of the leaflet instructions for device A than device B. Furthermore, when employing interval estimators (4.23) and (4.24), we obtain 95% confidence intervals to be [2.356, 5.615] and [2.267, 5.891]. Because both the lower limits of these resulting interval estimates fall above 1, there is significant evidence that the clarity of leaflet instructions for device B is worse than that for device A at the 5% level. This finding is certainly consistent with the finding that the leaflet instructions for device A are clearer than for device B, as claimed elsewhere (Ezzet and Whitehead, 1991; Senn, 1993).

4.5   Sample size determination

To assure that one can have an adequate opportunity to achieve the primary goal of a trial, we need to determine what the minimum required number of patients is for a desired power. For simplicity, we consider equal sample allocation (i.e., $n_1 = n_2 = n$).

4.5.1   Sample size for testing non-equality

Consider use of procedure (4.16) to test non-equality of treatments. We can show that the asymptotic variance $Var\left(\log\left(\widehat{GOR}_{BA}\right)\right)$ can be expressed as

$$V\left(\log\left(\widehat{GOR}_{BA}\right)\right)/n, \tag{4.25}$$

where $V\left(\log\left(\widehat{GOR}_{BA}\right)\right) = \left[\sum_{g=1}^{2} \left(\Pi_C^{(g)} + \Pi_D^{(g)}\right) / \left(\Pi_C^{(g)} \Pi_D^{(g)}\right)\right]/4$. Thus, when employing procedure (4.16) to test $H_0 : GOR_{BA} = 1$ versus $H_a : GOR_{BA} \neq 1$, we may obtain an approximate minimum required number n of patients per group for a desired power $1-\beta$ of detecting non-equality with a specified value $GOR^*_{BA} \neq 1$ at a nominal α-level as given by (Problem 4.7)

$$n = Ceil\left\{ (Z_{\alpha/2} + Z_\beta)^2 V\left(\log\left(\widehat{GOR}_{BA}\right)\right) / \left(\log\left(GOR^*_{BA}\right)\right)^2 \right\}, \tag{4.26}$$

where $Ceil\{x\}$ is the smallest integer $\geq x$ and $V\left(\log\left(\widehat{GOR}_{BA}\right)\right)$ is defined in (4.25).

4.5.2   Sample size for testing non-inferiority

On the basis of the test procedure (4.19) for testing $H_0 : GOR_{BA} \leq GOR_l$ (where $0 < GOR_l < 1$) versus $H_a : GOR_{BA} > GOR_l$, we can show that an approximate minimum required number n of patients per group for a desired power $1-\beta$ of detecting non-inferiority with a specified value $GOR^*_{BA} (> GOR_l)$ at a nominal α-level is given by

$$n = Ceil\left\{ (Z_\alpha + Z_\beta)^2 V\left(\log\left(\widehat{GOR}_{BA}\right)\right) / \left(\log(GOR_l) - \log(GOR^*_{BA})\right)^2 \right\}. \tag{4.27}$$

Note that if the resulting estimate n (4.27) is not large, then the sample size calculation formula (4.27) derived from the asymptotic test procedure (4.19) based on normal approximation can lose accuracy. In this case, we may consider using an exact sample size calculation procedure similar to that for dichotomous data under an AB/BA crossover trial (Lui and Chang, 2012b).

4.5.3   Sample size for testing equivalence

On the basis of procedure (4.21) for testing equivalence, we can show that the power function is approximately given by

$$\psi\left(GOR^*_{BA}\right) = \Phi\left(\frac{\log(GOR_u) - \log\left(GOR^*_{BA}\right)}{\sqrt{V\left(\log\left(\widehat{GOR}_{BA}\right)\right)/n}} - Z_\alpha \right) - \Phi\left(\frac{\log(GOR_l) - \log\left(GOR^*_{BA}\right)}{\sqrt{V\left(\log\left(\widehat{GOR}_{BA}\right)\right)/n}} + Z_\alpha \right),$$

$$\tag{4.28}$$

where $GOR_l < GOR^*_{BA} < GOR_u$ and $\Phi(X)$ is the cumulative standard normal distribution. On the basis of the power function $\psi\left(GOR^*_{BA}\right)$ (4.28), we cannot find the closed-form formula in calculation of the approximate minimum required number n of patients per group such that $\psi\left(GOR^*_{BA}\right) \geq 1-\beta$. However, we can easily apply the trial-and-error procedure to find an approximate minimum required sample size by searching for the smallest positive integer n satisfying $\psi\left(GOR^*_{BA}\right) \geq 1-\beta$.

   If the estimated minimum required number n of patients per group is large, we may approximate the power function $\psi\left(GOR^*_{BA}\right)$ (4.28) for $GOR_l < GOR^*_{BA} < 1$ by

$$1 - \Phi \left(\frac{\log(GOR_l) - \log\left(GOR_{BA}^*\right)}{\sqrt{V\left(\log\left(\widehat{GOR}_{BA}\right)\right)/n}} + Z_\alpha \right). \tag{4.29}$$

On the basis of (4.29), we obtain an approximate minimum required number n of patients per group for the desired power $(1 - \beta)$ of detecting equivalence with a specified GOR_{BA}^*, where $GOR_l < GOR_{BA}^* < 1$, at a nominal α-level as

$$n = Ceil\left\{ (Z_\alpha + Z_\beta)^2 V\left(\log\left(\widehat{GOR}_{BA}\right)\right) / \left(\log(GOR_l) - \log(GOR_{BA}^*)\right)^2 \right\}. \tag{4.30}$$

If the estimated minimum required number n of patients per group is large, we may approximate the power function $\psi\left(GOR_{BA}^*\right)$ (4.28) for $1 < GOR_{BA}^* < GOR_u$ by

$$\Phi \left(\frac{\log(GOR_u) - \log\left(GOR_{BA}^*\right)}{\sqrt{V\left(\log\left(\widehat{GOR}_{BA}\right)\right)/n}} - Z_\alpha \right). \tag{4.31}$$

On the basis of (4.31) we obtain an approximate minimum required number n of patients per group for a desired power $(1 - \beta)$ of detecting equivalence with a specified GOR_{BA}^*, where $1 < GOR_{BA}^* < GOR_u$, at a nominal α-level as

$$n = Ceil\left\{ (Z_\alpha + Z_\beta)^2 V\left(\log\left(\widehat{GOR}_{BA}\right)\right) / \left(\log(GOR_u) - \log(GOR_{BA}^*)\right)^2 \right\}. \tag{4.32}$$

When $GOR_{BA}^* = 1$, the power function $\psi\left(GOR_{BA}^*\right)$ (4.28) simply reduces to

$$\psi\left(GOR_{BA}^* = 1\right) = \Phi \left(\frac{\log(GOR_u)}{\sqrt{V\left(\log\widehat{GOR}_{BA}\right)/n}} - Z_\alpha \right) - \Phi \left(\frac{\log(GOR_l)}{\sqrt{V\left(\log\widehat{GOR}_{BA}\right)/n}} + Z_\alpha \right).$$

$$\tag{4.33}$$

When $\log(GOR_l) = -\log(GOR_u)$, we obtain an approximate minimum required number n of patients per group for the desired power $(1 - \beta)$ of detecting equivalence with a specified value $GOR_{BA}^* = 1$ at a nominal α-level based on (4.33) as

$$n = Ceil\left\{ (Z_\alpha + Z_{\beta/2})^2 V\left(\log\left(\widehat{GOR}_{BA}\right)\right) / \left(\log(GOR_u)\right)^2 \right\}. \tag{4.34}$$

Note that when deriving n (4.30) and n (4.32), we need to assume that the approximations of the power function $\psi\left(GOR_{BA}^*\right)$ (4.28) by (4.29) and (4.31) are accurate. When the predetermined equivalence margins GOR_l and GOR_l are away from 1, or the underlying $GOR_{BA}^*(\neq 1)$ of interest is chosen to be in the neighborhood of 1, the resulting minimum required number n of patients may not be large enough to assure these approximations to be accurate. In this case, because the power function (4.29) (or the power function (4.31)) is larger than $\psi\left(GOR_{BA}^*\right)$ (4.28), using n (4.30) (or n (4.32)) tends to underestimate the minimum required number of patients per group. Thus, we may use n (4.30) (or n (4.32)) as the initial estimate and apply a trial-and-error procedure to find the minimum positive integer n such that $\psi\left(GOR_{BA}^*\right) \geq 1-\beta$.

4.6 Hypothesis testing and estimation for the period effect

Using the same ideas as those for studying the relative treatment effect, we can easily obtain test procedures and interval estimators for the period effect. For example, on the basis of $\widehat{GOR}_P$ (4.12) with the logarithmic transformation and $\widehat{Var}\left(\log\left(\widehat{GOR}_P\right)\right)$ (4.13), we will reject $H_0 : GOR_P = 1$ (i.e., $\gamma = 0$) at the α-level if

$$\left|\log\left(\widehat{GOR}_P\right)\right| / \sqrt{\widehat{Var}\left(\log\left(\widehat{GOR}_P\right)\right)} > Z_{\alpha/2}. \tag{4.35}$$

Similarly, using $\widehat{GOR}_P$ (4.12) and $\widehat{Var}\left(\log\left(\widehat{GOR}_P\right)\right)$ (4.13), we can obtain an asymptotic $100(1-\alpha)\%$ confidence interval for GOR_P $(= \exp(\gamma))$ as

$$\left[\widehat{GOR}_P \exp\left(-Z_{\alpha/2}\sqrt{\widehat{Var}\left(\log\left(\widehat{GOR}_P\right)\right)}\right), \ \widehat{GOR}_P \exp\left(Z_{\alpha/2}\sqrt{\widehat{Var}\left(\log\left(\widehat{GOR}_P\right)\right)}\right)\right]. \tag{4.36}$$

When either $n_C^{(g)}$ or $n_D^{(g)}$ is not large, we may derive an exact $100(1-\alpha)\%$ confidence interval for GOR_P based on the following conditional distribution. Given the fixed total number $n_C^{(1)} + n_D^{(2)} = x_+$ of patients whose responses when receiving treatment B are higher than those when receiving treatment A, the random variable $n_C^{(1)} = x_1$ then follows the probability mass function:

$$P\left(n_C^{(1)} = x_1 | n_C^{(1)} + n_D^{(2)} = x_+, n_{dis}^{(1)}, n_{dis}^{(2)}, \Theta_P\right) = \binom{n_{dis}^{(1)}}{x_1}\binom{n_{dis}^{(2)}}{x_+ - x_1}\Theta_P^{x_1} / \sum_x \binom{n_{dis}^{(1)}}{x}\binom{n_{dis}^{(2)}}{x_+ - x}\Theta_P^x, \tag{4.37}$$

where $\Theta_P = (GOR_P)^2$ and the summation for x in the denominator is over the range $\max\left\{0, x_+ - n_{dis}^{(2)}\right\} \leq x \leq \min\left\{n_{dis}^{(1)}, x_+\right\}$. On the basis of the probability mass function (4.37), we can obtain an exact $100(1-\alpha)\%$ confidence interval for GOR_P, given an observed value $n_C^{(1)} = x_1$, as

$$\left[\Theta_{PL}^{1/2},\ \Theta_{PU}^{1/2}\right], \tag{4.38}$$

where

$$P\left(n_C^{(1)} \geq x_1 | n_C^{(1)} + n_D^{(2)} = x_+, n_{dis}^{(1)}, n_{dis}^{(2)}, \Theta_{PL}\right) = \alpha/2, \text{ and}$$

$$P\left(n_C^{(1)} \leq x_1 | n_C^{(1)} + n_D^{(2)} = x_+, n_{dis}^{(1)}, n_{dis}^{(2)}, \Theta_{PU}\right) = \alpha/2.$$

Example 4.3 Consider the data in Table 4.1 comparing the clarity of leaflet instructions for two devices. Suppose that we want to assess the period effect, and we obtain $\widehat{GOR}_P = 0.909$. When using interval estimators (4.36) and (4.38), we obtain the 95% confidence intervals to be [0.589, 1.404] and [0.562, 1.472]. Thus, the patient seems to feel clearer about the device instruction at period 2 versus period 1, but this period effect is not significant at the 5% level. This is because both of the resulting 95% confidence intervals cover 1.

Note that $\eta_{BA} = \gamma = 0$ if and only if $GOR^{(g)} = 1$ for both g. If both $n_C^{(g)}$ and $n_D^{(g)}$ are reasonably large, we can use $\widehat{GOR}^{(g)}$ (4.10) with the logarithmic transformation to test $H_0: \eta_{BA} = \gamma = 0$. We will reject $H_0: \eta_{BA} = \gamma = 0$ at the α-level if

$$\left[\log\left(\widehat{GOR}^{(1)}\right)\right]^2 / \widehat{Var}\left(\log\left(\widehat{GOR}^{(1)}\right)\right) + \left[\log\left(\widehat{GOR}^{(2)}\right)\right]^2 / \widehat{Var}\left(\log\left(\widehat{GOR}^{(2)}\right)\right) > \chi_\alpha^2(2),$$
$$\tag{4.39}$$

where $\widehat{Var}\left(\log\left(\widehat{GOR}^{(g)}\right)\right) = \left(\hat{\Pi}_C^{(g)} + \hat{\Pi}_D^{(g)}\right) / \left(n_g \hat{\Pi}_C^{(g)} \hat{\Pi}_D^{(g)}\right)$ and $\chi_\alpha^2(2)$ is the upper $100(\alpha)$th percentile of the chi-squared distribution with two degrees of freedom.

Recall that the conditional distribution of $n_C^{(g)}$, given $n_{dis}^{(g)}$ fixed, follows the binomial distribution with parameters $n_{dis}^{(g)}$ and $p^{(g)} = \Pi_C^{(g)} / \left(\Pi_C^{(g)} + \Pi_D^{(g)}\right)$ for $g = 1,\ 2$. Under $H_0: \eta_{BA} = \gamma = 0$, the probabilities of "success" $p^{(g)}$ for these two conditional binomial distributions are both equal to 1/2. Thus, we may reject $H_0: \eta_{BA} = \gamma = 0$ at the α-level (Problem 3.12) if

$$\left(n_C^{(1)} - n_D^{(1)}\right)^2 / n_{dis}^{(1)} + \left(n_C^{(2)} - n_D^{(2)}\right)^2 / n_{dis}^{(2)} > \chi_\alpha^2(2). \tag{4.40}$$

If $n_C^{(g)}$ or $n_D^{(g)}$ is small, we can apply the following exact test procedure. We will reject $H_0: \eta_{BA} = \gamma = 0$ at the α-level if we obtain observed values $(n_C^{(1)}, n_C^{(2)})$ such that

$$\sum_{\{(x,y)\in C\}} \binom{n_{dis}^{(1)}}{x} \binom{n_{dis}^{(2)}}{y} \left(\frac{1}{2}\right)^{n_{dis}^{(1)} + n_{dis}^{(2)}} < \alpha, \tag{4.41}$$

where

$$C = \left\{ (x,y) \middle| \binom{n_{dis}^{(1)}}{x} \binom{n_{dis}^{(2)}}{y} \left(\frac{1}{2}\right)^{n_{dis}^{(1)} + n_{dis}^{(2)}} \leq \binom{n_{dis}^{(1)}}{n_C^{(1)}} \binom{n_{dis}^{(2)}}{n_C^{(2)}} \left(\frac{1}{2}\right)^{n_{dis}^{(1)} + n_{dis}^{(2)}} \right\}.$$

Note that the above asymptotic test procedures and interval estimators derived for the GOR for paired samples or Agresti's α' depend on only the marginal frequencies $n_C^{(g)} \left(= \sum_{r=1}^{L-1} \sum_{s=r+1}^{L} n_{rs}^{(g)} \right)$ and $n_D^{(g)} \left(= \sum_{r=2}^{L} \sum_{s=1}^{r-1} n_{rs}^{(g)} \right)$ for $g = 1, 2$. Thus, all the above asymptotic test procedures and interval estimators are valid for use as long as $n_C^{(g)}$ and $n_D^{(g)}$ are adequately large despite some cell frequencies $n_{rs}^{(g)}$ being possibly small or even 0.

Ezzet and Whitehead (1991) proposed use of a random effects proportional odds model (Clayton and Cuzick, 1985) and required employment of a sophisticated iterative numerical procedure to find the estimate of treatment effect based on a likelihood involving non-closed form integrals. By contrast, following the general spirit of Agresti (1980), we use the GOR for paired samples as a summary measure of ordinal association. Because all asymptotic test procedures and estimators are, as shown here, in simple closed forms, we can easily do hypothesis testing or obtain an estimate of treatment effect by use of a pocket calculator. Furthermore, the exact test procedure derived here is of use when the number of patients in either group is small and all asymptotic test procedures derived from large sample theory are inappropriate. If the normal random effects proportional odds model holds, however, the test procedure based on the GOR proposed here is expected to be less efficient than Ezzet and Whitehead's likelihood-based approach. As noted by Agresti (1980, p. 60), however, the proportional odds model can be badly violated in many bivariate distributions. Because we make fewer assumptions, test procedures and estimators presented here should be applicable to more situations than those derived by assuming a specifically structural order between the ordinal levels of patient responses.

4.7   SAS codes for the proportional odds model with normal random effects

When assuming the proportional odds model with normal random effects (Ezzet and Whitehead, 1991) for the data in Table 4.1, we may use SAS's PROC GLIMMIX (SAS Institute, 2009) to do hypothesis testing and estimation (Jones and Kenward, 2014). To illustrate the use of this SAS procedure, we present the program codes in the following box, in which device A is "treat = 1" and device B is "treat = 2."

```
data step1;
ls = 80;
input patient treat period response;
datalines;
        1  1  1  1
        1  2  2  1
        2  1  1  1
        2  2  2  1
. . .
      286  2  1  4
      286  1  2  3
;;;;;
proc glimmix method = quad;
  class patient treat period;
  model response = treat period/ solution dist = multinomial
                       link = cumlogit;
  random intercept /subject = patient s cl;
  estimate 'treatment 2 versus treatment 1' treat -1 1;
  run;
```

We present the partial output of the above SAS procedure in the following box.

				Solutions for Fixed Effects				
Effect	response	treat	period	Estimate	Standard Error	DF	t Value	Pr > |t|
Intercept	1			0.1572	0.1797	285	0.87	0.3826
Intercept	2			3.3232	0.3145	285	10.57	<.0001
Intercept	3			4.5845	0.4465	285	10.27	<.0001
treat		1		1.2833	0.2134	282	6.01	<.0001
treat		2		0	.	.	.	.
period			1	-0.2052	0.1939	282	-1.06	0.2910
period			2	0	.	.	.	.

Since the p-value (< 0.0001) for "treat" is small, there is significant evidence that the clarity of leaflet instructions between devices A and B is different at the 5% level. Furthermore, because the parameter estimate for "treat" is 1.2833 (> 0), the leaflet instructions for device A are clearer than for device B (Ezzet and Whitehead, 1991; Senn, 1993). This is also consistent with the previous finding based on the GOR. Note that we have, as suggested by Jones and Kenward (2014), used "method = quad" in the above program. If we used the default estimation method in PROC GLIMMIX, we would have obtained the parameter estimate for "treat" as 1.067 with its estimated standard error 0.1807. The corresponding p-value is still < 0.0001. Although the above parameter estimates are not identical using different estimation methods for the data in Table 4.1, the conclusion is the same. Note also that the above estimate of period effect is -0.2050, which is < 0. This suggests that patients tend to feel clear at period 2 as compared with period 1, but the period effect is not significant at the 5% level. Again, this finding is the same as that obtained previously in Example 4.3.

Exercises

Problem 4.1. Under model (4.1), show that the GOR (or Agresti's α') of responses for paired samples between periods 2 and 1 for patient i in group g is given by (4.2).

Problem 4.2. Show that for a randomly selected patient from group g, the GOR of patient responses between periods 2 and 1 under model (4.1) is given by $GOR^{(g)} = \Pi_C^{(g)}/\Pi_D^{(g)} = \exp\left(\eta_{BA}\left(X_2^{(g)} - X_1^{(g)}\right) + \gamma\left(Z_2^{(g)} - Z_1^{(g)}\right)\right)$.

Problem 4.3. Show that from formulas (4.6) and (4.7), we can express the GOR of patient responses between treatments B and A and that between periods 2 and 1 as given by (4.8) and (4.9), respectively.

Problem 4.4. Using the delta method, show that the asymptotic variance of $\log\left(\widehat{GOR}_{BA}\right)$ is given by $Var\left(\log\left(\widehat{GOR}_{BA}\right)\right) = Var\left(\log\left(\widehat{GOR}_P\right)\right) = \left[\sum_{g=1}^{2}\left(\Pi_C^{(g)} + \Pi_D^{(g)}\right)/\left(n_g\Pi_C^{(g)}\Pi_D^{(g)}\right)\right]/4$.

Problem 4.5. Show that the conditional distribution of $n_C^{(g)}$, given $n_{dis}^{(g)}$ fixed, follows the binomial distribution with parameters $n_{dis}^{(g)}$ and $p^{(g)} = \Pi_C^{(g)}/\left(\Pi_C^{(g)} + \Pi_D^{(g)}\right)$ ($g = 1, 2$).

Problem 4.6. Show that $p^{(1)} = p^{(2)}$ (where $p^{(g)} = GOR^{(g)}/\left(1 + GOR^{(g)}\right)$) if and only if $GOR_{BA} = 1$.

Problem 4.7. On the basis of procedure (4.16) for testing $H_0 : GOR_{BA} = 1$ versus $H_a : GOR_{BA} \neq 1$, show that an approximate minimum required number n of patients per group for a desired power $1 - \beta$ of detecting non-equality with a specified value $GOR_{BA}^* \neq 1$ at a nominal α-level is given by (4.26).

5

AB/BA design in frequency data

When we study treatments for diseases such as epilepsy or asthma, one of most important clinical outcomes is the number of seizures in epilepsy or the number of exacerbations in asthma (Wilding *et al.*, 1997; Taylor *et al.*, 1998). Since the number of event occurrences is either 0 or a positive integer, and the sampling distribution of these occurrences is often skewed to the right, the normality assumption for continuous data is unlikely to be satisfied. Thus, test procedures and estimators derived under the normality assumption can be inappropriate for use in frequency data.

Assuming a random effects exponential multiplicative risk model for Poisson frequency data, we consider both asymptotic and exact methods under an AB/BA design (Lui and Chang, 2012d). We give procedures for testing non-equality of two treatments. We further give procedures for testing non-inferiority and equivalence between an experimental treatment and an active control treatment. We address interval estimation for the ratio of mean frequencies and sample size determination for testing non-equality, non-inferiority, and equivalence. We discuss hypothesis testing and estimation for the period effect. We also discuss estimation of the relative treatment effect in the presence of carry-over effects if we should unexpectedly encounter differential carry-over effects post–data collection. Note that an asymptotic distribution-free approach without assuming Poisson distribution under an AB/BA design has appeared elsewhere (Lui and Chang, 2012e). The interval estimators derived from this distribution-free method can lose accuracy or efficiency, however, when the number of patients in a trial is small and the underlying frequency actually follows the Poisson distribution (Lui and Chang, 2012d). Also, the exact test and exact interval estimator derived here under the Poisson assumption can be of use in small-sample cases. On

Crossover Designs: Testing, Estimation, and Sample Size, First Edition. Kung-Jong Lui.
© 2016 John Wiley & Sons, Ltd. Published 2016 by John Wiley & Sons, Ltd.
Companion website: www.wiley.com/go/lui/crossover

the other hand, if the Poisson assumption for event occurrences is seriously violated, test procedures and interval estimators derived under the Poisson assumption may lose efficiency (Lui and Chang, 2012e). The asymptotic distribution-free test procedures and interval estimators published elsewhere (Lui and Chang, 2012e) are applicable as long as the trial is of a large size.

Suppose that we compare an experimental treatment B with an active control treatment (or a placebo) A. Suppose further that we randomly assign n_1 patients to group ($g =$) 1 with A-then-B sequence, in which patients receive treatment A at period 1 and then cross over to receive treatment B at period 2, and n_2 patients to group ($g =$) 2 with B-then-A sequence, in which patients receive treatment B at period 1 and then cross over to receive treatment A at period 2. Let $Y_{iz}^{(g)}$ denote the frequency of event occurrences for patient i (= 1, 2, $\cdots$, n_g) assigned to group g (= 1, 2) at period z (= 1, 2). Let $X_{iz}^{(g)}$ represent the treatment-received covariate for the corresponding patient, and $X_{iz}^{(g)} = 1$ for the patient receiving treatment B, and = 0 otherwise. Let $Z_{iz}^{(g)}$ denote the period covariate and $Z_{iz}^{(g)} = 1$ for period 2 and = 0 otherwise. With an adequate wash-out period, we assume that there is no carry-over effect due to the treatment administered at period 1. We assume further that the frequency $Y_{iz}^{(g)}$ of event occurrences for patient i (= 1, 2, $\cdots$, n_g) assigned to group g (= 1, 2) at period z (= 1, 2) follows a Poisson distribution with mean that can be modeled as (Layard and Arveson, 1978; Lui and Chang, 2012d)

$$E\left(Y_{iz}^{(g)}\right) = \mu_i^{(g)} \exp\left(\eta_{BA} X_{iz}^{(g)} + \gamma Z_{iz}^{(g)}\right), \tag{5.1}$$

where $\mu_i^{(g)}$ represents the random effect due to the ith patient assigned to group g, and $\mu_i^{(g)}$'s are assumed to independently follow an unspecified probability density function $f_g(\mu)$, η_{BA} denotes the relative effect of treatment B to treatment A, and γ denotes the relative effect of period 2 to period 1. For a fixed period, the ratio of mean frequencies of event occurrences on a given patient between treatments B and A is equal to $RM_{BA} = \exp(\eta_{BA})$. Note that the ratio of mean frequencies RM_{AB} between treatments A and B is, by definition, equal to $1/RM_{BA}$. If there is no difference in effects between treatments A and B, the ratio of mean frequencies $RM_{BA} = 1$ (or equivalently, $\eta_{BA} = 0$). If treatment B tends to increase (or decrease) the frequency of event occurrences as compared with treatment A, then $RM_{BA} > 1$ (or $RM_{BA} < 1$). Similar interpretations as those for $RM_{BA} = \exp(\eta_{BA})$ are applicable to $RM_P = \exp(\gamma)$, which is the ratio of mean frequencies for period 2 versus period 1. Conditional upon each patient i in group ($g =$) 1, we can easily show that the conditional distribution of $Y_{i2}^{(1)}$, given $Y_{i+}^{(1)} = Y_{i1}^{(1)} + Y_{i2}^{(1)} = y_{i+}^{(1)}$ fixed, follows the binomial distribution with parameters $y_{i+}^{(1)}$ and $\exp(\eta_{BA} + \gamma)/(1 + \exp(\eta_{BA} + \gamma))$ (Problem 5.1). Because the sum of independent binomial random variables, each having the same constant probability of "success," follows the binomial distribution (Problem 5.2), the conditional probability mass function for the sum $Y_{+2}^{(1)}\left(= \sum_i Y_{i2}^{(1)}\right)$ of event occurrences over patients at period

2 in group $(g =)$ 1, given the random vector $\underline{y}_{+}^{(1)} = \left(y_{1+}^{(1)}, y_{2+}^{(1)}, \cdots, y_{n_1+}^{(1)}\right)'$ fixed, is given by

$$P\left(Y_{+2}^{(1)} = y_{+2}^{(1)} | \underline{y}_{+}^{(1)}, \eta_{BA}, \gamma\right) = \binom{y_{++}^{(1)}}{y_{+2}^{(1)}} p_1^{y_{+2}^{(1)}} (1-p_1)^{y_{++}^{(1)} - y_{+2}^{(1)}}, \tag{5.2}$$

where $y_{++}^{(1)} \left(= \sum_i y_{i+}^{(1)}\right)$ and $p_1 = \exp(\eta_{BA} + \gamma)/(1 + \exp(\eta_{BA} + \gamma))$.

Similarly, conditional upon each patient i in group $(g =)$ 2, we can show that the conditional distribution of $Y_{i2}^{(2)}$, given $Y_{i+}^{(2)} = Y_{i1}^{(2)} + Y_{i2}^{(2)} = y_{i+}^{(2)}$ fixed, follows the binomial distribution with parameters $y_{i+}^{(2)}$ and $\exp(\gamma)/(\exp(\eta_{BA}) + \exp(\gamma))$. Thus, the conditional probability mass function for the sum $Y_{+2}^{(2)} \left(= \sum_i Y_{i2}^{(2)}\right)$ of event occurrences over patients at period 2 in group $(g =)$ 2, given the random vector $\underline{y}_{+}^{(2)} = \left(y_{1+}^{(2)}, y_{2+}^{(2)}, \cdots, y_{n_2+}^{(2)}\right)'$ fixed, is given by

$$P\left(Y_{+2}^{(2)} = y_{+2}^{(2)} | \underline{y}_{+}^{(2)}, \eta_{BA}, \gamma\right) = \binom{y_{++}^{(2)}}{y_{+2}^{(2)}} p_2^{y_{+2}^{(2)}} (1-p_2)^{y_{++}^{(2)} - y_{+2}^{(2)}}, \tag{5.3}$$

where $y_{++}^{(2)} \left(= \sum_i y_{i+}^{(2)}\right)$ and $p_2 = \exp(\gamma)/(\exp(\eta_{BA}) + \exp(\gamma))$. Note that the conditional maximum likelihood estimator (CMLE) for p_g based on the binomial distribution (5.2) (for $g = 1$) or the binomial distribution (5.3) (for $g = 2$) is given by $\hat{p}_g = y_{+2}^{(g)}/y_{++}^{(g)}$ $(g = 1, 2)$. Note further that based on parameters p_g defined in (5.2) and (5.3), we can easily show that the ratio of mean frequencies between treatments B and A is equal to (Problem 5.3)

$$RM_{BA} = \{p_1(1-p_2)/[(1-p_1)p_2]\}^{1/2}. \tag{5.4}$$

By the functional invariance of the MLE (Casella and Berger, 1990), we obtain the CMLE for RM_{BA} as given by

$$\begin{aligned} \widehat{RM}_{BA} &= \{\hat{p}_1(1-\hat{p}_2)/[(1-\hat{p}_1)\hat{p}_2]\}^{1/2} \\ &= \left[\left(Y_{+2}^{(1)} Y_{+1}^{(2)}\right)/\left(Y_{+1}^{(1)} Y_{+2}^{(2)}\right)\right]^{1/2}. \end{aligned} \tag{5.5}$$

Note that $\widehat{RM}_{BA}$ (5.5) is actually the same estimator as that suggested by Senn (2002) using different arguments from those presented here. Using the delta method (Agresti, 1990; Lui, 2004), we obtain the asymptotic variance for $\log\left(\widehat{RM}_{BA}\right)$ based on the conditional binomial distributions (5.2) and (5.3) as given by (Problem 5.4)

$$Var\left(\log\left(\widehat{RM}_{BA}\right)\right) = \left\{1/\left[y_{++}^{(1)}p_1(1-p_1)\right] + 1/\left[y_{++}^{(2)}p_2(1-p_2)\right]\right\}/4. \quad (5.6)$$

When substituting $\hat{p}_g\left(=y_{+2}^{(g)}/y_{++}^{(g)}\right)$ for p_g in (5.6), we obtain the estimated asymptotic conditional variance $\widehat{Var}\left(\log\left(\widehat{RM}_{BA}\right)\right) = [1/Y_{+2}^{(1)} + 1/Y_{+1}^{(1)} + 1/Y_{+1}^{(2)} + 1/Y_{+2}^{(2)}]/4$, which is again identical to that suggested elsewhere (Senn, 2002). Note that the CMLE for $RM_{AB}(=1/RM_{BA})$ is $\widehat{RM}_{AB} = 1/\widehat{RM}_{BA}$ and the asymptotic variance $\widehat{Var}\left(\log\left(\widehat{RM}_{AB}\right)\right)$ is equal to $\widehat{Var}\left(\log\left(\widehat{RM}_{BA}\right)\right)$.

Given the total frequency $Y_{+2}^{(+)}\left(=Y_{+2}^{(1)}+Y_{+2}^{(2)}\right)=y_{+2}^{(+)}$ over the two groups at period 2 as well as random vectors $\underline{y}_{-+}^{(1)}$ and $\underline{y}_{-+}^{(2)}$ fixed, we can easily show that the conditional probability mass function for $Y_{+2}^{(1)}=y_1$ is distributed as the following non-central hypergeometric distribution (Agresti, 1990):

$$P\left(Y_{+2}^{(1)}=y_1|y_{+2}^{(+)},\underline{y}_{-+}^{(1)},\underline{y}_{-+}^{(2)},RM_{BA}^2\right)$$

$$= \binom{y_{++}^{(1)}}{y_1}\binom{y_{++}^{(2)}}{y_{+2}^{(+)}-y_1}(RM_{BA}^2)^{y_1}/\sum_y\binom{y_{++}^{(1)}}{y}\binom{y_{++}^{(2)}}{y_{+2}^{(+)}-y}(RM_{BA}^2)^y, \quad (5.7)$$

where the summation of y in (5.7) is over $\max\left\{0,y_{+2}^{(+)}-y_{++}^{(2)}\right\}\leq y\leq\min\left\{y_{++}^{(1)},y_{+2}^{(+)}\right\}$. Note that the conditional probability mass function (5.7) does not depend on the nuisance parameter γ and reduces to the central hypergeometric distribution when $RM_{BA}=1$ as

$$P\left(Y_{+2}^{(1)}=y_1|y_{+2}^{(+)},\underline{y}_{-+}^{(1)},\underline{y}_{-+}^{(2)},RM_{BA}^2=1\right) = \binom{y_{++}^{(1)}}{y_1}\binom{y_{++}^{(2)}}{y_{+2}^{(+)}-y_1}/\binom{y_{++}^{(+)}}{y_{+2}^{(+)}}, \quad (5.8)$$

where $y_{++}^{(+)}=y_{++}^{(1)}+y_{++}^{(2)}$ and $\max\left\{0,y_{+2}^{(+)}-y_{++}^{(2)}\right\}\leq y_1\leq\min\left\{y_{++}^{(1)},y_{+2}^{(+)}\right\}$.

5.1   Testing non-equality of treatments

Suppose that we wish to study whether there is a difference in effects between treatments A and B by testing the null hypothesis $H_0:RM_{BA}=1$ (i.e., $\eta_{BA}=0$) versus the alternative hypothesis $H_a:RM_{BA}\neq1$ (i.e., $\eta_{BA}\neq0$). On the basis of $\widehat{RM}_{BA}$ (5.5) with the logarithmic transformation, we will reject $H_0:RM_{BA}=1$ at the α-level if

$$|\log\left(\widehat{RM}_{BA}\right)|/\sqrt{\widehat{Var}_{H_0}\left(\log\left(\widehat{RM}_{BA}\right)\right)}>Z_{\alpha/2}, \quad (5.9)$$

where $\widehat{Var}_{H_0}\left(\log\left(\widehat{RM}_{BA}\right)\right) = \left(1/y_{++}^{(1)} + 1/y_{++}^{(2)}\right)/[4\hat{p}(1-\hat{p})]$, $\hat{p} = \left(Y_{+2}^{(1)} + Y_{+2}^{(2)}\right)/\left(y_{++}^{(1)} + y_{++}^{(2)}\right)$, the pooled-sample proportion calculated under $H_0: RM_{BA} = 1$, and Z_α is the upper $100(\alpha)$th percentile of the standard normal distribution.

To alleviate the concern that a test procedure is based on the possibly skewed sampling distribution of $\widehat{RM}_{BA}$ (5.5), we may also employ the idea of Fieller's theorem (Casella and Berger, 1990). We define $Z(\psi_{BA}) = \hat{p}_1(1-\hat{p}_2) - \psi_{BA}(1-\hat{p}_1)\hat{p}_2$, where $\psi_{BA} = RM_{BA}^2$. We can see that the expectation $E(Z(\psi_{BA})) = 0$. Furthermore, given ψ_{BA} fixed, we can show that the estimated variance of $Z(\psi_{BA})$ based on the conditional binomial distributions (5.2) and (5.3) is given by (Problem 5.5)

$$\widehat{Var}(Z(\psi_{BA})) = \widehat{Var}(\hat{p}_1(1-\hat{p}_2)) + \psi_{BA}^2 \widehat{Var}((1-\hat{p}_1)\hat{p}_2) \tag{5.10}$$
$$- 2\psi_{BA}\widehat{Cov}(\hat{p}_1(1-\hat{p}_2), (1-\hat{p}_1)\hat{p}_2),$$

where

$$\widehat{Var}(\hat{p}_1(1-\hat{p}_2)) = \left[\hat{p}_1(1-\hat{p}_1)/y_{++}^{(1)}\right]\left[\hat{p}_2(1-\hat{p}_2)/y_{++}^{(2)}\right] + (\hat{p}_1)^2\left[\hat{p}_2(1-\hat{p}_2)/y_{++}^{(2)}\right]$$
$$+ (1-\hat{p}_2)^2\left[\hat{p}_1(1-\hat{p}_1)/y_{++}^{(1)}\right],$$

$$\widehat{Var}((1-\hat{p}_1)\hat{p}_2) = \left[\hat{p}_1(1-\hat{p}_1)/y_{++}^{(1)}\right]\left[\hat{p}_2(1-\hat{p}_2)/y_{++}^{(2)}\right] + (1-\hat{p}_1)^2\left[\hat{p}_2(1-\hat{p}_2)/y_{++}^{(2)}\right]$$
$$+ (\hat{p}_2)^2\left[\hat{p}_1(1-\hat{p}_1)/y_{++}^{(1)}\right], \text{ and}$$

$$\widehat{Cov}(\hat{p}_1(1-\hat{p}_2), (1-\hat{p}_1)\hat{p}_2) = -\hat{p}_1(1-\hat{p}_1)\hat{p}_2(1-\hat{p}_2)\left(y_{++}^{(1)} + y_{++}^{(2)} - 1\right)/\left(y_{++}^{(1)}y_{++}^{(2)}\right).$$

On the basis of $\widehat{Var}(Z(\psi_{BA}))$ (5.10), we will reject $H_0: RM_{BA} = 1$ at the α-level if

$$|Z(1)|/\sqrt{\widehat{Var}_{H_0}(Z(1))} > Z_{\alpha/2}, \tag{5.11}$$

where $\widehat{Var}_{H_0}(Z(1))$ is obtained by substituting $\hat{p}\left(= \left(Y_{+2}^{(1)} + Y_{+2}^{(2)}\right)/\left(y_{++}^{(1)} + y_{++}^{(2)}\right)\right)$ for $\hat{p}_g$ ($g = 1, 2$), and the value 1 for ψ_{BA} in $\widehat{Var}(Z(\psi_{BA}))$ (5.10).

Under $H_0: RM_{BA} = 1$ (or equivalently, $\eta_{BA} = 0$) we can easily see that $p_1 = p_2$. Thus, we may employ the commonly used procedure for testing non-equality of proportions between two independent binomial samples. Given the totals $y_{++}^{(g)}$ being large for both g, we will reject $H_0: RM_{BA} = 1$ at the α-level if

$$|\hat{p}_1 - \hat{p}_2|/\sqrt{\hat{p}(1-\hat{p})\left(1/y_{++}^{(1)} + 1/y_{++}^{(2)}\right)} > Z_{\alpha/2}. \tag{5.12}$$

If $y_{+1}^{(g)}$ or $y_{+2}^{(g)}$ (for $g = 1, 2$) is small, then asymptotic test procedures (5.9), (5.11), and (5.12) may not perform well. In this case, we may consider use of Fisher's exact test procedure. On the basis of the conditional distribution (5.8), we will reject $H_0 : RM_{BA} = 1$ at the α-level if we obtain an observed value for $Y_{+2}^{(1)} = y_1$ (where $\max\left\{0, y_{+2}^{(+)} - y_{++}^{(2)}\right\} \le y_1 \le \min\left\{y_{++}^{(1)}, y_{+2}^{(+)}\right\}$) such that

$$
P\left(Y \ge y_1 \mid y_{+2}^{(+)}, y_{-+}^{(1)}, y_{-+}^{(2)}, RM_{BA}^2 = 1\right) = \sum_{y \ge y_1} \binom{y_{++}^{(1)}}{y}\binom{y_{++}^{(2)}}{y_{+2}^{(+)} - y} \bigg/ \binom{y_{++}^{(+)}}{y_{+2}^{(+)}} \le \alpha/2, \text{ or}
$$

$$
P\left(Y \le y_1 \mid y_{+2}^{(+)}, y_{-+}^{(1)}, y_{-+}^{(2)}, RM_{BA}^2 = 1\right) = \sum_{y \le y_1} \binom{y_{++}^{(1)}}{y}\binom{y_{++}^{(2)}}{y_{+2}^{(+)} - y} \bigg/ \binom{y_{++}^{(+)}}{y_{+2}^{(+)}} \le \alpha/2.
$$

$$(5.13)$$

On the basis of Monte Carlo simulations, Lui and Chang (2012d) found that all the test procedures (5.9), (5.11), (5.12), and (5.13) can perform well even when the number of patients $n(= n_1 = n_2)$ per group is moderate. All three asymptotic test procedures (5.9), (5.11), and (5.12) are generally more powerful than the exact test procedure (5.13). Thus, unless the number of patients per group is small and the normal approximation on which asymptotic test procedures (5.9), (5.11), and (5.12) are based is invalid, we may wish to employ the asymptotic test procedure rather than the exact test procedure to avoid the loss of power.

Example 5.1   Consider the double-blind crossover trial studying the effect of the beta-agonist salmeterol (50 µg twice daily) (treatment B) versus a placebo (treatment A) in asthma patients (Wilding *et al.*, 1997; Senn, 2002). One hundred and one patients were randomized to one of the two groups distinguished by the sequence of treatment-receipt: placebo for 24 weeks-then-salmeterol for 24 weeks, or salmeterol for 24 weeks-then-placebo for 24 weeks. A four-week washout period between the two treatment periods was employed. There were only 87 patients who completed the trial. Note that using procedures (5.9), (5.11), (5.12), and (5.13), we need only the information on the sum $Y_{+z}^{(g)}$ (for $z = 1, 2$, and $g = 1, 2$) rather than the individual frequency $Y_{iz}^{(g)}$. We summarize in Table 5.1 the data regarding these sums of exacerbations on 87 patients with complete information. When applying asymptotic test procedures (5.9), (5.11), and (5.12) and the exact test procedure (5.13) to test nonequality, we obtain the corresponding p-values 0.010, 0.014, 0.014, and 0.028, respectively. All these suggest that there may be significant evidence that taking salmeterol can reduce, as compared with taking placebo, the mean number of exacerbations in asthma patients at the 5% level.

Example 5.2   Consider the data in Table 5.2, which are actually taken from a two-center double-dummy three-period crossover trial in which there were 165 patients randomly assigned to receive salbutamol, salmeterol, or placebo (Taylor *et al.*,

Table 5.1   Totals of exacerbations $\left(Y_{+1}^{(g)}, Y_{+2}^{(g)}\right)$ over patients at the two periods between two groups (g = 1, 2): placebo-then-salmeterol and salmeterol-then-placebo under an AB/BA crossover trial.

	Period I	Period II	Total
Placebo-then-salmeterol (g = 1)	15	6	21
Salmeterol-then-placebo (g = 2)	14	23	37
Total	29	29	58

Table 5.2   Totals of exacerbations $\left(Y_{+1}^{(g)}, Y_{+2}^{(g)}\right)$ over patients at the first two periods between two groups (g = 1, 2): placebo-then-salbutamol and salbutamol-then-placebo. These data are taken as part of a double-blind three-period crossover trial comparing salbutamol and salmeterol with a placebo.

	Period I	Period II	Total
Placebo-then-salbutamol (g = 1)	5	4	9
Salbutamol-then-placebo (g = 2)	23	24	47
Total	28	28	56

1998). There were five patients excluded from the data analysis because of the incomplete information on the number of exacerbations. For the purpose of illustration, we include in Table 5.2 only the data regarding 160 patients between the two groups with the treatment sequences: placebo-then-salbutamol and salbutamol-then-placebo for the first two periods. When using test procedures (5.9), (5.11), and (5.12), we obtain the p-values 0.715, 0.716, and 0.716, respectively. Thus, as compared with the placebo, there is no significant evidence that taking salbutamol can reduce the number of exacerbations at the 5% level.

5.2   Testing non-inferiority of an experimental treatment to an active control treatment

Suppose that we want to assess whether an experimental treatment B is non-inferior to an active control treatment A. Suppose further that the higher the mean frequency, the better is the treatment. Thus, to detect the non-inferiority of treatment B to treatment A, we want to test the null hypothesis $H_0 : RM_{BA} \leq RM_l$ (where $0 < RM_l < 1$) versus the alternative hypothesis $H_a : RM_{BA} > RM_l$, where RM_l is the maximum clinically acceptable low margin such that treatment B can be regarded as non-inferior to treatment A when $RM_{BA} > RM_l$. When the observed frequencies $Y_{+1}^{(g)}$ and $Y_{+2}^{(g)}$ are reasonably large for both groups g, we may apply $\widehat{RM}_{BA}$ (5.5) with the logarithmic transformation and the estimated asymptotic variance $\widehat{Var}\left(\log\left(\widehat{RM}_{BA}\right)\right)$ to test $H_0 : RM_{BA} \leq RM_l$ versus $H_a : RM_{BA} > RM_l$. We will reject H_0 at the α-level and claim that treatment B is non-inferior to treatment A if

$$\left(\log\left(\widehat{RM}_{BA}\right) - \log(RM_l)\right) / \sqrt{\widehat{Var}\left(\log\left(\widehat{RM}_{BA}\right)\right)} > Z_\alpha. \tag{5.14}$$

Furthermore, consider use of the test statistic $Z(\psi_{BA})(=\hat{p}_1(1-\hat{p}_2)-\psi_{BA}(1-\hat{p}_1)\hat{p}_2)$ and $\widehat{Var}(Z(\psi_{BA}))$ (5.8) to detect non-inferiority. We may also reject $H_0 : RM_{BA} \leq RM_l$ at the α-level if

$$Z(\psi_l)/\sqrt{\widehat{Var}(Z(\psi_l))} > Z_\alpha, \tag{5.15}$$

where $\psi_l = RM_l^2$. Note that both test procedures (5.14) and (5.15) are derived on the basis of large-sample theory. If either of the observed frequencies $Y_{+1}^{(g)}$ and $Y_{+2}^{(g)}$ (for $g = 1, 2$) is small, these test procedures can be inappropriate. In this case, we may consider use of the following exact test procedure based on the conditional distribution (5.7). When testing $H_0 : RM_{BA} \leq RM_l$ versus $H_a : RM_{BA} > RM_l$, we calculate the p-value for an observed $Y_{+2}^{(1)} = y_1$ (where $\max\left\{0, y_{+2}^{(+)} - y_{++}^{(2)}\right\} \leq y_1 \leq \min\left\{y_{++}^{(1)}, y_{+2}^{(+)}\right\}$) as given by

$$P\left(Y \geq y_1 | y_{+2}^{(+)}, y_{-+}^{(1)}, y_{-+}^{(2)}, RM_l^2\right)$$

$$= \sum_{y \geq y_1} \binom{y_{++}^{(1)}}{y} \binom{y_{++}^{(2)}}{y_{+2}^{(+)} - y} (RM_l^2)^y / \left[\sum_y \binom{y_{++}^{(1)}}{y} \binom{y_{++}^{(2)}}{y_{+2}^{(+)} - y} (RM_l^2)^y\right]. \tag{5.16}$$

If the p-value (5.16) is less than α, we will reject $H_0 : RM_{BA} \leq RM_l$ at the α-level and claim that treatment B is non-inferior to treatment A.

On the basis of Monte Carlo simulations, Lui and Chang (2012d) have found that (5.14), (5.15), and the exact test procedure (5.16) can perform well with respect to Type I error in a variety of situations. On the other hand, the test procedure (5.14) on the basis of $\widehat{RM}_{BA}$ (5.5) with the logarithmic transformation can be preferable to the other two procedures with respect to power. Furthermore, the exact test procedure (5.16) is generally, as what one would expect, of the least power among the three test procedures considered here.

When the undesirable outcome, such as the number of seizures or the number of exacerbations, is of interest, a high mean frequency of these events represents a bad outcome. To test the non-inferiority of treatment B to treatment A, we want to test $H_0 : RM_{BA} \geq RM_u$ (where $RM_u > 1$) versus $H_a : RM_{BA} < RM_u$. This is equivalent to testing $H_0 : RM_{AB} \leq 1/RM_u$ versus $H_a : RM_{AB} > 1/RM_u$. Using the same procedure as (5.14) with switching treatments between A and B and $RM_l = 1/RM_u$, we will reject H_0 at the α-level and claim that treatment B is non-inferior to treatment A if the test statistic

$$\left(\log\left(\widehat{RM}_{AB}\right) - \log(1/RM_u)\right) / \sqrt{\widehat{Var}\left(\log\left(\widehat{RM}_{AB}\right)\right)} > Z_\alpha. \qquad (5.17)$$

Similarly, we can easily modify test procedures (5.15) and (5.16) to test non-inferiority in the situation in which the event occurrence of interest represents an undesirable outcome.

5.3 Testing equivalence between an experimental treatment and an active control treatment

Using the intersection-union test (Casella and Berger, 1990), we can modify the above test procedures (5.14)–(5.16) for testing non-inferiority to accommodate testing equivalence between two treatments. When assessing equivalence between treatment B and treatment A, we want to test $H_0 : RM_{BA} \leq RM_l$ or $RM_{BA} \geq RM_u$ versus $H_a : RM_l < RM_{BA} < RM_u$, where RM_l and RM_u are the maximum clinically acceptable margins such that treatment B can be regarded as equivalent to treatment A when $RM_l < RM_{BA} < RM_u$ holds. Note that the inequality $RM_l < RM_{BA} < RM_u$ holds if and only if $1/RM_l > RM_{AB} > 1/RM_u$ holds. Thus, it is desirable to choose $RM_u = 1/RM_l$ to avoid the situation in which our claim that treatments A and B are equivalent depends on which treatment is called treatment A or treatment B.

On the basis of $\widehat{RM}_{BA}$ (5.5) with the logarithmic transformation, we will reject $H_0 : RM_{BA} \leq RM_l$ or $RM_{BA} \geq RM_u$ at the α-level and claim that treatment B is equivalent to treatment A if

$$\left(\log\left(\widehat{RM}_{BA}\right) - \log(RM_l)\right) / \sqrt{\widehat{Var}\left(\log\left(\widehat{RM}_{BA}\right)\right)} > Z_\alpha \quad \text{and}$$

$$\left(\log\left(\widehat{RM}_{BA}\right) - \log(RM_u)\right) / \sqrt{\widehat{Var}\left(\log\left(\widehat{RM}_{BA}\right)\right)} < -Z_\alpha. \qquad (5.18)$$

Similarly, on the basis of $Z(\psi_{BA})$ and its asymptotic variance $\widehat{Var}(Z(\psi_{BA}))$ (5.10), we will reject the null hypothesis $H_0 : RM_{BA} \leq RM_l$ or $RM_{BA} \geq RM_u$ at the α-level if the test statistic

$$Z(\psi_l) / \sqrt{\widehat{Var}(Z(\psi_l))} > Z_\alpha, \quad \text{and}$$

$$Z(\psi_u) / \sqrt{\widehat{Var}(Z(\psi_u))} < -Z_\alpha, \qquad (5.19)$$

where $\psi_l = RM_l^2$ and $\psi_u = RM_u^2$.

When $Y_{+1}^{(g)}$ or $Y_{+2}^{(g)}$ is small, asymptotic test procedures (5.18) and (5.19) can be inappropriate. In this case, we may consider using the exact test procedure based on the conditional distribution (5.7). Given an observed frequency $Y_{+2}^{(1)} = y_1$, we will reject $H_0 : RM_{BA} \leq RM_l$ or $RM_{BA} \geq RM_u$ at the α-level and claim that the two treatments are equivalent if the following two inequalities simultaneously hold:

$$P\left(Y \geq y_1 | y_{+2}^{(+)}, y_{-+}^{(1)}, y_{-+}^{(2)}, RM_l^2\right) < \alpha, \quad \text{and}$$

$$P\left(Y \leq y_1 | y_{+2}^{(+)}, y_{-+}^{(1)}, y_{-+}^{(2)}, RM_u^2\right) < \alpha. \tag{5.20}$$

5.4   Interval estimation of the ratio of mean frequencies

On the basis of the CMLE $\widehat{RM}_{BA}$ (5.5) and the estimated asymptotic variance $\widehat{Var}\left(\log\left(\widehat{RM}_{BA}\right)\right)$, we obtain an asymptotic $100(1 - \alpha)\%$ confidence interval for RM_{BA} as

$$\left[\widehat{RM}_{BA} \exp\left(-Z_{\alpha/2}\sqrt{\widehat{Var}\left(\log\left(\widehat{RM}_{BA}\right)\right)}\right), \ \widehat{RM}_{BA} \exp\left(Z_{\alpha/2}\sqrt{\widehat{Var}\left(\log\left(\widehat{RM}_{BA}\right)\right)}\right)\right]. \tag{5.21}$$

Furthermore, consider use of $Z(\psi_{BA})$ and its asymptotic variance $\widehat{Var}(Z(\psi_{BA}))$ (5.10). We have the probability $P\left((Z(\psi_{BA}))^2/\widehat{Var}(Z(\psi_{BA})) \leq Z_{\alpha/2}^2\right) \approx 1 - \alpha$ as both $y_{++}^{(g)}$'s are large. This leads us to consider the following quadratic equation (Problem 5.6):

$$A\psi_{BA}^2 - 2B\psi_{BA} + C \leq 0, \tag{5.22}$$

where

$$A = ((1-\hat{p}_1)\hat{p}_2)^2 - Z_{\alpha./2}^2 \widehat{Var}((1-\hat{p}_1)\hat{p}_2),$$

$$B = \hat{p}_1(1-\hat{p}_2)(1-\hat{p}_1)\hat{p}_2 - Z_{\alpha/2}^2 \widehat{Cov}(\hat{p}_1(1-\hat{p}_2),(1-\hat{p}_1)\hat{p}_2), \quad \text{and}$$

$$C = (\hat{p}_1(1-\hat{p}_2))^2 - Z_{\alpha/2}^2 \widehat{Var}(\hat{p}_1(1-\hat{p}_2)).$$

If $A > 0$ and $B^2 - AC > 0$, we obtain an asymptotic $100(1 - \alpha)\%$ confidence interval for RM_{BA} as given by

$$\left[\max\left\{\left(B-\sqrt{B^2-AC}\right)/A, 0\right\}^{1/2}, \ \left(\left(B+\sqrt{B^2-AC}\right)/A\right)^{1/2}\right], \tag{5.23}$$

where $\max\{a, b\}$ denotes the maximum of a and b. If $Y_{+1}^{(g)}$ or $Y_{+2}^{(g)}$ is small for $g = 1, 2$, we may derive the interval estimator based on the exact conditional distribution (5.7). Given an observed $Y_{+2}^{(1)} = y_1$, we obtain an exact $100(1 - \alpha)\%$ confidence interval for RM_{BA} as given by

$$[RM_{BAL}, RM_{BAU}], \tag{5.24}$$

where $P\left(Y \geq y_1 | y_{+2}^{(+)}, y_{-+}^{(1)}, y_{-+}^{(2)}, RM_{BAL}^2\right) = \alpha/2$, and $P\left(Y \leq y_1 | y_{+2}^{(+)}, y_{-+}^{(1)}, y_{-+}^{(2)}, RM_{BAU}^2\right) = \alpha/2$.

Note that we can easily write a numerical iterative procedure to solve the above equations to obtain the exact $100(1 - \alpha)\%$ confidence limits RM_{BAL} and RM_{BAU} in (5.24). We can also apply SAS's PROC FREQ (SAS Institute, 2009) to obtain the exact $100(1 - \alpha)\%$ confidence limits for RM_{BA}^2. We then take the square roots of these limits to obtain the corresponding limits as given in (5.24).

When evaluating and comparing the performance of interval estimators (5.21), (5.23), and (5.24) based on Monte Carlo simulation, Lui and Chang (2012d) noted that 95% confidence intervals using these interval estimators can all perform well with respect to the coverage probability in a variety of situations. Also, the interval estimator (5.21) is generally more precise than the others with respect to the average length. This is certainly consistent with the previous finding that the corresponding procedure (5.14) based on $\widehat{RM}_{BA}$ with the logarithmic transformation is more powerful than the other two procedures for testing non-inferiority. However, note that the exact interval estimator (5.24) can be of use when the number of patients per group is small and asymptotic interval estimators are not theoretically valid for use.

Note that the asymptotic interval estimators derived elsewhere (Lui and Chang, 2012e) without assuming the frequency of events to follow any parametric distribution can perform well when the number of patients per group is large ($n \geq 50$). When the number of patients per group is moderate ($n = 30$) and the underlying frequency follows the Poisson distribution, the asymptotic distribution-free interval estimators may lose accuracy or efficiency as compared with the asymptotic interval estimator (5.21) accounting for the Poisson assumption (Lui and Chang, 2012e). The exact interval estimator (5.24) can be of use when the number of patients per group is so small that all asymptotic interval estimators, including the interval estimator (5.21), are inappropriate.

Example 5.3   Consider the data in Table 5.1 comparing the beta-agonist salmeterol (50 µg twice daily) (treatment B) with a placebo (treatment A) for reducing exacerbations in asthma patients (Wilding *et al.*, 1997; Senn, 2002). Given these data, we obtain the CMLE $\widehat{RM}_{BA} = 0.493$. When employing interval estimators (5.21), (5.23), and (5.24), we obtain the 95% confidence intervals for RM_{BA} as given by [0.277, 0.880], [0.167, 0.931], and [0.252, 0.937], respectively. We can see that the resulting 95% confidence interval of using (5.21) has the shortest length among these three interval estimators. Because all the upper limits of these resulting 95% confidence

Table 5.3   Totals of exacerbations $\left(Y_{+1}^{(g)}, Y_{+2}^{(g)} \right)$ over patients at the first two periods between two groups (g = 1, 2): salbutamol-then-salmeterol and salmeterol-then-salbutamol. These data are taken as part of an original three-period crossover trial comparing salbutamol and salmeterol with a placebo.

	Period I	Period II	Total
Salbutamol-then-salmeterol (g = 1)	12	1	13
Salmeterol-then-salbutamol (g = 2)	3	13	16
Total	15	14	29

intervals fall below 1, we may claim that taking salmeterol reduces the mean number of exacerbations in asthma patients as compared with the placebo. These results are certainly consistent with the previous findings based on procedures for testing non-equality of treatments.

Example 5.4   Consider in Table 5.3 the data taken as a part of a two-center double-dummy three-period crossover trial (Taylor *et al.*, 1998). For illustration purpose, we include in Table 5.3 only partial data of the first two periods regarding 160 patients with complete information on the number of exacerbations between salbutamol (treatment A) and salmeterol (treatment B). Given these data, we obtain the CMLE $\widehat{RM}_{BA} = 0.139$. When employing interval estimators (5.21), (5.23), and (5.24), we obtain the 95% confidence intervals for RM_{BA} as given by [0.042, 0.459], [0.000, 0.447], and [0.020, 0.504], respectively. Because all the upper limits of these resulting 95% confidence intervals fall below 1, we may claim that taking salmeterol reduces the mean number of exacerbations in asthma patients as compared with salbutamol at the 5% level.

5.5   Sample size determination

In designing a trial, it is of essential importance to obtain an adequate number of patients needed for achieving the primary goal of our study. In the following discussion, we consider equal sample allocation (i.e., $n_1 = n_2 = n$) for simplicity.

5.5.1   Sample size for testing non-equality

Note that we can re-express the test statistic $\log\left(\widehat{RM}_{BA} \right)$ as

$$(1/2) \left[\log\left(Y_{+2}^{(1)}/Y_{+1}^{(1)} \right) - \log\left(Y_{+2}^{(2)}/Y_{+1}^{(2)} \right) \right]. \tag{5.25}$$

Let m denote the expectation $E\left(\mu_i^{(g)}\right)$ of the underlying random effects. Since $E\left(y_{++}^{(1)}\right) = nm\left(1 + e^{(\eta_{BA} + \gamma)}\right)$ and $E\left(y_{++}^{(2)}\right) = nm(e^{\eta_{BA}} + e^{\gamma})$ (Problem 5.7), the asymptotic variance $Var\left(\log\left(\widehat{RM}_{BA}\right)\right)$ (5.6) can be for a large n approximated by

$$Var\left(\log\left(\widehat{RM}_{BA}\right)\right) = V(m, \eta_{BA}, \gamma)/n, \tag{5.26}$$

where

$$V(m, \eta_{BA}, \gamma) = \left\{1/\left[m\left(1 + e^{(\eta_{BA} + \gamma)}\right)p_1(1 - p_1)\right] + 1/\left[m\left(e^{\eta_{BA}} + e^{\gamma}\right)p_2(1 - p_2)\right]\right\}/4.$$

Under $H_0 : RM_{BA} = 1$ (or $\eta_{BA} = 0$), the variance component $V(m, \eta_{BA}, \gamma)$ in (5.26) can be further approximated by $V_{H_0}(m, \eta_{BA}, \gamma) = [1/(m(1 + e^{\eta_{BA} + \gamma})) + 1/(m(e^{\eta_{BA}} + e^{\gamma}))]/[4\bar{p}(1 - \bar{p})]$, where $\bar{p}$ is the pooled proportions of p_1 and p_2, and is given by $\bar{p} = \left(e^{(\eta_{BA} + \gamma)} + e^{\gamma}\right)/\left(e^{(\eta_{BA} + \gamma)} + 1 + e^{\gamma} + e^{\eta_{BA}}\right)$.

Thus, an approximate minimum required number of patients n per group for a desired power $1 - \beta$ of detecting a specified $\eta_{BA}(\neq 0)$ at the α-level based on the test procedure (5.9) is given by (Lui, 2013)

$$n = Ceil\left\{\left(Z_{\alpha/2}\sqrt{V_{H_0}(m, \eta_{BA}, \gamma)} + Z_{\beta}\sqrt{V(m, \eta_{BA}, \gamma)}\right)^2/(\eta_{BA})^2\right\}, \tag{5.27}$$

where $Ceil\{x\}$ denotes the smallest integer larger than or equal to x.

5.5.2   Sample size for testing non-inferiority

On the basis of the test procedure (5.14), we can show that an approximate minimum required number of patients n per group for a desired power $1 - \beta$ of detecting non-inferiority with a specified value $RM_{BA}^*(> RM_l)$ at a nominal α-level is given by (Problem 5.8)

$$n = Ceil\left\{(Z_{\alpha} + Z_{\beta})^2 V(m, \eta_{BA}, \gamma)/\left(\log(RM_l) - \log\left(RM_{BA}^*\right)\right)^2\right\}, \tag{5.28}$$

where $V(m, \eta_{BA}, \gamma)$ is defined in (5.26). Note that if the resulting estimate n (5.28) is not large, then the sample size calculation formula (5.28) derived from the asymptotic test procedure (5.14) based on normal approximation can lose accuracy. In this case, we may employ the exact sample size determination procedure analogous to that for testing non-equality published elsewhere (Lui, 2013).

5.5.3 Sample size for testing equivalence

When the number n of patients per group is reasonably large, we may obtain the power function for testing equivalence based on the test procedure (5.18) as given by

$$\psi\left(RM_{BA}^*\right) = \Phi\left(\frac{\log(RM_u) - \log\left(RM_{BA}^*\right)}{\sqrt{V(m,\eta_{BA},\gamma)/n}} - Z_\alpha\right) - \Phi\left(\frac{\log(RM_l) - \log\left(RM_{BA}^*\right)}{\sqrt{V(m,\eta_{BA},\gamma)/n}} + Z_\alpha\right),$$

(5.29)

where $RM_l < RM_{BA}^* < RM_u$ and $\Phi(X)$ is the cumulative standard normal distribution. On the basis of the power function $\psi\left(RM_{BA}^*\right)$ (5.29), we cannot find the closed-form formula in calculation of the minimum required number n of patients per group such that $\psi\left(RM_{BA}^*\right) \geq 1 - \beta$. However, we can apply the trial-and-error procedure to find the approximate minimum required sample size by searching for the smallest positive integer n satisfying $\psi\left(RM_{BA}^*\right) \geq 1 - \beta$.

5.6 Hypothesis testing and estimation for the period effect

Under model (5.1), the ratio of mean frequencies between periods 2 and 1 for a fixed treatment on a given patient is equal to $RM_P = \exp(\gamma)$. On the basis of conditional distributions (5.2) and (5.3), we can show that the ratio of mean frequencies between periods 2 and 1 is (Problem 5.9)

$$RM_P = \{p_1 p_2 / [(1 - p_1)(1 - p_2)]\}^{1/2}.$$

(5.30)

Thus, we can estimate the ratio of mean frequencies RM_P between periods 2 and 1 by

$$\widehat{RM}_p = \{\hat{p}_1 \hat{p}_2 / [(1 - \hat{p}_1)(1 - \hat{p}_2)]\}^{1/2}$$

$$= \left[\left(Y_{+2}^{(1)} Y_{+2}^{(2)}\right) / \left(Y_{+1}^{(1)} Y_{+1}^{(2)}\right)\right]^{1/2}.$$

(5.31)

We can easily show that an asymptotic variance $Var\left(\log\left(\widehat{RM}_P\right)\right)$ for $\widehat{RM}_p$ (5.31) with the logarithmic transformation based on the conditional distributions (5.2) and (5.3) is the same as $Var\left(\log\left(\widehat{RM}_{BA}\right)\right)$ (Problem 5.10). On the basis of the above results, we can do hypothesis testing and interval estimation for RM_P. For example, suppose that we wish to study whether there is a difference in effects between periods 2 and 1 by testing $H_0 : RM_P = 1$ (i.e., $\gamma = 0$) versus $H_a : RM_P \neq 1$ (i.e., $\gamma \neq 0$). Note that $RM_P = 1$ if and only if $p_1 = 1 - p_2$ (Problem 5.11). On the basis of $\widehat{RM}_P$ (5.31) with the logarithmic transformation, we will reject $H_0 : RM_{BA} = 1$ at the α-level if

$$|\log(\widehat{RM}_P)|/\sqrt{\widehat{Var}_{H_0}\left(\log(\widehat{RM}_P)\right)} > Z_{\alpha/2},$$ (5.32)

where $\widehat{Var}_{H_0}\left(\log(\widehat{RM}_P)\right) = \left(1/y_{++}^{(1)} + 1/y_{++}^{(2)}\right)/[4\hat{p}^*(1-\hat{p}^*)]$, and $\hat{p}^* = \left(Y_{+2}^{(1)} + Y_{+1}^{(2)}\right)/\left(y_{++}^{(1)} + y_{++}^{(2)}\right)$, the pooled sample proportion calculated under $H_0 : RM_P = 1$. Furthermore, we can obtain an estimated asymptotic variance $\widehat{Var}\left(\log(\widehat{RM}_P)\right)$ as given by $[1/Y_{+2}^{(1)} + 1/Y_{+1}^{(1)} + 1/Y_{+1}^{(2)} + 1/Y_{+2}^{(2)}]/4$. Based on $\widehat{RM}_P$ (5.31) and $\widehat{Var}\left(\log(\widehat{RM}_P)\right)$, we obtain an asymptotic $100(1-\alpha)\%$ confidence interval for RM_P as

$$\left[\widehat{RM}_P \exp\left(-Z_{\alpha/2}\sqrt{\widehat{Var}\left(\log(\widehat{RM}_P)\right)}\right), \ \widehat{RM}_P \exp\left(Z_{\alpha/2}\sqrt{\widehat{Var}\left(\log(\widehat{RM}_P)\right)}\right)\right].$$ (5.33)

When $Y_{+1}^{(g)}$ or $Y_{+2}^{(g)}$ is small, we may consider deriving an exact $100(1-\alpha)\%$ confidence interval for RM_P based on the following conditional distribution. Given the total frequencies $Y_{+2}^{(1)} + Y_{+1}^{(2)} = y_+$ of events for patients receiving treatment B over the two groups fixed, the random frequency $Y_{+2}^{(1)} = y_{+2}^{(1)}$ then follows the probability mass function:

$$P\left(Y_{+2}^{(1)} = y_1 | Y_{+2}^{(1)} + Y_{+1}^{(2)} = y_+, y_+^{(1)}, y_+^{(2)}, \Psi_P\right)$$
$$= \binom{y_{++}^{(1)}}{y_1}\binom{y_{++}^{(2)}}{y_+ - y_1}\Psi_P^{y_1} \Big/ \sum_y \binom{y_{++}^{(1)}}{y}\binom{y_{++}^{(2)}}{y_+ - y}\Psi_P^y,$$ (5.34)

where $\Psi_P = p_1 p_2/[(1-p_1)(1-p_2)] = RM_P^2$, and the summation for y in the denominator of (5.34) is over $\max\{0, y_+ - y_{++}^{(2)}\} \le y \le \min\{y_{++}^{(1)}, y_+\}$. On the basis of the probability mass function (5.34), we obtain for an observed value y_1 an exact $100(1-\alpha)\%$ confidence interval for RM_P as given by

$$\left[\psi_{PL}^{1/2}, \ \psi_{PU}^{1/2}\right],$$ (5.35)

where

$$P\left(Y \ge y_1 | Y_{+2}^{(1)} + Y_{+1}^{(2)} = y_+, y_+^{(1)}, y_+^{(2)}, \psi_{PL}\right) = \alpha/2, \quad \text{and}$$
$$P\left(Y \le y_1 | Y_{+2}^{(1)} + Y_{+1}^{(2)} = y_+, y_+^{(1)}, y_+^{(2)}, \psi_{PU}\right) = \alpha/2.$$

Finally, we note that we wish to simultaneously test the null hypothesis $H_0 : \eta_{BA} = \gamma = 0$ versus $H_a : \eta_{BA} \neq 0$ or $\gamma \neq 0$. When $Y_{+1}^{(g)}$ and $Y_{+2}^{(g)}$ are reasonably large for both g, we will reject $H_0 : \eta_{BA} = \gamma = 0$ at the α-level if the following test statistic (Problem 5.12)

$$\left(Y_{+2}^{(1)} - Y_{+1}^{(1)}\right)^2 / y_{++}^{(1)} + \left(Y_{+2}^{(2)} - Y_{+1}^{(2)}\right)^2 / y_{++}^{(2)} > \chi_\alpha^2(2), \qquad (5.36)$$

where $\chi_\alpha^2(2)$ is the upper $100(\alpha)$th percentile of the central chi-squared distribution with two degrees of freedom. If $Y_{+1}^{(g)}$ or $Y_{+2}^{(g)}$ is small, we may apply the following exact test procedure. We will reject $H_0 : \eta_{BA} = \gamma = 0$ at the α-level if we obtain an observed vector $\left(y_{+2}^{(1)}, y_{+2}^{(2)}\right)$ such that

$$\sum_{\{(x,y) \in C\}} \binom{y_{++}^{(1)}}{x} \binom{y_{++}^{(2)}}{y} \left(\frac{1}{2}\right)^{y_{++}^{(1)} + y_{++}^{(2)}} < \alpha, \qquad (5.37)$$

where $C = \left\{ (x,y) \mid \binom{y_{++}^{(1)}}{x} \binom{y_{++}^{(2)}}{y} \left(\frac{1}{2}\right)^{y_{++}^{(1)} + y_{++}^{(2)}} \leq \binom{y_{++}^{(1)}}{y_{+2}^{(1)}} \binom{y_{++}^{(2)}}{y_{+2}^{(2)}} \left(\frac{1}{2}\right)^{y_{++}^{(1)} + y_{++}^{(2)}} \right\}.$

5.7   Estimation of the relative treatment effect in the presence of differential carry-over effects

The purpose of this section is to illustrate the point that it is senseless to carry out an AB/BA design when there are carry-over effects in frequency data. To extend model (5.1) to account for the carry-over effect due to treatments A and B, we assume that the random frequency $Y_{iz}^{(g)}$ of event occurrences on patient i ($= 1, 2, \ldots, n_g$) assigned to group g ($= 1, 2$) at period z ($= 1, 2$) follows the random effects multiplicative risk model with mean given by

$$E\left(Y_{iz}^{(g)}\right) = \mu_i^{(g)} \exp\left(\eta_{BA} X_{iz}^{(g)} + \gamma Z_{iz}^{(g)} + \lambda_A I_{\{g=1\}} Z_{iz}^{(g)} + \lambda_B \left(1 - I_{\{g=1\}}\right) Z_{iz}^{(g)}\right), \qquad (5.38)$$

where $I_{\{g=1\}}$ denotes the indicator function for group 1, and $I_{\{g=1\}} = 1$ for $g = 1$, and $= 0$ otherwise; λ_A and λ_B denote the carry-over effect due to treatments A and B, respectively, and all the other parameters, covariates, and random effects are defined and assumed to be the same as those in model (5.1). We can show that under model (5.38) (Problem 5.15)

$$[p_1(1-p_2)/[(1-p_1)p_2] = \exp(2\eta_{BA} + (\lambda_A - \lambda_B)). \qquad (5.39)$$

Thus, $\widehat{RM}_{BA}$ ($= \{\hat{p}_1(1-\hat{p}_2)/[(1-\hat{p}_1)\hat{p}_2]\}^{1/2}$) (5.5) is no longer a consistent estimator for the ratio of mean frequencies RM_{BA} unless $\lambda_A = \lambda_B$. We can further see that $\widehat{RM}_{BA}$ (5.5) will tend to overestimate (or underestimate) RM_{BA} if $\lambda_A > \lambda_B$ (or $\lambda_A < \lambda_B$).

Define $W_i^{(g)} = Y_{i1}^{(g)} Y_{i2}^{(g)}$ for $g = 1, 2$. We can show that (Problem 5.16)

$$E\left(W_i^{(1)}\right) = \exp(\eta_{BA} + \gamma + \lambda_A)E\left(\left(\mu_i^{(1)}\right)^2\right), \quad \text{and}$$
$$E\left(W_i^{(2)}\right) = \exp(\eta_{BA} + \gamma + \lambda_B)E\left(\left(\mu_i^{(2)}\right)^2\right). \tag{5.40}$$

Because we randomly assign patients to either group 1 or group 2, we may assume that $E\left(\left(\mu_i^{(1)}\right)^2\right) = E\left(\left(\mu_i^{(2)}\right)^2\right)$. On the basis of (5.40), we can see that

$$E\left(W_i^{(1)}\right)/E\left(W_i^{(1)}\right) = \exp(\lambda_A - \lambda_B). \tag{5.41}$$

Thus, $E\left(W_i^{(1)}\right) = E\left(W_i^{(2)}\right)$ if and only if $\lambda_A = \lambda_B$. This may lead us to consider testing $H_0 : \lambda_A = \lambda_B$ by using statistics $\bar{W}^{(1)}$ and $\bar{W}^{(2)}$, where $\bar{W}^{(g)} = \sum_i W_i^{(g)}/n_g$. We will reject $H_0 : \lambda_A = \lambda_B$ at the α-level if

$$\left(\log\left(\bar{W}^{(1)}/\bar{W}^{(2)}\right)\right)^2/\widehat{Var}\left(\log\left(\bar{W}^{(1)}/\bar{W}^{(2)}\right)\right) > \chi_\alpha^2(1), \tag{5.42}$$

where $\widehat{Var}\left(\log\left(\bar{W}^{(1)}/\bar{W}^{(2)}\right)\right) = \widehat{Var}\left(\log\left(\bar{W}^{(1)}\right)\right) + \widehat{Var}\left(\log\left(\bar{W}^{(2)}\right)\right)$, $\widehat{Var}\left(\log\left(\bar{W}^{(g)}\right)\right) = \left(\sum_i \left(W_i^{(g)}\right)^2 - \left(\sum_i W_i^{(g)}\right)^2/n_g\right)/\left[\left(\bar{W}^{(g)}\right)^2 n_g(n_g - 1)\right]$. As for testing whether there are differential carry-over effects in continuous data (Chapter 2), the test procedure (5.42) is expected to lack power. Note that we can also estimate $\exp(\lambda_A - \lambda_B)$ by using $\left(\bar{W}^{(1)}/\bar{W}^{(2)}\right)$. To adjust the bias of the estimator $\widehat{RM}_{BA}$ (5.5) under model (5.38), we may consider

$$\widehat{RM}_{BA}^* = \left\{\hat{p}_1(1 - \hat{p}_2)\bar{W}^{(2)}/\left[(1 - \hat{p}_1)\hat{p}_2\bar{W}^{(1)}\right]\right\}^{1/2}. \tag{5.43}$$

Using the delta method, we can easily obtain the estimated asymptotic variance of $\widehat{RM}_{BA}^*$. We may also consider the estimator based on only the data at period 1 to avoid the bias due to differential carry-over effects between treatments A and B as given by (Problem 5.17)

$$\widehat{RM}_{BA}^{**} = \bar{Y}_{+1}^{(2)}/\bar{Y}_{+1}^{(1)}. \tag{5.44}$$

Using Monte Carlo simulations, we have found that $\widehat{RM}_{BA}^{**}$ (5.44) can generally outperform $\widehat{RM}_{BA}^*$ (5.43) with respect to the mean squared error. Because $\widehat{RM}_{BA}^{**}$ is the commonly used estimator in parallel groups design, the gain in efficiency of using the crossover design will completely disappear when one needs to adjust the bias due to carry-over effects under the AB/BA design. Thus, there is really no reason or justification to carry out an AB/BA design in the presence of carry-over effects.

Exercises

Problem 5.1. Suppose that X_1 and X_2 are independently distributed as a Poisson distribution with means λ_1 and λ_2, respectively. Show that the conditional distribution of X_1, given $X_1 + X_2 = x_+$ fixed, follows the binomial distribution with parameters x_+ and $\lambda_1/(\lambda_1 + \lambda_2)$.

Problem 5.2. Show that the sum of independent binomial random variables $Y = X_1 + X_2 + \cdots + X_n$, each X_i having the binomial distribution with parameters m_i ($i = 1, 2, \cdots, n$) and the same constant probability of success p, follows the binomial distribution with parameters $\sum_i m_i$ and p.

Problem 5.3. Given p_g (for $g = 1, 2$) defined in (5.2) and (5.3), show that $RM_{BA}^2 = p_1(1-p_2)/[(1-p_1)p_2]$.

Problem 5.4. Using the delta method, show that the asymptotic variance for $\log\left(\widehat{RM}_{BA}\right)$ based on the conditional binomial distributions (5.2) and (5.3) is given by $Var\left(\log\left(\widehat{RM}_{BA}\right)\right) = \{1/\left[y_{++}^{(1)}p_1(1-p_1)\right] + 1/\left[y_{++}^{(2)}p_2(1-p_2)\right]\}/4$.

Problem 5.5. Show that the estimated variance of $Z(\psi_{BA})$ based on the conditional distributions (5.2) and (5.3) is given by (5.10).

Problem 5.6. Show that $(Z(\psi_{BA}))^2/\widehat{Var}(Z(\psi_{BA})) \leq Z_{\alpha/2}^2$ is equivalent to the quadratic equation $A\psi_{BA}^2 - 2B\psi_{BA} + C \leq 0$ defined in (5.22).

Problem 5.7. Under model (5.1), show that $E\left(y_{++}^{(1)}\right) = nm\left(1 + e^{(\eta_{BA} + \gamma)}\right)$ and $E\left(y_{++}^{(2)}\right) = nm(e^{\eta_{BA}} + e^{\gamma})$, where $m = E\left(\mu_i^{(g)}\right)$.

Problem 5.8. Based on the test procedure (5.14), show that the approximate minimum required number n of patients per group for a desired power $1 - \beta$ of detecting non-inferiority with a specified value $RM_{BA}^*(>RM_l)$ at a nominal α-level is given by (5.28).

Problem 5.9. Show that the square of the ratio of mean frequencies between periods 2 and 1 under model (5.1) is $RM_P^2(= \exp(2\gamma)) = p_1 p_2/[(1-p_1)(1-p_2)]$, where p_1 and p_2 are defined in (5.2) and (5.3).

Problem 5.10. Show that the asymptotic variance for $\log\left(\widehat{RM}_p\right)$ under the conditional distributions (5.2) and (5.3) is given by (5.6).

Table 5.4   Totals of exacerbations $\left(Y^{(g)}_{+1}, Y^{(g)}_{+2}\right)$ over patients at the first two periods between two groups (g = 1, 2): placebo-then-salmeterol and salmeterol-then-placebo. These data are taken as part of a double-blind three-period crossover trial comparing salbutamol and salmeterol with a placebo.

	Period I	Period II	Total
Placebo-then-salmeterol (g = 1)	26	12	38
Salmeterol-then-placebo (g = 2)	9	14	23
Total	35	26	61

Problem 5.11.   Show that $RM_P(= \exp(\gamma)) = 1$ if and only if $p_1 = 1 - p_2$, where p_1 and p_2 are defined in (5.2) and (5.3).

Problem 5.12.   Show that we can apply the test procedure (5.36) to simultaneously test $H_0 : \eta_{BA} = \gamma = 0$ at the α-level.

Problem 5.13.   Given the data in Table 5.2, what are the 95% confidence intervals for RM_P in use of interval estimators (5.33) and (5.35)?

Problem 5.14.   Consider the data in Table 5.4 regarding the number of exacerbations at the first two periods between the two groups: placebo-then-salmeterol and salmeterol-then-placebo (Taylor *et al.*, 1998).

(a) What is the CMLE $\widehat{RM}_{BA}$?

(b) When we use procedures (5.9), (5.11), (5.12), and (5.13) to test non-equality, what are the p-values?

(c) When we use interval estimators (5.21), (5.23), and (5.24), what are the 95% confidence intervals for RM_{BA}?

(d) What is the estimate $\widehat{RM}_P$ for period 2 versus period 1, and is there evidence that the period effect is different from 0 at the 5% level?

Problem 5.15.   Show that $[p_1(1-p_2)/[(1-p_1)p_2] = \exp(2\eta_{BA} + (\lambda_A - \lambda_B))$ in the presence of carry-over effects under model (5.38).

Problem 5.16.   Show that $E\left(W^{(1)}_i\right) = \exp(\eta_{BA} + \gamma + \lambda_A)E\left(\left(u^{(1)}_i\right)^2\right)$, and $E\left(W^{(2)}_i\right) = \exp(\eta_{BA} + \gamma + \lambda_B)E\left(\left(u^{(2)}_i\right)^2\right)$ under model (5.38), where $W^{(g)}_i = Y^{(g)}_{i1}Y^{(g)}_{i2}$. Thus, we have $E\left(W^{(1)}_i\right)/E\left(W^{(2)}_i\right) = \exp(\lambda_A - \lambda_B)$.

Problem 5.17. Show that $E\left(Y_{i1}^{(1)}\right) = E\left(u_i^{(1)}\right)$; $E\left(Y_{i2}^{(1)}\right) = \exp(\gamma + \eta_{BA} + \lambda_A)\, E\left(u_i^{(1)}\right)$; $E\left(Y_{i1}^{(2)}\right) = \exp(\eta_{BA})E\left(u_i^{(2)}\right)$; and $E\left(Y_{i2}^{(2)}\right) = \exp(\gamma + \lambda_B)E\left(u_i^{(2)}\right)$. Because we randomly assign patients to groups with different treatment-receipt sequences, we may assume that $E\left(u_i^{(1)}\right) = E\left(u_i^{(2)}\right)$. On the basis of the above results, we can show that $\left(E\left(Y_{i2}^{(1)}\right)E\left(Y_{i1}^{(1)}\right)\right) / \left(E\left(Y_{i2}^{(2)}\right)E\left(Y_{i1}^{(2)}\right)\right) = \exp(\lambda_A - \lambda_B)$. Thus, we can use $\left(\bar{Y}_{+2}^{(1)}\bar{Y}_{+1}^{(1)}\right) / \left(\bar{Y}_{+2}^{(2)}\bar{Y}_{+1}^{(2)}\right)$ to estimate $\exp(\lambda_A - \lambda_B)$ as well. From (5.39), we may consider the estimator for RM_{BA} by $\left\{\hat{p}_1(1-\hat{p}_2)/[(1-\hat{p}_1)\hat{p}_2]/\left[\left(\bar{Y}_{+2}^{(1)}\bar{Y}_{+1}^{(1)}\right)/\left(\bar{Y}_{+2}^{(2)}\bar{Y}_{+1}^{(2)}\right)\right]\right\}^{1/2}$. Show that this estimator with adjusting the bias due to differential carry-over effects reduces to the same estimator as $\widehat{RM}_{BA}^{**}$ (5.44), which ignores all the data at period 2. Note also that we can apply $\log\left(\left(\bar{Y}_{+2}^{(1)}\bar{Y}_{+1}^{(1)}\right)/\left(\bar{Y}_{+2}^{(2)}\bar{Y}_{+1}^{(2)}\right)\right)$ and its estimated asymptotic variance to test $H_0 : \lambda_A = \lambda_B$. However, we do not recommend use of this test procedure to verify the assumption of no carry-over effect due to the same concern as that noted elsewhere (Freeman, 1989).

6

Three-treatment three-period crossover design in continuous data

In an RCT, we may want to simultaneously study more than two treatments for various reasons. For example, we may consider a minimum of three dose levels in a dose-finding trial. This is because we commonly expect a nonlinear dose response and wish to investigate departure from linearity (Senn, 2002). When studying whether the combination of two therapies A and B is superior to therapy A or B alone in a double-blind trial, we may have at least three treatment arms: A and placebo, B and placebo, as well as A and B combination. When employing a gold standard trial to assess equivalence between an experimental treatment and a standard treatment, or compare an experimental treatment with a placebo, by definition, we have a new treatment, a standard treatment, and a placebo.

In this chapter, we focus attention on continuous data in which there are three treatments under a three-period crossover trial. For example, consider the data in Table 6.1 taken from a double-blind three-period crossover trial comparing two treatments, including a single dose of formoterol solution aerosol (12 µg) and a single dose of salbutamol suspension aerosol (100 µg), with a placebo for patients suffering from exercise-induced asthma on the forced expiratory volume in one second (FEV_1) (Tsoy et al., 1990; Senn and Hildebrand, 1991; Senn, 2002). The patients were asked to perform an exercise test 2 h after each of the three treatments. The values in Table 6.1 represented the lowest of a number of determinations of FEV_1 observed in the period after the exercise test. We want to compare the effects of the two treatments with that of the placebo on FEV_1 (in ml).

Crossover Designs: Testing, Estimation, and Sample Size, First Edition. Kung-Jong Lui.
© 2016 John Wiley & Sons, Ltd. Published 2016 by John Wiley & Sons, Ltd.
Companion website: www.wiley.com/go/lui/crossover

Table 6.1 FEV_1 (in ml) for the six groups with treatment-receipt sequences: C-A-B ($g = 1$), C-B-A ($g = 2$), A-C-B ($g = 3$), A-B-C ($g = 4$), B-C-A ($g = 5$), and B-A-C ($g = 6$) over the three periods.

	Period I	Period II	Period III
C-A-B ($g = 1$)	900	1900	2900
	1500	2600	2000
	1200	2200	2700
	2400	2600	3800
	1900	2700	2800
C-B-A ($g = 2$)	2200	2500	2400
	2200	3200	3300
	800	1400	1000
	950	1320	1480
	1700	2600	2400
	1400	2500	2200
A-C-B ($g = 3$)	2200	1100	2600
	2800	2000	2800
	2400	1700	3400
A-B-C ($g = 4$)	2100	3200	1000
	1600	2300	1600
	1600	1400	800
	3100	3200	1000
	2800	3100	2000
B-C-A ($g = 5$)	3100	1800	2400
	2800	1600	2200
	3100	1600	1400
	2300	1500	2200
	3000	1700	2600
	3100	2100	2800
B-A-C ($g = 6$)	3500	3200	2900
	3400	2800	2200
	2300	2200	1700
	2300	1300	1400
	3000	2400	1800

A, salbutamol; B, formoterol; C, placebo.

Under a random effects linear additive risk model allowing the variance of patient responses to vary between treatments, we provide procedures for testing non-equality of treatments based on the weighted-least-squares (WLS) method (Fleiss, 1981; Senn, 2002; Lui, 2004). We give procedures for testing non-inferiority and equivalence between an experimental treatment and an active control treatment. We discuss interval estimation of the mean difference between treatments. We address hypothesis testing and estimation for period effects. We develop procedures for testing treatment-by-period interactions.

Assuming constant variance across treatments, we present SAS codes of PROC MIXED and PROC GLIMMIX (SAS Institute, 2009), as well as compare the results obtained by using the ordinary linear regression method (for fixed patient effects) and the general linear mixed model (for random patient effects) (Senn, 2002, pp. 175–178) with those obtained by use of the WLS method. We discuss in exercises the use of a Latin square to reduce the number of groups with different treatment-receipt sequences. This is especially of use when there are four or more treatments under comparison in a crossover design.

Suppose that we compare two experimental treatments A and B with a placebo C (or a standard treatment A, a new treatment B, and a placebo C in a gold standard design) under a three-period crossover trial. We use the treatment-receipt sequence U-V-W to denote that a patient receives treatments U, V, and W at periods 1, 2, and 3, respectively. Suppose that we randomly assign n_g patients to group $g = 1$ with C-A-B treatment-receipt sequence; $= 2$ with C-B-A treatment-receipt sequence; $= 3$ with A-C-B treatment receipt sequence; $= 4$ with A-B-C treatment-receipt sequence; $= 5$ with B-C-A treatment-receipt sequence; and $= 6$ with B-A-C treatment-receipt sequence. For patient i ($=1, 2, \cdots, n_g$) assigned to group g ($=1, 2, 3, 4, 5, 6$), let $Y_{iz}^{(g)}$ denote the patient response at period z ($=1, 2, 3$). Let $X_{iz1}^{(g)}$ denote the treatment-received covariate for treatment A, and $X_{iz1}^{(g)} = 1$ if the corresponding patient at period z receives treatment A, and $= 0$ otherwise. Similarly, let $X_{iz2}^{(g)}$ denote the treatment-received covariate for treatment B, and $X_{iz2}^{(g)} = 1$ if the corresponding patient at period z receives treatment B, and $= 0$ otherwise. Furthermore, we let $Z_{iz1}^{(g)}$ and $Z_{iz2}^{(g)}$ denote the indicator functions of period covariates with setting $Z_{iz1}^{(g)} = 1$ for period $z = 2$, and $= 0$ otherwise; and $Z_{iz2}^{(g)} = 1$ for period $z = 3$, and $= 0$ otherwise. As commonly assumed for a crossover design, we assume with an adequate washout period that there is no carry-over effect due to the treatment administered at an earlier period on the patient response. We assume further that the patient response $Y_{iz}^{(g)}$ on patient i ($=1, 2, \cdots, n_g$) assigned to group g ($=1, 2, \cdots, 6$) at period z ($=1, 2, 3$) follows the random effects linear additive risk model (Grizzle, 1965) as given by

$$
\begin{aligned}
Y_{iz}^{(g)} = {} & \mu_i^{(g)} + \eta_{AC} X_{iz1}^{(g)} + \eta_{BC} X_{iz2}^{(g)} + \gamma_1 Z_{iz1}^{(g)} + \gamma_2 Z_{iz2}^{(g)} \\
& + \varepsilon_{izA}^{(g)} X_{iz1}^{(g)} + \varepsilon_{izB}^{(g)} X_{iz2}^{(g)} + \varepsilon_{izC}^{(g)} \left(1 - X_{iz1}^{(g)} \right) \left(1 - X_{iz2}^{(g)} \right),
\end{aligned}
\tag{6.1}
$$

where $\mu_i^{(g)}$ represents the random effect due to the ith patient assigned to group g, and all $\mu_i^{(g)}$'s are assumed to independently follow an unspecified probability density function $f_g(\mu)$ with variance σ_μ^2; η_{AC} and η_{BC} denote the respective effect of treatments A and B relative to treatment C; and γ_1 and γ_2 denote the respective effect for periods 2 and 3 versus period 1; and random errors $\varepsilon_{izT}^{(g)}$'s (for $T = $ A, B, and C) are assumed to be independently distributed as a normal distribution with mean 0 and variance σ_{eT}^2 and to be independent of $\mu_i^{(g)}$'s. Note that under model (6.1), the variances of random errors $\varepsilon_{iT}^{(g)}$'s are allowed to vary among treatments A, B, and C. Thus, this model can account for situations in which the treatment can affect both mean and variance of patient responses. When the effects between treatments A and C on the patient response are equal to each other, η_{AC} is equal to 0. If the response of a randomly selected patient receiving treatment A tends to be, at a given fixed period, higher than that of the patient receiving treatment C, $\eta_{AC} > 0$. If the response of a randomly selected patient receiving treatment A tends to be, at a given fixed period, lower than that of the patient receiving treatment C, $\eta_{AC} < 0$. Similar interpretations as those for parameter η_{AC} are applicable to parameter η_{BC}. Note that the mean difference between treatments B and A for a fixed period on a given patient is simply $\eta_{BA} = \eta_{BC} - \eta_{AC}$. When $\eta_{BA} = 0$, the effects between treatments B and A on the mean response of a patient are the same. When $\eta_{BA} > 0$ (or $\eta_{BA} < 0$), treatment B tends to increase (or decrease) the mean response of a patient as compared with treatment A.

For patient i in group g, define $d_i^{(g)}(z_1, z_2) = Y_{iz_2}^{(g)} - Y_{iz_1}^{(g)}$ (for $z_1 \neq z_2$, z_1 and $z_2 = 1, 2, 3$), denoting the difference in responses between periods z_2 and z_1. For brevity, let "+" denote the summation over that subscript. For example, $Y_{+z}^{(g)} = \sum_{i=1}^{n_g} Y_{iz}^{(g)}$ denotes the sum of responses over patients at period z (=1, 2, 3) in group g (=1, 2, $\cdots$, 6). We define $\bar{Y}_{+z}^{(g)} = \sum_{i=1}^{n_g} Y_{iz}^{(g)}/n_g$ as the average of responses at period z over patients in group g. We further define $\bar{d}^{(g)}(z_1, z_2) = \sum_{i=1}^{n_g} d_i^{(g)}(z_1, z_2)/n_g = \bar{Y}_{+z_2}^{(g)} - \bar{Y}_{+z_1}^{(g)}$. Under model (6.1), we can show that the following three estimators are all unbiased estimators for η_{AC} (Problem 6.1):

$$\hat{\eta}_{AC1} = \left(\bar{d}^{(1)}(1,2) - \bar{d}^{(3)}(1,2) \right)/2,$$

$$\hat{\eta}_{AC2} = \left(\bar{d}^{(2)}(1,3) - \bar{d}^{(4)}(1,3) \right)/2, \text{ and} \qquad (6.2)$$

$$\hat{\eta}_{AC3} = \left(\bar{d}^{(5)}(2,3) - \bar{d}^{(6)}(2,3) \right)/2.$$

The variances for $\hat{\eta}_{ACk}$ (for $k = 1, 2, 3$) are given by (Problem 6.2)

$$Var(\hat{\eta}_{AC1}) = \left[\sigma_{AC}^2(1/n_1 + 1/n_3) \right]/4,$$
$$Var(\hat{\eta}_{AC2}) = \left[\sigma_{AC}^2(1/n_2 + 1/n_4) \right]/4, \text{ and} \qquad (6.3)$$
$$Var(\hat{\eta}_{AC3}) = \left[\sigma_{AC}^2(1/n_5 + 1/n_6) \right]/4,$$

where $\sigma_{AC}^2 = \sigma_{eA}^2 + \sigma_{eC}^2$.

On the basis of (6.2) and (6.3), we obtain the WLS estimator for η_{AC} as

$$\hat{\eta}_{AC}^{(WLS)} = \sum_{k=1}^{3} W_k \hat{\eta}_{ACk} / \left(\sum_{i=1}^{3} W_k \right), \qquad (6.4)$$

where $W_1 = n_1 n_3/(n_1 + n_3)$, $W_2 = n_2 n_4/(n_2 + n_4)$, and $W_3 = n_5 n_6/(n_5 + n_6)$. Note that $\hat{\eta}_{AC}^{(WLS)}$ is an unbiased estimator of η_{AC}. We can further show that the variance for $\hat{\eta}_{AC}^{(WLS)}$ (6.4) is (Problem 6.3)

$$Var\left(\hat{\eta}_{AC}^{(WLS)}\right) = \sigma_{AC}^2 / \left(4\sum_{k=1}^{3} W_k\right). \tag{6.5}$$

Furthermore, we can estimate the variance σ_{AC}^2 by the pooled-sample variance:

$$\hat{\sigma}_{AC}^2 = \left[\sum_{i=1}^{n_1} \left(d_i^{(1)}(1,2) - \bar{d}^{(1)}(1,2)\right)^2 + \sum_{i=1}^{n_3} \left(d_i^{(3)}(1,2) - \bar{d}^{(3)}(1,2)\right)^2 \right.$$
$$+ \sum_{i=1}^{n_2} \left(d_i^{(2)}(1,3) - \bar{d}^{(2)}(1,3)\right)^2 + \sum_{i=1}^{n_4} \left(d_i^{(4)}(1,3) - \bar{d}^{(4)}(1,3)\right)^2$$
$$\left. + \sum_{i=1}^{n_5} \left(d_i^{(5)}(2,3) - \bar{d}^{(5)}(2,3)\right)^2 + \sum_{i=1}^{n_6} \left(d_i^{(6)}(2,3) - \bar{d}^{(6)}(2,3)\right)^2\right] / (n_+ - 6), \tag{6.6}$$

where $n_+ = \sum_{i=1}^{6} n_i$ denotes the total number of patients in the trial. Therefore, when substituting $\hat{\sigma}_{AC}^2$ (6.6) for σ_{AC}^2 in $Var(\hat{\eta}_{AC})$ (6.5), we obtain the variance estimator $\widehat{Var}\left(\hat{\eta}_{AC}^{(WLS)}\right)$. We can show that the statistic

$$t_{AC} = \left(\hat{\eta}_{AC}^{(WLS)} - \eta_{AC}\right) / \sqrt{\widehat{Var}(\hat{\eta}_{AC})} \tag{6.7}$$

follows a t-distribution with $n_+ - 6$ degrees of freedom (Problem 6.4). Note that the unbiased estimator for η_{AC} suggested by Senn and Hildebrand (1991) is the linear combination of $\hat{\eta}_{ACk}$ with equal weights (i.e., $W_1 = W_2 = W_3 = 1/3$) as given by

$$\hat{\eta}_{AC}^{(SH)} = \sum_{k=1}^{3} \hat{\eta}_{ACk}/3. \tag{6.8}$$

We can show that the variance of $\hat{\eta}_{AC}^{(SH)}$ is given by (Problem 6.5)

$$Var\left(\hat{\eta}_{AC}^{(SH)}\right) = \left(\sum_{g=1}^{6} \sigma_{AC}^2 / n_g\right)/36. \tag{6.9}$$

Because we use optimal weights W_k to minimize the variance of $\hat{\eta}_{AC}^{(WLS)}$ among all linear combinations of $\hat{\eta}_{ACk}$, $Var\left(\hat{\eta}_{AC}^{(WLS)}\right)$ (6.5) is smaller than or equal to $Var\left(\hat{\eta}_{AC}^{(SH)}\right)$ (6.9). When $n_1 = n_2 = \cdots = n_6$ (i.e., balanced cases), we can easily see that $\hat{\eta}_{AC}^{(WLS)} = \hat{\eta}_{AC}^{(SH)}$ and $Var\left(\hat{\eta}_{AC}^{(WLS)}\right) = Var\left(\hat{\eta}_{AC}^{(SH)}\right)$. When we randomly assign patients with equal probability to groups with different treatment-receipt sequences, all n_g's are expected to be approximately equal to one another. Thus, the gain in efficiency by using the WLS estimator $\hat{\eta}_{AC}^{(WLS)}$ (6.4) instead of Senn and Hildebrand's estimator $\hat{\eta}_{AC}^{(SH)}$ (6.8) is likely to be minimal. Note that we form the strata, each consisting of two groups according to the pair of periods at which the two treatments under comparison are in reverse order so that we can remove period effects when taking a difference $\bar{d}^{(g)}(z_1, z_2) - \bar{d}^{(g')}(z_1, z_2)$ (for $g \neq g'$) under model (6.1). Thus, the above weights W_k are optimal only among linear combinations of $\hat{\eta}_{ACk}$ based on the strata defined here. It is still possible that one may find an estimator with variance even smaller than $\hat{\eta}_{AC}^{(WLS)}$ (Senn, 2002). Since $\hat{\eta}_{AC}^{(WLS)}$ (6.4) has variance smaller than $\hat{\eta}_{AC}^{(SH)}$ (6.8), however, the improvement in efficiency by using the estimator with optimal weights among all linear combinations of "basic estimators" (Senn, 2002) instead of the WLS estimator presented here can be expected to be even minimal in most randomized trials.

Example 6.1   Consider the data in Table 6.1 regarding FEV_1 (in ml) obtained from a three-period double-blind crossover trial comparing the experimental treatment (B) of formoterol solution aerosol (12 µg), the standard treatment (A) of salbutamol suspension aerosol (100 µg), and placebo (C) in exercise-induced asthma (Tsoy *et al.*, 1990; Senn and Hildebrand, 1991; Senn, 2002). We use these data to illustrate the difference between estimators $\hat{\eta}_{AC}^{(WLS)}$ (6.4) and $\hat{\eta}_{AC}^{(SH)}$ (6.8) and the possible efficiency gained by use of the former instead of the latter. We obtain $\hat{\eta}_{AC}^{(WLS)} = 676.82$ ml and $\hat{\eta}_{AC}^{(SH)} = 694.17$ ml, as well as $\widehat{Var}\left(\hat{\eta}_{AC}^{(WLS)}\right) = 6{,}557.01$ ml^2 and $\widehat{Var}\left(\hat{\eta}_{AC}^{(SH)}\right) = 6{,}763.99$ ml^2. The difference between these two resulting point estimates is small relative to the magnitude of their variances. To measure the efficiency between these two estimators, we calculate the variance ratio $Var\left(\hat{\eta}_{AC}^{(WLS)}\right)/Var\left(\hat{\eta}_{AC}^{(SH)}\right)$ and obtain it to be 96.94%. In other words, the gain of efficiency in use of $\hat{\eta}_{AC}^{(WLS)}$ instead of $\hat{\eta}_{AC}^{(SH)}$ is only 3.06% ($\approx 1 - 96.94\%$).

Using the same ideas as for deriving t_{AC} (6.7), we may consider the following three unbiased estimators (Problem 6.6) for η_{BC} under model (6.1) as

$$\hat{\eta}_{BC1} = \left(\bar{d}^{(1)}(1,3) - \bar{d}^{(6)}(1,3)\right)/2,$$

$$\hat{\eta}_{BC2} = \left(\bar{d}^{(2)}(1,2) - \bar{d}^{(5)}(1,2)\right)/2, \text{ and} \qquad (6.10)$$

$$\hat{\eta}_{BC3} = \left(\bar{d}^{(3)}(2,3) - \bar{d}^{(4)}(2,3)\right)/2.$$

The variances for $\hat{\eta}_{BCk}$ (for $k = 1, 2, 3$) are given by (Problem 6.7)

$$Var(\hat{\eta}_{BC1}) = \left[\sigma_{BC}^2(1/n_1 + 1/n_6)\right]/4,$$
$$Var(\hat{\eta}_{BC2}) = \left[\sigma_{BC}^2(1/n_2 + 1/n_5)\right]/4, \text{ and} \qquad (6.11)$$
$$Var(\hat{\eta}_{BC3}) = \left[\sigma_{BC}^2(1/n_3 + 1/n_4)\right]/4,$$

where $\sigma_{BC}^2 = \sigma_{eB}^2 + \sigma_{eC}^2$.

On the basis of (6.10) and (6.11), we obtain the WLS estimator for η_{BC} as

$$\hat{\eta}_{BC}^{(WLS)} = \sum\nolimits_{k=1}^{3} W_k^* \hat{\eta}_{BCk} / \left(\sum\nolimits_{i=1}^{3} W_k^*\right), \qquad (6.12)$$

where $W_1^* = n_1 n_6 / (n_1 + n_6)$, $W_2^* = n_2 n_5 / (n_2 + n_5)$, and $W_3^* = n_3 n_4 / (n_3 + n_4)$. Again, the WLS estimator $\hat{\eta}_{BC}^{(WLS)}$ (6.12) is an unbiased estimator of η_{BC}. We can further show that the variance for $\hat{\eta}_{BC}^{(WLS)}$ (6.12) is

$$Var\left(\hat{\eta}_{BC}^{(WLS)}\right) = \sigma_{BC}^2 / \left(4 \sum_{k=1}^{3} W_k^*\right). \tag{6.13}$$

Furthermore, we can estimate the variance σ_{BC}^2 by the unbiased pooled-sample variance:

$$\hat{\sigma}_{BC}^2 = \left[\sum_{i=1}^{n_1} \left(d_i^{(1)}(1,3) - \bar{d}^{(1)}(1,3) \right)^2 + \sum_{i=1}^{n_6} \left(d_i^{(6)}(1,3) - \bar{d}^{(6)}(1,3) \right)^2 \right.$$
$$+ \sum_{i=1}^{n_2} \left(d_i^{(2)}(1,2) - \bar{d}^{(2)}(1,2) \right)^2 + \sum_{i=1}^{n_5} \left(d_i^{(5)}(1,2) - \bar{d}^{(5)}(1,2) \right)^2$$
$$\left. + \sum_{i=1}^{n_3} \left(d_i^{(3)}(2,3) - \bar{d}^{(3)}(2,3) \right)^2 + \sum_{i=1}^{n_4} \left(d_i^{(4)}(2,3) - \bar{d}^{(4)}(2,3) \right)^2 \right] / (n_+ - 6). \tag{6.14}$$

Therefore, when substituting $\hat{\sigma}_{BC}^2$ (6.14) for σ_{BC}^2 in $Var\left(\hat{\eta}_{BC}^{(WLS)}\right)$ (6.13), we obtain the variance estimator $\widehat{Var}\left(\hat{\eta}_{BC}^{(WLS)}\right)$. Thus, we have

$$t_{BC} = \left(\hat{\eta}_{BC}^{(WLS)} - \eta_{BC}\right) / \sqrt{\widehat{Var}\left(\hat{\eta}_{BC}^{(WLS)}\right)}, \tag{6.15}$$

which follows a t-distribution with $n_+ - 6$ degrees of freedom.

When estimating the mean difference in effects between treatments B and A, we may consider the following three unbiased estimators (Problem 6.8) for η_{BA} under model (6.1) as

$$\hat{\eta}_{BA1} = \left(\bar{d}^{(1)}(2,3) - \bar{d}^{(2)}(2,3) \right) / 2,$$
$$\hat{\eta}_{BA2} = \left(\bar{d}^{(3)}(1,3) - \bar{d}^{(5)}(1,3) \right) / 2, \text{ and} \tag{6.16}$$
$$\hat{\eta}_{BA3} = \left(\bar{d}^{(4)}(1,2) - \bar{d}^{(6)}(1,2) \right) / 2.$$

The variances for $\hat{\eta}_{BAk}$ (for $k = 1, 2, 3$) are given by (Problem 6.9)

$$Var(\hat{\eta}_{BA1}) = \left[\sigma_{BA}^2 (1/n_1 + 1/n_2) \right] / 4,$$
$$Var(\hat{\eta}_{BA2}) = \left[\sigma_{BA}^2 (1/n_3 + 1/n_5) \right] / 4, \text{ and} \tag{6.17}$$
$$Var(\hat{\eta}_{BA3}) = \left[\sigma_{BA}^2 (1/n_4 + 1/n_6) \right] / 4,$$

where $\sigma_{BA}^2 = \sigma_{eB}^2 + \sigma_{eA}^2$.

On the basis of (6.16) and (6.17), we obtain the WLS estimator for η_{BA} as

$$\hat{\eta}_{BA}^{(WLS)} = \sum_{k=1}^{3} W_k^{**} \hat{\eta}_{BAk} / \left(\sum_{i=1}^{3} W_k^{**} \right), \tag{6.18}$$

where $W_1^{**} = n_1 n_2 / (n_1 + n_2)$, $W_2^{**} = n_3 n_5 / (n_3 + n_5)$, and $W_3^{**} = n_4 n_6 / (n_4 + n_6)$. We can further show that the variance for $\hat{\eta}_{BA}^{(WLS)}$ (6.18) is

$$Var\left(\hat{\eta}_{BA}^{(WLS)} \right) = \sigma_{BA}^2 / \left(4 \sum_{k=1}^{3} W_k^{**} \right). \tag{6.19}$$

Furthermore, we can estimate the variance σ_{BA}^2 by the unbiased pooled-sample variance:

$$\hat{\sigma}_{BA}^2 = \left[\sum_{i=1}^{n_1} \left(d_i^{(1)}(2,3) - \bar{d}^{(1)}(2,3) \right)^2 + \sum_{i=1}^{n_2} \left(d_i^{(2)}(2,3) - \bar{d}^{(2)}(2,3) \right)^2 \right.$$

$$+ \sum_{i=1}^{n_3} \left(d_i^{(3)}(1,3) - \bar{d}^{(3)}(1,3) \right)^2 + \sum_{i=1}^{n_5} \left(d_i^{(5)}(1,3) - \bar{d}^{(5)}(1,3) \right)^2$$

$$\left. + \sum_{i=1}^{n_4} \left(d_i^{(4)}(1,2) - \bar{d}^{(4)}(1,2) \right)^2 + \sum_{i=1}^{n_6} \left(d_i^{(6)}(1,2) - \bar{d}^{(6)}(1,2) \right)^2 \right] / (n_+ - 6). \tag{6.20}$$

Therefore, when substituting $\hat{\sigma}_{BA}^2$ (6.20) for σ_{BA}^2 in $Var\left(\hat{\eta}_{BA}^{(WLS)} \right)$ (6.19), we obtain the variance estimator $\widehat{Var}\left(\hat{\eta}_{BA}^{(WLS)} \right)$. On the basis of the above results, we can show that the following statistic:

$$t_{BA} = \left(\hat{\eta}_{BA}^{(WLS)} - \eta_{BA} \right) / \sqrt{\widehat{Var}\left(\hat{\eta}_{BA}^{(WLS)} \right)}, \tag{6.21}$$

follows a t-distribution with $n_+ - 6$ degrees of freedom.

6.1   Testing non-equality between treatments and placebo

Suppose that treatments A and B represent two new experimental treatments, and treatment C represents the placebo. We may often be interested in finding out whether either treatment A or treatment B differs from the placebo, while whether there is a difference between treatments A and B is not our primary concern (Dunnett, 1964). Thus, we consider testing $H_0 : \eta_{AC} = \eta_{BC} = 0$ versus $H_a : \eta_{AC} \neq 0$ or $\eta_{BC} \neq 0$. On the basis of t_{AC} (6.7) and t_{BC} (6.15) with use of Bonferroni's inequality to adjust the inflation due to multiple tests in Type I error, we will reject $H_0 : \eta_{AC} = \eta_{BC} = 0$ at the α-level if either of the following two inequalities holds:

$$|\hat{\eta}_{AC}^{(WLS)}| / \sqrt{\widehat{\text{var}}\left(\hat{\eta}_{AC}^{(WLS)}\right)} > t_{\alpha/4, n_+ - 6}, \text{ or}$$

$$|\hat{\eta}_{BC}^{(WLS)}| / \sqrt{\widehat{\text{var}}\left(\hat{\eta}_{BC}^{(WLS)}\right)} > t_{\alpha/4, n_+ - 6}, \tag{6.22}$$

where $t_{\alpha,df}$ is the upper $100(\alpha)$th percentile of the t-distribution with df degrees of freedom.

Example 6.2 Consider the data in Table 6.1 again. When employing the test procedure (6.22), we obtain p-values for using both the individual test $|\hat{\eta}_{AC}^{(WLS)}| / \sqrt{\widehat{\text{var}}\left(\hat{\eta}_{AC}^{(WLS)}\right)}$ and $|\hat{\eta}_{BC}^{(WLS)}| / \sqrt{\widehat{\text{var}}\left(\hat{\eta}_{BC}^{(WLS)}\right)}$ to be < 0.001. Because $\hat{\eta}_{AC}^{(WLS)} =$ 676.82 ml > 0 and $\hat{\eta}_{BC}^{(WLS)} = 1093.90$ ml > 0, there is significant evidence that both the experimental treatment of formoterol solution aerosol and the standard treatment of salbutamol suspension aerosol can, as compared with placebo, increase FEV_1.

If treatments A and B represent two different doses of a treatment, it may be of interest to find out whether there is a dose effect. Also, after finding out that the two new treatments are significantly better than the placebo C, we may also want to study whether there is a difference between these two new treatments A and B. In this case, we consider testing $H_0 : \eta_{BA} = 0$ versus $H_a : \eta_{BA} \neq 0$. On the basis of t_{BA} (6.21), we will reject $H_0 : \eta_{BA} = 0$ at the α-level if

$$|\hat{\eta}_{BA}^{(WLS)}| / \sqrt{\widehat{Var}\left(\hat{\eta}_{BA}^{(WLS)}\right)} > t_{\alpha/2, n_+ - 6}. \tag{6.23}$$

Example 6.3 Consider the data in Table 6.1. If we are interested in finding out whether there is a difference between formoterol solution aerosol and salbutamol suspension aerosol, then we may employ the test procedure (6.23). We obtain the p-value to be < 0.001. Because $\hat{\eta}_{BA}^{(WLS)} = 417.610$ ml > 0, there is significant evidence that using formoterol solution aerosol tends to increase FEV_1 as compared with salbutamol suspension aerosol.

6.2   Testing non-inferiority of an experimental treatment to an active control treatment

When treatment A represents an active control (or a standard) treatment and treatment B represents an experimental treatment, it can be of interest to study whether the experimental treatment B is non-inferior to the active control treatment A, especially when the former has few side effects or less expense than the latter. For simplicity, we shall assume $\sigma_{eA}^2 = \sigma_{eB}^2$ in the present and next sections.

Suppose that the larger the patient response, the better is the patient outcome. Thus, when assessing the non-inferiority of treatment B to treatment A with respect to the mean difference in therapeutic efficacy, we want to test $H_0 : \eta_{BA} \le \eta_l$ versus $H_a : \eta_{BA} > \eta_l$, where η_l ($\eta_l < 0$) is the maximum clinically acceptable low margin such that treatment B can be regarded as non-inferior to treatment A when $\eta_{BA} > \eta_l$ holds. On the basis of t_{BA} (6.21), we will reject $H_0 : \eta_{BA} \le \eta_l$ at the α-level and claim that treatment B is non-inferior to treatment A if

$$\left(\hat{\eta}_{BA}^{(WLS)} - \eta_l \right) / \sqrt{\widehat{\mathrm{var}} \left(\hat{\eta}_{BA}^{(WLS)} \right)} > t_{\alpha, n_+ - 6}. \tag{6.24}$$

6.3   Testing equivalence between an experimental treatment and an active control treatment

When an experimental treatment is found to be much more effective than an active control treatment, we may have the concern that the former can be more toxic than the latter. In this case, we may wish to test equivalence rather than non-inferiority. Using the intersection-union test (Casella and Berger, 1990), we can modify procedures for testing non-inferiority to accommodate testing equivalence. Suppose that we want to test $H_0 : \eta_{BA} \le \eta_l$ or $\eta_{BA} \ge \eta_u$ versus $H_a : \eta_l < \eta_{BA} < \eta_u$, where η_l ($\eta_l < 0$) and η_u ($\eta_u > 0$) are the maximum clinically acceptable lower and upper margins such that treatment B can be regarded as equivalent to treatment A when $\eta_l < \eta_{BA} < \eta_u$ holds. On the basis of t_{BA} (6.21), we will reject $H_0 : \eta_{BA} \le \eta_l$ or $\eta_{BA} \ge \eta_u$ at the α-level if

$$
\begin{aligned}
& \left(\hat{\eta}_{BA}^{(WLS)} - \eta_l \right) / \sqrt{\widehat{\mathrm{var}} \left(\hat{\eta}_{BA}^{(WLS)} \right)} > t_{\alpha, n_+ - 6}, \text{ and} \\
& \left(\hat{\eta}_{BA}^{(WLS)} - \eta_u \right) / \sqrt{\widehat{\mathrm{var}} \left(\hat{\eta}_{BA}^{(WLS)} \right)} < -t_{\alpha, n_+ - 6}.
\end{aligned}
\tag{6.25}
$$

Note that we may wish to choose $\eta_u = -\eta_l$ to avoid the undesirable cases in which the claim of two treatments to be equivalent depends on which treatment is named A or which treatment is named B. For testing bioequivalence (instead of therapeutic equivalence) between treatments A and B, we often consider the AUC, the maximum concentration $C_{\max}$, or the time to reach its peak $T_{\max}$ as a measure of the patient response. Because the values of these variables are positive and their sampling distributions are frequently skewed, we may employ the logarithmic transformation to alleviate the skewness. In these cases, we will apply the test procedure (6.25) to $\log \left(Y_{iz}^{(g)} \right)$ (instead of $Y_{iz}^{(g)}$) (see Chapter 2).

6.4   Interval estimation of the mean difference

When assessing the magnitude of the mean difference between treatment A and treatment C, we want to obtain an interval estimator for η_{AC}. On the basis of t_{AC} (6.7), we obtain a 100(1 − α)% confidence interval for η_{AC} as

$$\left[\hat{\eta}_{AC}^{(WLS)} - t_{\alpha/2, n_+ - 6} \sqrt{\widehat{Var} \left(\hat{\eta}_{AC}^{(WLS)} \right)}, \hat{\eta}_{BA}^{(WLS)} + t_{\alpha/2, n_+ - 6} \sqrt{\widehat{Var} \left(\hat{\eta}_{BA}^{(WLS)} \right)} \right]. \tag{6.26}$$

Similarly, when assessing the magnitude of the mean difference between treatments B and A, we want to obtain an interval estimator for η_{BA}. On the basis of t_{BA} (6.21), we obtain a $100(1 - \alpha)\%$ confidence interval for η_{BA} as

$$\left[\hat{\eta}_{BA}^{(WLS)} - t_{\alpha/2, n_+ - 6} \sqrt{\widehat{Var}\left(\hat{\eta}_{BA}^{(WLS)} \right)}, \hat{\eta}_{BA}^{(WLS)} + t_{\alpha/2, n_+ - 6} \sqrt{\widehat{Var}\left(\hat{\eta}_{BA}^{(WLS)} \right)} \right]. \quad (6.27)$$

Note that procedure (6.25) for testing equivalence between treatments A and B is equivalent to claiming that these two treatments are equivalent if the resulting $100(1 - 2\alpha)\%$ confidence interval using interval estimator (6.27) lies entirely in the equivalence interval (η_l, η_u).

Example 6.4   When applying interval estimator (6.27) to the data in Table 6.1, we obtain the 95% confidence interval for η_{BA} (in ml) as [226.57, 608.65]. Because the resulting lower confidence limit falls above 0, there is significant evidence that using formoterol solution aerosol tends to increase FEV_1 as compared with salbutamol suspension aerosol. This is consistent with the previous result based on hypothesis testing (see Example 6.3). For the reader's interest, we also apply the interval estimator for η_{BA} based on the simple average of $\hat{\eta}_{BAk}$ (for $k = 1, 2, 3$) with equal weights (Senn and Hildebrand, 1991). We obtain the 95% confidence interval for η_{BA} (in ml) as [237.89, 623.23], which is slightly wider than that obtained by use of (6.27) based on $\hat{\eta}_{BA}^{(WLS)}$.

Conditional upon each strata ($k = 1, 2, 3$) defined here, we may employ the Mann–Whitney–Wilcoxon rank sum test as done in Chapter 2 if readers wish to apply a nonparametric test procedure. If there are no treatment-by-period interactions, we can also apply a weighted sum of Wilcoxon rank sum tests across strata to obtain a summary test for testing non-equality between two treatments (Lehmann, 1975, pp. 132–141). The codes using SAS packages for nonparametric methods appear elsewhere (Senn, 2002, pp. 193–194).

6.5 Hypothesis testing and estimation for period effects

The parameters γ_1 and γ_2, representing period effects under model (6.1) can sometimes be of interest in a crossover trial. Thus, we discuss hypothesis testing and estimation for period effects γ_1 and γ_2.

When estimating γ_1 between periods 2 and 1, we can show that the following statistics under model (6.1) are all unbiased estimators for γ_1 (Problem 6.10):

$$\hat{\gamma}_{11} = \left(\bar{d}^{(1)}(1,2) + \bar{d}^{(3)}(1,2) \right) / 2,$$

$$\hat{\gamma}_{12} = \left(\bar{d}^{(2)}(1,2) + \bar{d}^{(5)}(1,2) \right) / 2, \text{ and} \quad (6.28)$$

$$\hat{\gamma}_{13} = \left(\bar{d}^{(4)}(1,2) + \bar{d}^{(6)}(1,2) \right) / 2.$$

The variances for $\hat{\gamma}_{1k}$ (for $k = 1, 2, 3$) are given by (Problem 6.11)

$$
\begin{aligned}
Var(\hat{\gamma}_{11}) &= \left[\sigma_{AC}^2(1/n_1 + 1/n_3)\right]/4, \\
Var(\hat{\gamma}_{12}) &= \left[\sigma_{BC}^2(1/n_2 + 1/n_5)\right]/4, \text{ and} \\
Var(\hat{\gamma}_{13}) &= \left[\sigma_{BA}^2(1/n_4 + 1/n_6)\right]/4.
\end{aligned}
\tag{6.29}
$$

On the basis of (6.28) and (6.29), we may consider the weighted linear (WL) combination of $\hat{\gamma}_{1k}$ for γ_1 as given by

$$
\hat{\gamma}_1^{(WL)} = \sum_{k=1}^3 WP_k \hat{\gamma}_{1k} / \left(\sum_{i=1}^3 WP_k\right),
\tag{6.30}
$$

where $WP_1 = n_1 n_3/(n_1 + n_3)$, $WP_2 = n_2 n_5/(n_2 + n_5)$, and $WP_3 = n_4 n_6/(n_4 + n_6)$. Note that $\hat{\gamma}_1^{(WL)}$ is an unbiased estimator of γ_1 under model (6.1). Note also that $\hat{\gamma}_1^{(WL)}$ is no longer the WLS estimator unless all variances σ_{AC}^2, σ_{BC}^2, and σ_{BA}^2 are equal to one another (i.e., $\sigma_{eA}^2 = \sigma_{eB}^2 = \sigma_{eC}^2$). We can further show that the variance for $\hat{\gamma}_1^{(WL)}$ (6.30) is (Problem 6.12)

$$
Var\left(\hat{\gamma}_1^{(WL)}\right) = \left(WP_1\sigma_{AC}^2 + WP_2\sigma_{BC}^2 + WP_3\sigma_{BA}^2\right)/\left[4\left(\sum_{k=1}^3 WP_k\right)^2\right].
\tag{6.31}
$$

As noted by Senn and Hildebrand (1991), the t-statistic is most robust providing that the calculation of a variance estimator in the denominator is based on the same set of observations for calculation of a test statistic in the numerator. Thus, when estimating σ_{AC}^2, σ_{BC}^2, and σ_{AC}^2 in (6.31), we will employ the following three variance estimators based on the data only for the first two periods:

$$
\hat{\sigma}_{AC}^2(1,2) = \left[\sum_{i=1}^{n_1}\left(d_i^{(1)}(1,2) - \bar{d}^{(1)}(1,2)\right)^2 + \sum_{i=1}^{n_3}\left(d_i^{(3)}(1,2) - \bar{d}^{(3)}(1,2)\right)^2\right]/(n_1 + n_3 - 2),
$$

$$
\hat{\sigma}_{BC}^2(1,2) = \left[\sum_{i=1}^{n_2}\left(d_i^{(2)}(1,2) - \bar{d}^{(2)}(1,2)\right)^2 + \sum_{i=1}^{n_5}\left(d_i^{(5)}(1,2) - \bar{d}^{(5)}(1,2)\right)^2\right]/(n_2 + n_5 - 2), \text{ and}
$$

$$
\hat{\sigma}_{BA}^2(1,2) = \left[\sum_{i=1}^{n_4}\left(d_i^{(4)}(1,2) - \bar{d}^{(4)}(1,2)\right)^2 + \sum_{i=1}^{n_6}\left(d_i^{(6)}(1,2) - \bar{d}^{(6)}(1,2)\right)^2\right]/(n_4 + n_6 - 2).
\tag{6.32}
$$

Thus, we can estimate $Var\left(\hat{\gamma}_1^{(WL)}\right)$ by the unbiased variance estimator

$$
\widehat{Var}\left(\hat{\gamma}_1^{(WL)}\right) = \left(a_1\hat{\sigma}_{AC}^2(1,2) + a_2\hat{\sigma}_{BC}^2(1,2) + a_3\hat{\sigma}_{BA}^2(1,2)\right),
\tag{6.33}
$$

where $a_k = WP_k / \left[4\left(\sum_{k=1}^3 WP_k\right)^2\right]$, $k = 1, 2, 3$. When testing $H_0 : \gamma_1 = 0$, we will reject $H_0 : \gamma_1 = 0$ at the α-level if

$$
|\hat{\gamma}_1^{(WL)}| / \sqrt{\widehat{Var}\left(\hat{\gamma}_1^{(WL)}\right)} > t_{\alpha/2, df^*},
\tag{6.34}
$$

where the degrees of freedom df^* is calculated as the closest integer to (Satterthwaite, 1946; Fleiss, 1986a) $\left[a_1\hat{\sigma}^2_{AC}(1,2)+a_2\hat{\sigma}^2_{BC}(1,2)+a_3\hat{\sigma}^2_{BA}(1,2)\right]^2/\left[a_1^2\hat{\sigma}^4_{AC}(1,2)/(n_1+n_3-2)+a_2^2\hat{\sigma}^4_{BC}(1,2)/(n_2+n_5-2)+a_3^2\hat{\sigma}^4_{BA}(1,2)/(n_4+n_6-2)\right]$.

Similarly, we may obtain an approximate $100(1-\alpha)\%$ confidence interval for γ_1 as

$$\left[\hat{\gamma}_1^{(WL)}-t_{\alpha/2,df^*}\sqrt{\widehat{Var}\left(\hat{\gamma}_1^{(WL)}\right)},\hat{\gamma}_1^{(WL)}+t_{\alpha/2,df^*}\sqrt{\widehat{Var}\left(\hat{\gamma}_1^{(WL)}\right)}\right]. \qquad (6.35)$$

Following similar arguments as those in the above, we can study γ_2 between periods 3 and 1 as well (Problem 6.13).

Example 6.5 Consider the data in Table 6.1 to illustrate the use of procedure (6.34) for testing $H_0:\gamma_1=0$ and interval estimator (6.35) for γ_1. When using test procedure (6.34), we obtain the p-value 0.078. Because $\hat{\gamma}_1^{(WL)}=-122.20\text{ ml}<0$, though the FEV_1 seems to decrease at period 2 versus period 1, this period effect is not significant at the 5% level. When employing interval estimator (6.35), we obtain the 95% confidence interval for γ_1 as $[-259.87, 15.46]$.

6.6 Procedures for testing treatment-by-period interactions

When employing a summary test or assessing a summary treatment effect across strata, we commonly need to assume that there is no interaction between treatment and strata. Otherwise, if the treatment effect is positive in some strata and negative in other strata, we can see that, for example, the value of $\hat{\eta}_{AC}^{(WLS)}$ $(=\sum_k W_k\hat{\eta}_{ACk}/\sum_k W_k)$ can be small due to cancelation of the positive and negative values $\hat{\eta}_{ACk}$ between strata. Thus, a summary test procedure can lack power. Furthermore, if the relative treatment effect varies between strata, we may want to present findings for each stratum separately to avoid providing readers with possibly misleading conclusions. It can be of interest and importance to study whether there are treatment-by-period interactions.

To account for treatment-by-period interactions, we extend model (6.1) to include terms representing these interactions as given by

$$\begin{aligned}
Y_{iz}^{(g)} &= \mu_i^{(g)}+\eta_{AC}X_{iz1}^{(g)}+\eta_{BC}X_{iz2}^{(g)}+\gamma_1 Z_{iz1}^{(g)}+\gamma_2 Z_{iz2}^{(g)}\\
&\quad +\lambda_{11}X_{iz1}^{(g)}Z_{iz1}^{(g)}+\lambda_{12}X_{iz1}^{(g)}Z_{iz2}^{(g)}+\lambda_{21}X_{iz2}^{(g)}Z_{iz1}^{(g)}+\lambda_{22}X_{iz2}^{(g)}Z_{iz2}^{(g)}\\
&\quad +\varepsilon_{izA}^{(g)}X_{iz1}^{(g)}+\varepsilon_{izB}^{(g)}X_{iz2}^{(g)}+\varepsilon_{izC}^{(g)}\left(1-X_{iz1}^{(g)}\right)\left(1-X_{iz2}^{(g)}\right),
\end{aligned} \qquad (6.36)$$

where λ_{1j}'s $(j=1,2)$ represent the interactions between treatment A (versus placebo C) and periods, and λ_{2j}'s $(j=1,2)$ represent the interactions between treatment

B (versus placebo C) and periods, respectively. When $\lambda_{11} = \lambda_{12} = 0$, the mean response difference between treatment A and treatment C (for a fixed period) on a given patient is constant over periods. Similarly, when $\lambda_{21} = \lambda_{22} = 0$, the mean response difference (for a fixed period) on a given patient between treatment B and treatment C is constant over periods. Furthermore, when $\lambda_{11} = \lambda_{21}$ and $\lambda_{12} = \lambda_{22}$, the mean response difference (for a fixed period) on a given patient between treatment B and treatment A is constant over periods.

Under model (6.36), we can show that (Problem 6.14)

$$E(\hat{\eta}_{AC1}) = \eta_{AC} + \lambda_{11}/2,$$
$$E(\hat{\eta}_{AC2}) = \eta_{AC} + \lambda_{12}/2, \text{ and} \qquad (6.37)$$
$$E(\hat{\eta}_{AC3}) = \eta_{AC} + (\lambda_{11} + \lambda_{12})/2,$$

where $\hat{\eta}_{ACk}$'s are defined in (6.2). Because $E(\hat{\eta}_{AC1}) = E(\hat{\eta}_{AC2}) = E(\hat{\eta}_{AC3})$ if and only if $\lambda_{11} = \lambda_{12} = 0$, we can apply the following WLS procedure for testing the homogeneity of mean differences across strata (i.e., $E(\hat{\eta}_{AC1}) = E(\hat{\eta}_{AC2}) = E(\hat{\eta}_{AC3})$) to test $H_0 : \lambda_{11} = \lambda_{12} = 0$. We will reject $H_0 : \lambda_{11} = \lambda_{12} = 0$ at the α-level (Problem 6.15) if

$$2\left[\sum_{k=1}^{3} W_k(\hat{\eta}_{ACk})^2 - \left(\sum_{k=1}^{3} W_k \hat{\eta}_{ACk}\right)^2 / \left(\sum_{i=1}^{3} W_k\right)\right] / \hat{\sigma}_{AC}^2 > F_{\alpha,2,n_+ - 6}, \qquad (6.38)$$

where $F_{\alpha,2,n_+ - 6}$ is the upper $100(\alpha)$th percentile of the F-distribution with 2 and $n_+ - 6$ degrees of freedom. Similarly, we can show that the expectations of $\hat{\eta}_{BCk}$ (6.10) under model (6.36) (Problem 6.16) are

$$E(\hat{\eta}_{BC1}) = \eta_{BC} + \lambda_{22}/2,$$
$$E(\hat{\eta}_{BC2}) = \eta_{BC} + \lambda_{21}/2, \text{ and} \qquad (6.39)$$
$$E(\hat{\eta}_{BC3}) = \eta_{BC} + (\lambda_{21} + \lambda_{22})/2.$$

Therefore, $E(\hat{\eta}_{BC1}) = E(\hat{\eta}_{BC2}) = E(\hat{\eta}_{BC3})$ if and only if $\lambda_{21} = \lambda_{22} = 0$. Following the same arguments as before, we will reject $H_0 : \lambda_{21} = \lambda_{22} = 0$ at the α-level if

$$2\left[\sum_{k=1}^{3} W_k^*(\hat{\eta}_{BCk})^2 - \left(\sum_{k=1}^{3} W_k^* \hat{\eta}_{BCk}\right)^2 / \left(\sum_{i=1}^{3} W_k^*\right)\right] / \hat{\sigma}_{BC}^2 > F_{\alpha,2,n_+ - 6}. \qquad (6.40)$$

Finally, we can show that the expectations of $\hat{\eta}_{BAk}$ (6.16) for $k = 1, 2, 3$ under model (6.36) are (Problem 6.17)

$$E(\hat{\eta}_{BA1}) = \eta_{BA} + [(\lambda_{22} - \lambda_{12}) + (\lambda_{21} - \lambda_{11})]/2,$$
$$E(\hat{\eta}_{BA2}) = \eta_{BA} + (\lambda_{22} - \lambda_{12})/2, \text{ and} \qquad (6.41)$$
$$E(\hat{\eta}_{BA3}) = \eta_{BA} + (\lambda_{21} - \lambda_{11})/2.$$

Thus, we will reject $H_0 : \lambda_{11} = \lambda_{21}$ and $\lambda_{12} = \lambda_{22}$ at the α-level if

$$2\left[\sum_{k=1}^{3} W_k^{**}(\hat{\eta}_{BAk})^2 - \left(\sum_{k=1}^{3} W_k^{**}\hat{\eta}_{BAk}\right)^2 \bigg/ \left(\sum_{i=1}^{3} W_k^{**}\right)\right] \bigg/ \hat{\sigma}_{BA}^2 > F_{\alpha,2,n_+ -6}. \qquad (6.42)$$

Example 6.6   Consider the data in Table 6.1. When applying test procedure (6.42) to test $H_0 : \lambda_{11} = \lambda_{21}$ and $\lambda_{12} = \lambda_{22}$, we obtain the p-value as 0.494. Thus, there is no significant evidence to claim that the relative effect of treatment B to treatment A varies across periods at the 0.05 level.

6.7   SAS program codes and results for constant variance

When patient effects $\mu_i^{(g)}$ are assumed to be fixed (or random), and random errors $\varepsilon_{iT}^{(g)}$'s ($T =$ A, B, and C) are independent and identically distributed as a normal distribution with constant variance σ_e^2 ($=\sigma_{eA}^2 = \sigma_{eB}^2 = \sigma_{eC}^2$), we use SAS's PROC MIXED and PROC GLIMMIX (SAS Institute, 2009) for comparison of test results and parameter estimates between using various methods. When patient effects are regarded as fixed, we may employ the ordinal least squares regression by treating all patients, periods, and treatments as classification variables (Senn, 2002, pp. 176–178). We present the SAS codes of PROC MIXED in the following box when analyzing the data in Table 6.1. Note that formoterol, salbutamol, and placebo are coded as "f," "s," and "p" for the "treat" covariate.

```
data step1;
input patient period treat$ fev1;
cards;
    1    1    f    3500
    1    2    s    3200
    1    3    p    2900
   10    1    f    3400
   10    2    s    2800
   10    3    p    2200
..... .
;;;;
proc mixed;
  class patient period treat;
  model fev1=patient period treat;
  estimate "for-sal" treat 1 0 -1;
  estimate "for-pla" treat 1 -1 0;
  estimate "sal-pla" treat 0 -1 1;
run;
```

We obtain the following outputs:

Label	Estimate	Error	DF	t Value	Pr > |t|
for-sal	422.62	88.2647	56	4.79	<.0001
for-pla	1103.46	87.8208	56	12.56	<.0001
sal-pla	680.84	87.9690	56	7.74	<.0001

By contrast, the corresponding estimates with their estimated standard error (SE) using the WLS methods under model (6.1) are $\hat{\eta}_{BA}^{(WLS)} = 417.61$ (SE = 92.56); $\hat{\eta}_{BC}^{(WLS)} = 1093.90$ (SE = 88.20); and $\hat{\eta}_{AC}^{(WLS)} = 676.82$ (SE = 80.98). We can see that these estimates are similar to those obtained in the above box under the model with fixed patient effects and constant error variance between treatments.

When patient effects are assumed to independently follow a normal distribution, we may apply PROC MIXED or PROC GLIMMIX. We present the SAS codes of using PROC GLIMMIX in the following box.

```
data step1;
input patient period treat$ fev1 group;
cards;
    1    1    f    3500    1
    1    2    s    3200    1
    1    3    p    2900    1
   10    1    f    3400    1
   10    2    s    2800    1
   10    3    p    2200    1
....
;;;;
  proc glimmix;
    class patient period treat group;
    model fev1=period treat/solution
                        dist=normal
                        link=id;
    random intercept/subject=patient;
    estimate "for-sal" treat 1 0 -1;
    estimate "for-pla" treat 1 -1 0;
    estimate "sal-pla" treat 0 -1 1;
  run;
```

For brevity, we include only a partial output of PROC GLIMMIX below.

```
                    Solutions for Fixed Effects
                                Standard
Effect      treat period Estimate   Error    DF   t Value   Pr > |t|
Intercept                2306.91   113.23    29    20.37    <.0001
period              1    42.7659   88.2647   56     0.48    0.6299
period              2   -66.9569   87.9690   56    -0.76    0.4498
period              3       0         .       .      .        .
treat        f           422.62    88.2647   56     4.79    <.0001
treat        p          -680.84    87.9690   56    -7.74    <.0001
treat        s              0         .       .      .        .
                             Estimates
                                Standard
    Label        Estimate      Error      DF    t Value   Pr > |t|
    for-sal       422.62      88.2647     56     4.79     <.0001
    for-pla      1103.46      87.8208     56    12.56     <.0001
    sal-pla       680.84      87.9690     56     7.74     <.0001
```

We can see that the estimates of the relative treatment effect are identical to those previously obtained with treating patient effects as fixed in use of PROC MIXED. As noted by Senn (2002, pp. 178–179), because all patients have complete information from three periods and there are no carry-over effects, the results between using PROC GLIMMIX assuming random patient effects and PROC MIXED assuming fixed patient effects are expected to be the same. However, when there are missing data (such as in an incomplete block crossover design, considered in Chapter 10), there will be some inter-patient information to recover. The parameter estimates between a random effects and a fixed effects models can be different.

Exercises

Problem 6.1.   Show that the three estimators given in (6.2) are all unbiased estimators for η_{AC} under model (6.1).

Problem 6.2.   Show that the variances for $\hat{\eta}_{ACk}$ (for $k = 1, 2, 3$) are given by formulas in (6.3).

Problem 6.3.   Show that the variance for $\hat{\eta}_{AC}^{(WLS)}$ (6.4) is given by $Var\left(\hat{\eta}_{AC}^{(WLS)}\right) = \sigma_{AC}^2 / \left(4\sum_{k=1}^{3} W_k\right)$.

Problem 6.4.   Show that $t_{AC} = \left(\hat{\eta}_{AC}^{(WLS)} - \eta_{AC}\right) / \sqrt{\widehat{Var}(\hat{\eta}_{AC})}$ follows a t-distribution with $n_+ - 6$ degrees of freedom.

Problem 6.5. Show that the variance of $\hat{\eta}_{AC}^{(SH)}$ is given by $Var\left(\hat{\eta}_{AC}^{(SH)}\right) = \left(\sum_{g=1}^{6} \sigma_{AC}^2/n_g\right)/36$.

Problem 6.6. Show that the three estimators given in (6.10) are all unbiased estimators for η_{BC} under model (6.1).

Problem 6.7. Show that the variances for $\hat{\eta}_{BCk}$ (for $k = 1, 2, 3$) in (6.10) are given by formulas in (6.11).

Problem 6.8. Show that the three estimators in (6.16) are all unbiased estimators for η_{BA} under model (6.1).

Problem 6.9. Show that the variances for $\hat{\eta}_{BAk}$ (for $k = 1, 2, 3$) are given by variance formulas in (6.17).

Problem 6.10. Show that the three estimators in (6.28) are all unbiased estimators of γ_1.

Problem 6.11. Show that the variances for $\hat{\gamma}_{1k}$ (for $k = 1, 2, 3$) in (6.28) are given by formulas in (6.29).

Problem 6.12. Show that the variance for $\hat{\gamma}_1^{(WL)}$ (6.30) is given by

$$Var\left(\hat{\gamma}_1^{(WL)}\right) = \left(WP_1\sigma_{AC}^2 + WP_2\sigma_{BC}^2 + WP_3\sigma_{BA}^2\right) \Bigg/ \left[4\left(\sum_{k=1}^{3} WP_k\right)^2\right].$$

Problem 6.13.

(a) Show that the following three estimators under model (6.1) are all unbiased estimators for γ_2: $\hat{\gamma}_{21} = \left(\bar{d}^{(1)}(1,3) + \bar{d}^{(6)}(1,3)\right)/2$, $\hat{\gamma}_{22} = \left(\bar{d}^{(2)}(1,3) + \bar{d}^{(4)}(1,3)\right)/2$, and $\hat{\gamma}_{23} = \left(\bar{d}^{(3)}(1,3) + \bar{d}^{(5)}(1.3)\right)/2$.

(b) Show that the variance for $\hat{\gamma}_{2k}$ for $k = 1$, 2, 3, is given by $Var(\hat{\gamma}_{21}) = \left[\sigma_{BC}^2(1/n_1 + 1/n_6)\right]/4$, $Var(\hat{\gamma}_{22}) = \left[\sigma_{AC}^2(1/n_2 + 1/n_4)\right]/4$, and $Var(\hat{\gamma}_{23}) = \left[\sigma_{BA}^2(1/n_3 + 1/n_5)\right]/4$.

(c) Show that the WL combination $\hat{\gamma}_2^{(WL)} = \sum_{k=1}^{3} WP_k^*\hat{\gamma}_{2k} \Big/ \left(\sum_{i=1}^{3} WP_k^*\right)$, where $WP_1^* = n_1n_6/(n_1 + n_6)$, $WP_2^* = n_2n_4/(n_2 + n_4)$, and $WP_3^* = n_3n_5/(n_3 + n_5)$ is an unbiased estimator of γ_2 under model (6.1).

(d) Show that the variance for $\hat{\gamma}_2^{(WL)}$ is $Var\left(\hat{\gamma}_2^{(WL)}\right) = \left(WP_1^*\sigma_{BC}^2 + WP_1^*\sigma_{AC}^2 + WP_3^*\sigma_{BA}^2\right) \Big/ \left[4\left(\sum_{k=1}^{3} WP_k^*\right)^2\right].$

(e) When one wants to estimate σ_{BC}^2, σ_{AC}^2, and σ_{BA}^2, show that the following three variance estimators based on the data for the first and third periods are all unbiased:

$$\hat{\sigma}^2_{BC}(1,3) = \left[\sum_{i=1}^{n_1}\left(d_i^{(1)}(1,3)-\bar{d}^{(1)}(1,3)\right)^2 + \sum_{i=1}^{n_6}\left(d_i^{(6)}(1,3)-\bar{d}^{(6)}(1,3)\right)^2\right]/(n_1+n_6-2),$$

$$\hat{\sigma}^2_{AC}(1,3) = \left[\sum_{i=1}^{n_2}\left(d_i^{(2)}(1,3)-\bar{d}^{(2)}(1,3)\right)^2 + \sum_{i=1}^{n_4}\left(d_i^{(4)}(1,3)-\bar{d}^{(4)}(1,3)\right)^2\right]/(n_2+n_4-2), \text{ and}$$

$$\hat{\sigma}^2_{BA}(1,3) = \left[\sum_{i=1}^{n_3}\left(d_i^{(3)}(1,3)-\bar{d}^{(3)}(1,3)\right)^2 + \sum_{i=1}^{n_5}\left(d_i^{(5)}(1,3)-\bar{d}^{(5)}(1,3)\right)^2\right]/(n_3+n_5-2).$$

Thus, we can estimate $Var\left(\hat{\gamma}_2^{(WL)}\right)$ by the unbiased variance estimator $\widehat{Var}\left(\hat{\gamma}_2^{(WL)}\right) =$

$\left(a_1^*\hat{\sigma}^2_{BC}(1,3) + a_2^*\hat{\sigma}^2_{AC}(1,3) + a_3^*\hat{\sigma}^2_{BA}(1,3)\right)$, where $a_k^* = WP_k^*/\left[4\left(\sum_{k=1}^{3}WP_k^*\right)^2\right]$, $k =$

1, 2, 3. When testing $H_0 : \gamma_2 = 0$, we will reject $H_0 : \gamma_2 = 0$ at the α-level if

$|\hat{\gamma}_2^{(WL)}|/\sqrt{\widehat{Var}\left(\hat{\gamma}_2^{(WL)}\right)} > t_{\alpha/2,df^{**}}$, where the degrees of freedom df^{**} are calculated as

the closest integer to $\left[a_1^*\hat{\sigma}^2_{BC}(1,3) + a_2^*\hat{\sigma}^2_{AC}(1,3) + a_3^*\hat{\sigma}^2_{BA}(1,3)\right]^2/\left[\left(a_1^*\right)^2\hat{\sigma}^4_{BC}(1,3)/(n_1+$

$n_6-2) + \left(a_2^*\right)^2\hat{\sigma}^4_{AC}(1,3)/(n_2+n_4-2) + \left(a_3^*\right)^2\hat{\sigma}^4_{BA}(1,3)/(n_3+n_5-2)\right]$.

Problem 6.14. Under model (6.36), show that the expectations given in (6.37) hold.

Problem 6.15. Show that under $H_0 : \lambda_{11} = \lambda_{12} = 0$, the test statistic
$4\left[\sum_{k=1}^{3}W_k(\hat{\eta}_{ACk})^2 - \left(\sum_{k=1}^{3}W_k\hat{\eta}_{ACk}\right)^2/\left(\sum_{i=1}^{3}W_k\right)\right]/\sigma^2_{AC}$ follows the central
χ^2-distribution with 2 degrees of freedom. (Hint: See Graybill, 1976, p. 135. Note
that the random vector $\hat{\underline{\eta}}_{AC} = [\hat{\eta}_{AC1}\ \hat{\eta}_{AC2}\ \hat{\eta}_{AC3}]'$ follows the trivariate normal distribution with mean vector $\underline{\eta}_{AC} = [E(\hat{\eta}_{AC1})\ E(\hat{\eta}_{AC2})\ E(\hat{\eta}_{AC3})]'$ and covariance

matrix $\ \underline{\underline{\Sigma}} = \begin{bmatrix} \dfrac{\sigma^2_{AC}}{4W_1} & 0 & 0 \\ 0 & \dfrac{\sigma^2_{AC}}{4W_2} & 0 \\ 0 & 0 & \dfrac{\sigma^2_{AC}}{4W_3} \end{bmatrix}$. Define $\ \underline{\underline{A}} = \begin{bmatrix} W_1 & 0 & 0 \\ 0 & W_2 & 0 \\ 0 & 0 & W_3 \end{bmatrix} - \dfrac{1}{\sum_{k=1}^{3}W_k}\begin{bmatrix} W_1 \\ W_2 \\ W_3 \end{bmatrix}$

$[W_1\ W_2\ W_3]$. We can show that $4\left[\sum_{k=1}^{3}W_k(\hat{\eta}_{ACk})^2 - \left(\sum_{k=1}^{3}W_k\hat{\eta}_{ACk}\right)^2/\right.$

$\left.\left(\sum_{i=1}^{3}W_k\right)\right]/\sigma^2_{AC} = \hat{\underline{\eta}}'_{AC}\left(4\underline{\underline{A}}/\sigma^2_{AC}\right)\hat{\underline{\eta}}_{AC}$. Prove that $\underline{\underline{\Sigma A}}\left(4/\sigma^2_{AC}\right)$ is an idempotent

matrix with rank of two.)

Problem 6.16. Show that the expectations given in (6.39) hold under model (6.36).

Problem 6.17. Show that the expectations of $\hat{\eta}_{BAk}$ (for $k = 1, 2, 3$) in (6.41) hold
under model (6.36).

Problem 6.18. Suppose that there are four treatments, including three experimental
treatments A, B, and C, as well as one control treatment or placebo D, under

comparison. If we employ the four-treatment four-period crossover design with the complete set of treatment-receipt sequences, there will be 24 (=4!) groups with different treatment-receipt sequences. This number of groups can be too large to be of use in practice. Thus, we may consider employing a Latin square to reduce the number of groups with different treatment-receipt sequences. Suppose that we choose to employ one of the Latin squares [in group I, e.g., (I, 3) on p. 163 by Senn (2002)] and randomly assign n_g patients to group g = 1 with A-C-B-D treatment-receipt sequence; = 2 with B-D-A-C treatment-receipt sequence; = 3 with C-A-D-B treatment receipt sequence; and = 4 with D-B-C-A treatment-receipt sequence. For patient i (=1, 2, $\cdots$, n_g) assigned to group g (=1, 2, 3, 4), let $Y_{iz}^{(g)}$ denote the patient response at period z (=1, 2, 3, 4). We assume that the patient response $Y_{iz}^{(g)}$ on patient i (=1, 2, $\cdots$, n_g) assigned to group g (=1, 2, 3, 4) at period z (=1, 2, 3, 4) corresponds to the following random effects linear additive risk model:

$$Y_{iz}^{(g)} = \mu_i^{(g)} + \eta_{AD}X_{iz1}^{(g)} + \eta_{BD}X_{iz2}^{(g)} + \eta_{CD}X_{iz3}^{(g)} + \gamma_1 Z_{iz1}^{(g)} + \gamma_2 Z_{iz2}^{(g)} + \gamma_3 Z_{iz3}^{(g)}$$
$$+ \varepsilon_{izA}^{(g)}X_{iz1}^{(g)} + \varepsilon_{izB}^{(g)}X_{iz2}^{(g)} + \varepsilon_{izC}^{(g)}X_{iz3}^{(g)} + \varepsilon_{izD}^{(g)}\left(1 - X_{iz1}^{(g)}\right)\left(1 - X_{iz2}^{(g)}\right)\left(1 - X_{iz3}^{(g)}\right),$$

where $X_{iz1}^{(g)}$, $X_{iz2}^{(g)}$, and $X_{iz3}^{(g)}$ denote the indicator functions of treatment-receipt for treatments A, B, and C and = 1 if the patient in group g at period z receives the corresponding treatment, and = 0 otherwise; $Z_{iz1}^{(g)}$, $Z_{iz2}^{(g)}$, and $Z_{iz3}^{(g)}$ denote the indicator functions of periods 2, 3, and 4 by setting $Z_{iz1}^{(g)} = 1$ for period $z = 2$, and = 0 otherwise; $Z_{iz2}^{(g)} = 1$ for period $z = 3$, and = 0 otherwise; and $Z_{iz3}^{(g)} = 1$ for period $z = 4$, and = 0 otherwise; $\mu_i^{(g)}$ represents the random effect due to the underlying characteristics of the ith patient assigned to group g, and all $\mu_i^{(g)}$'s are assumed to independently follow an unspecified probability density function $f_g(\mu)$ with variance σ_μ^2; η_{AD}, η_{BD}, and η_{CD} denote the respective effect of treatments A, B, and C relative to treatment (or placebo) D; γ_1, γ_2, and γ_3 denote the respective effect for periods 2, 3, and 4 versus period 1; and random errors $\varepsilon_{izT}^{(g)}$'s (for T = A, B, C, and D) are assumed to be independent and distributed as a normal distribution with mean 0 and variance σ_{eT}^2 and independent of $\mu_i^{(g)}$'s. Using similar ideas as those presented here, discuss how to obtain unbiased estimators for the relative treatment effects η_{AD}, η_{BD}, and η_{CD} based on the WLS method and derive their respective variance estimators. (Hint: For any pair of treatments in a given treatment-receipt sequence under comparison, we can find another treatment-receipt sequence in which these two treatments appear in the reverse order of the same pair of periods. This provides a clue about how to form strata in derivation of the WLS estimator. For example, suppose that we want to estimate η_{AD}. We can easily see that both $\left[\left(\bar{Y}_{+4}^{(4)} - \bar{Y}_{+1}^{(4)}\right) - \left(\bar{Y}_{+4}^{(1)} - \bar{Y}_{+1}^{(1)}\right)\right]/2$ and $\left[\left(\bar{Y}_{+3}^{(2)} - \bar{Y}_{+2}^{(2)}\right) - \left(\bar{Y}_{+3}^{(3)} - \bar{Y}_{+2}^{(3)}\right)\right]/2$ are unbiased estimators of η_{AD}. Therefore, we can obtain the WLS estimator for η_{AD} based on these two estimators. Similarly, we can obtain the WLS unbiased estimators for η_{BD} and η_{CD} and the difference between these parameters.)

7

Three-treatment three-period crossover design in dichotomous data

It is desirable to reduce in an RCT the number of patients receiving an inert placebo, especially when there is a treatment known to be effective for a disease. To make the best of the information on patients receiving a placebo, it can be appealing to compare more than one experimental treatment with a placebo in a single trial instead of several trials, each having its own placebo arm. In a gold standard trial, by definition, there are three treatment arms: a new treatment, a standard treatment, and a placebo. In a dose-finding trial, we may want to compare the patient responses at a minimum of two different doses with those of patients receiving a placebo for detecting a nonlinear dose response curve (Senn, 2002).

In this chapter, we focus discussions on comparing two experimental treatments with a placebo (or an active control treatment) in a three-period crossover trial with dichotomous responses. For example, consider the data in Table 7.1 taken from a three-period crossover trial comparing two different doses of analgesic with a placebo for the relief of primary dysmenorrhea (Jones and Kenward, 1987). Patients were randomly assigned to one of the six groups with different treatment-receipt sequences. At the end of each of the three treatment periods, each patient rated the treatment as giving either no relief (coded as 0) or some relief (coded as 1). Thus, each patient could have exactly one of the eight response patterns: $(1, 1, 1)$, $(1, 1, 0)$, $\cdots$, $(0, 0, 0)$. For example, the pattern $(1, 1, 1)$ represents that the patient has the relief of pain at all three periods, while the pattern $(1, 1, 0)$ represents that the patient has relief at the first two periods and no relief at the third period.

Crossover Designs: Testing, Estimation, and Sample Size, First Edition. Kung-Jong Lui.
© 2016 John Wiley & Sons, Ltd. Published 2016 by John Wiley & Sons, Ltd.
Companion website: www.wiley.com/go/lui/crossover

Table 7.1 Frequency of patients with response vector ($Y_{i1}^{(g)} = r$, $Y_{i2}^{(g)} = s$, $Y_{i3}^{(g)} = t$), where r, s, and $t = 1$ for relief, $= 0$ otherwise, at the three periods in group g ($= 1, 2, 3, 4, 5, 6$) determined by different treatment-receipt sequences.

Response vector ($Y_{i1}^{(g)} = r$, $Y_{i2}^{(g)} = s$, $Y_{i3}^{(g)} = t$)								
	(1, 1, 1)	(1, 1, 0)	(1, 0, 1)	(0, 1, 1)	(1, 0, 0)	(0, 1, 0)	(0, 0, 1)	(0, 0, 0)
C-A-B (g = 1)	1	1	0	9	0	2	2	0
C-B-A (g = 2)	4	0	0	9	1	0	0	2
A-C-B (g = 3)	1	0	8	3	1	1	1	0
A-B-C (g = 4)	1	8	0	0	1	1	1	0
B-C-A (g = 5)	1	1	7	2	0	0	0	3
B-A-C (g = 6)	0	4	3	1	5	0	0	1

A, lower dose of the analgesic; B, higher dose of the analgesic; C, placebo.

Under a random effects logistic regression model, we provide asymptotic and exact procedures for testing non-equality of treatments (Lui, Cumberland, and Chang, 2014). We further provide procedures for testing non-inferiority and equivalence between either of two experimental treatments and an active control treatment with respect to the OR of patient responses (Garrett, 2003). We address interval estimation of the OR of patient responses between treatments. We discuss hypothesis testing and estimation for period effects. We show that one can simply apply the commonly used WLS procedure for testing the homogeneity of OR (Fleiss, 1981) to study whether there are treatment-by-period interactions. When assuming random effects to independently follow a normal distribution, we present SAS codes of PROC GLIMMIX (SAS Institute, 2009) using the marginal-likelihood approach and compare the results with those obtained by use of the conditional method focused on here. We also discuss in exercises the use of a Latin square to reduce the number of groups with different treatment-receipt sequences. This is of use especially when there are four or more treatments under comparison in a crossover design.

Suppose that we compare two experimental treatments A and B with treatment C (that can be a placebo or an active control treatment) in a three-period crossover design. For brevity, we use U-V-W to denote the treatment-receipt sequence that a patient receives treatments U, V, and W at periods 1, 2, and 3, respectively. Suppose that we randomly assign n_g patients to group $g = 1$ with C-A-B treatment-receipt sequence; $= 2$ with C-B-A treatment-receipt sequence; $= 3$ with A-C-B treatment-receipt sequence; $= 4$ with A-B-C treatment-receipt sequence; $= 5$ with B-C-A treatment-receipt sequence; and $= 6$ with B-A-C treatment-receipt sequence. Given an adequate washout period, we assume that there is no carry-over effect due to the treatment administered at an earlier period on the patient response. For patient $i (= 1, 2, \cdots, n_g)$ assigned to group $g (= 1, 2, 3, 4, 5, 6)$, let $Y_{iz}^{(g)}$ denote the binary outcome at period $z (= 1, 2, 3)$, and $Y_{iz}^{(g)} = 1$ for a positive response, and $= 0$ otherwise. Let $X_{iz1}^{(g)}$ denote the indicator function of treatment-receipt for treatment A, and $X_{iz1}^{(g)} = 1$ if patient i in group g at period z receives treatment A, and $= 0$ otherwise. Similarly, let $X_{iz2}^{(g)}$ denote the indicator function of treatment-receipt for treatment B, and $X_{iz2}^{(g)} = 1$ if patient i in group g at period z receives treatment B, and $= 0$ otherwise. We further let $Z_{iz1}^{(g)}$ and $Z_{iz2}^{(g)}$ represent the indicator functions of the period covariate, defining $Z_{iz1}^{(g)} = 1$ for period $z = 2$, and $= 0$ otherwise; as well as $Z_{iz2}^{(g)} = 1$ for period $z = 3$, and $= 0$ otherwise. We assume that the probability of a positive response for patient i in group g at period z is given by the following random effects logistic regression model:

$$
P\left(Y_{iz}^{(g)} = 1 | X_{iz1}^{(g)}, X_{iz2}^{(g)}, Z_{iz1}^{(g)}, Z_{iz2}^{(g)}\right)
$$
$$
= \frac{\exp\left(\mu_i^{(g)} + \eta_{AC} X_{iz1}^{(g)} + \eta_{BC} X_{iz2}^{(g)} + \gamma_1 Z_{iz1}^{(g)} + \gamma_2 Z_{iz2}^{(g)}\right)}{1 + \exp\left(\mu_i^{(g)} + \eta_{AC} X_{iz1}^{(g)} + \eta_{BC} X_{iz2}^{(g)} + \gamma_1 Z_{iz1}^{(g)} + \gamma_2 Z_{iz2}^{(g)}\right)}, \tag{7.1}
$$

where $\mu_i^{(g)}$ denotes the random effect due to the ith patient in group g, and all $\mu_i^{(g)}$'s are assumed to independently follow an unspecified probability density function $f_g(\mu)$; η_{AC} and η_{BC} denote the respective effects of treatments A and B relative to treatment C; and γ_1 and γ_2 represent the respective effects of periods 2 and 3 versus period 1. Under model (7.1), the OR of a positive response for a fixed period on a given patient between treatments A and C is equal to $\varphi_{AC} = \exp(\eta_{AC})$. Similarly, the OR of a positive response for a fixed period on a given patient between treatments B and C is given by $\varphi_{BC} = \exp(\eta_{BC})$. Thus, the OR of a positive response for a fixed period on a given patient between treatments B and A is, by definition, equal to $\varphi_{BA} = \exp(\eta_{BC} - \eta_{AC})$. Note that we do not assume $\mu_i^{(g)}$ here to follow any specified parametric distribution, such as a normal distribution, and hence our approach is semiparametric. Let $n_{rst}^{(g)}$ denote in group g (= 1, 2, 3, 4, 5, 6) the number of patients among n_g patients with response vector $(Y_{i1}^{(g)} = r, Y_{i2}^{(g)} = s, Y_{i3}^{(g)} = t)$, where $r = 1, 0, s = 1, 0, t = 1, 0$. The random frequencies $\{n_{rst}^{(g)} \mid r = 1, 0, s = 1, 0, \text{ and } t = 1, 0\}$ then follow the multinomial distribution with parameters n_g and $\{\pi_{rst}^{(g)} \mid r = 1, 0, s = 1, 0, t = 1, 0\}$, where $\pi_{rst}^{(g)}$ denotes the cell probability that a randomly selected patient i from group g has the response vector $(Y_{i1}^{(g)} = r, Y_{i2}^{(g)} = s, Y_{i3}^{(g)} = t)$ over three periods. For example, the parameter $\pi_{101}^{(g)}$ denotes the cell probability that a randomly selected patient from group g has a positive response at period 1, a negative response at period 2, and a positive response at period 3. For brevity, let "+" denote the summation over that subscript in the following discussion. For example, the parameter $\pi_{01+}^{(g)}$ denotes in group g the probability of a randomly selected patient with a negative response at period 1 and a positive response at period 2 and is equal to $\pi_{01+}^{(g)} = \pi_{011}^{(g)} + \pi_{010}^{(g)}$. We can express the OR (= φ_{AC}) of a positive response between treatments A and C under model (7.1) as (Problem 7.1)

$$\varphi_{AC} = \left[\left(\pi_{01+}^{(1)} \pi_{10+}^{(3)} \right) / \left(\pi_{10+}^{(1)} \pi_{01+}^{(3)} \right) \right]^{1/2}$$
$$= \left[\left(\pi_{0+1}^{(2)} \pi_{1+0}^{(4)} \right) / \left(\pi_{1+0}^{(2)} \pi_{0+1}^{(4)} \right) \right]^{1/2} \tag{7.2}$$
$$= \left[\left(\pi_{+01}^{(5)} \pi_{+10}^{(6)} \right) / \left(\pi_{+10}^{(5)} \pi_{+01}^{(6)} \right) \right]^{1/2},$$

regardless of the probability density function for $f_g(\mu)$. Similarly, we can show that the OR of a positive response between treatments B and C under model (7.1) is (Problem 7.2)

$$\varphi_{BC} = \left[\left(\pi_{0+1}^{(1)} \pi_{1+0}^{(6)} \right) / \left(\pi_{1+0}^{(1)} \pi_{0+1}^{(6)} \right) \right]^{1/2}$$
$$= \left[\left(\pi_{01+}^{(2)} \pi_{10+}^{(5)} \right) / \left(\pi_{10+}^{(2)} \pi_{01+}^{(5)} \right) \right]^{1/2} \tag{7.3}$$
$$= \left[\left(\pi_{+01}^{(3)} \pi_{+10}^{(4)} \right) / \left(\pi_{+10}^{(3)} \pi_{+01}^{(4)} \right) \right]^{1/2}.$$

Also, the OR of a positive response between treatments B and A under model (7.1) is (Problem 7.3)

$$
\begin{aligned}
\varphi_{BA}\left(=\exp(\eta_{BC}-\eta_{AC})\right) &= \left[\left(\pi_{+01}^{(1)}\pi_{+10}^{(2)}\right)/\left(\pi_{+10}^{(1)}\pi_{+01}^{(2)}\right)\right]^{1/2} \\
&= \left[\left(\pi_{0+1}^{(3)}\pi_{1+0}^{(5)}\right)/\left(\pi_{1+0}^{(3)}\pi_{0+1}^{(5)}\right)\right]^{1/2} \qquad (7.4) \\
&= \left[\left(\pi_{01+}^{(4)}\pi_{10+}^{(6)}\right)/\left(\pi_{10+}^{(4)}\pi_{01+}^{(6)}\right)\right]^{1/2}.
\end{aligned}
$$

Note that we can estimate $\pi_{rst}^{(g)}$ by the unbiased consistent sample proportion estimator $\hat{\pi}_{rst}^{(g)} = n_{rst}^{(g)}/n_g$. From these, we can obtain unbiased consistent estimators for the marginal probabilities: $\hat{\pi}_{rs+}^{(g)} = \hat{\pi}_{rs1}^{(g)} + \hat{\pi}_{rs0}^{(g)}$, $\hat{\pi}_{r+t}^{(g)} = \hat{\pi}_{r1t}^{(g)} + \hat{\pi}_{r0t}^{(g)}$, and $\hat{\pi}_{+st}^{(g)} = \hat{\pi}_{1st}^{(g)} + \hat{\pi}_{0st}^{(g)}$.

For convenience, we define $(f_{11k}, f_{12k}, f_{21k}, f_{22k})$ (for $k = 1, 2, 3$) as the vector of random cell frequencies for the three 2×2 tables corresponding to equations in (7.2), each table k ($= 1, 2, 3$) consisting of frequency f_{ijk} in cell (i, j) (for $i, j = 1, 2$) defined as

$$
\begin{aligned}
&\left(f_{111} = n_{01+}^{(1)}, f_{121} = n_{01+}^{(3)}, f_{211} = n_{10+}^{(1)}, f_{221} = n_{10+}^{(3)}\right), \\
&\left(f_{112} = n_{0+1}^{(2)}, f_{122} = n_{0+1}^{(4)}, f_{212} = n_{1+0}^{(2)}, f_{222} = n_{1+0}^{(4)}\right), \text{ and} \qquad (7.5) \\
&\left(f_{113} = n_{+01}^{(5)}, f_{123} = n_{+01}^{(6)}, f_{213} = n_{+10}^{(5)}, f_{223} = n_{+10}^{(6)}\right).
\end{aligned}
$$

On the basis of (7.2) and (7.5), we may obtain the WLS estimator for φ_{AC} as given by (Fleiss, 1981)

$$
\hat{\varphi}_{AC}^{(WLS)} = \sum_k W_k \left(\widehat{OR}_k\right)^{1/2} / \sum_k W_k, \qquad (7.6)
$$

where $\widehat{OR}_k = (f_{11k}f_{22k})/(f_{12k}f_{21k})$, and $W_k = 1/\widehat{Var}\left(\log\left(\widehat{OR}_k\right)\right) = [1/f_{11k} + 1/f_{12k} + 1/f_{21k} + 1/f_{22k}]^{-1}$.

Similarly, we define $\left(f_{11k}^*, f_{12k}^*, f_{21k}^*, f_{22k}^*\right)$ (for $k = 1, 2, 3$) as the vector of random cell frequencies for the three 2×2 tables corresponding to equations in (7.3), each table k ($= 1, 2, 3$) consisting of frequency f_{ijk}^* in cell (i, j) (for $i, j = 1, 2$) defined as

$$
\begin{aligned}
&\left(f_{111}^* = n_{0+1}^{(1)}, f_{121}^* = n_{0+1}^{(6)}, f_{211}^* = n_{1+0}^{(1)}, f_{221}^* = n_{1+0}^{(6)}\right), \\
&\left(f_{112}^* = n_{01+}^{(2)}, f_{122}^* = n_{01+}^{(5)}, f_{212}^* = n_{10+}^{(2)}, f_{222}^* = n_{10+}^{(5)}\right), \text{ and} \qquad (7.7) \\
&\left(f_{113}^* = n_{+01}^{(3)}, f_{123}^* = n_{+01}^{(4)}, f_{213}^* = n_{+10}^{(3)}, f_{223}^* = n_{+10}^{(4)}\right).
\end{aligned}
$$

On the basis of (7.3) and (7.7), we may obtain the WLS estimator for φ_{BC} as

$$\hat{\varphi}_{BC}^{(WLS)} = \sum_k W_k^* \left(\widehat{OR}_k^*\right)^{1/2} / \sum_k W_k^*, \tag{7.8}$$

where $\widehat{OR}_k^* = \left(f_{11k}^* f_{22k}^*\right)/\left(f_{12k}^* f_{21k}^*\right)$, and $W_k^* = 1/\widehat{Var}\left(\log\left(\widehat{OR}_k^*\right)\right) = \left[1/f_{11k}^* + 1/f_{12k}^* + 1/f_{21k}^* + 1/f_{22k}^*\right]^{-1}$.

Similarly, we define $\left(f_{11k}^{**}, f_{12k}^{**}, f_{21k}^{**}, f_{22k}^{**}\right)$ (for $k = 1, 2, 3$) as the vector of random cell frequencies for the three 2×2 tables corresponding to equations in (7.4), each table k ($= 1, 2, 3$) consisting of frequency f_{ijk}^{**} in cell (i, j) (for $i, j = 1, 2$) defined as

$$\left(f_{111}^{**} = n_{+01}^{(1)}, f_{121}^{**} = n_{+01}^{(2)}, f_{211}^{**} = n_{+10}^{(1)}, f_{221}^{**} = n_{+10}^{(2)}\right),$$

$$\left(f_{112}^{**} = n_{0+1}^{(3)}, f_{122}^{**} = n_{0+1}^{(5)}, f_{212}^{**} = n_{1+0}^{(3)}, f_{222}^{**} = n_{1+0}^{(5)}\right), \text{ and} \tag{7.9}$$

$$\left(f_{113}^{**} = n_{01+}^{(4)}, f_{123}^{**} = n_{01+}^{(6)}, f_{213}^{**} = n_{10+}^{(4)}, f_{223}^{**} = n_{10+}^{(6)}\right).$$

On the basis of (7.4) and (7.9), we may obtain the WLS estimator for φ_{BA} as

$$\hat{\varphi}_{BA}^{(WLS)} = \sum_k W_k^{**} \left(\widehat{OR}_k^{**}\right)^{1/2} / \sum_k W_k^{**}, \tag{7.10}$$

where $\widehat{OR}_k^{**} = \left(f_{11k}^{**} f_{22k}^{**}\right)/\left(f_{12k}^{**} f_{21k}^{**}\right)$, and $W_k^{**} = \widehat{Var}\left(\log\left(\widehat{OR}_k^{**}\right)\right)^{-1} = \left[1/f_{11k}^{**} + 1/f_{12k}^{**} + 1/f_{21k}^{**} + 1/f_{22k}^{**}\right]^{-1}$.

Note that the conditional probability distribution of f_{11k}, given $f_{+1k}, f_{+2k}, f_{1+k}$, and f_{2+k} fixed, in table k ($= 1, 2, 3$) is given by

$$P\left(f_{11k} | f_{+1k}, f_{+2k}, f_{1+k}, f_{2+k}, \varphi_{AC}^2\right) = \frac{\binom{f_{+1k}}{f_{11k}}\binom{f_{+2k}}{f_{1+k}-f_{11k}}(\varphi_{AC}^2)^{f_{11k}}}{\sum_{x_k}\binom{f_{+1k}}{x_k}\binom{f_{+2k}}{f_{1+k}-x_k}(\varphi_{AC}^2)^{x_k}}, \tag{7.11}$$

where the summation of x_k in the denominator is calculated over $a_k \le x_k \le b_k$, $a_k = \max\{0, f_{1+k} - f_{+2k}\}$, and $b_k = \min\{f_{+1k}, f_{1+k}\}$ for $k = 1, 2, 3$. Thus, the joint conditional probability mass function of the random vector $f_{-11} = (f_{111}, f_{112}, f_{113})'$ is given by

$$P\left(f_{111}, f_{112}, f_{113} | f_{-+1}, f_{-+2}, f_{1+}, f_{2+}, \varphi_{AC}^2\right) = \prod_{k=1}^3 \frac{\binom{f_{+1k}}{f_{11k}}\binom{f_{+2k}}{f_{1+k}-f_{11k}}(\varphi_{AC}^2)^{f_{11k}}}{\sum_{x_k}\binom{f_{+1k}}{x_k}\binom{f_{+2k}}{f_{1+k}-x_k}(\varphi_{AC}^2)^{x_k}}, \tag{7.12}$$

where $f_{-w+} = (f_{w+1}, f_{w+2}, f_{w+3})'$ for $w = 1, 2$, and $f_{-+v} = (f_{+v1}, f_{+v2}, f_{+v3})'$ for $v = 1, 2$. The probability mass function for a specified value f_{11+}^0 $(= f_{111}^0 + f_{112}^0 + f_{113}^0)$ based on (7.12) is then given by

$$P\left(f_{11+} = f_{11+}^0 \mid f_{-+1}, f_{-+2}, f_{-1+}, f_{-2+}, \varphi_{AC}^2\right)$$

$$= \sum_{f_{-11} \in C(f_{11+}^0)} \prod_{k=1}^{3} \frac{\binom{f_{+1k}}{f_{11k}} \binom{f_{+2k}}{f_{1+k} - f_{11k}} (\varphi_{AC}^2)^{f_{11k}}}{\sum_{x_k} \binom{f_{+1k}}{x_k} \binom{f_{+2k}}{f_{1+k} - x_k} (\varphi_{AC}^2)^{x_k}}, \tag{7.13}$$

where $C(f_{11+}^0) = \{(f_{111}, f_{112}, f_{113})' \mid f_{111} + f_{112} + f_{113} = f_{11+}^0, a_k \leq f_{11k} \leq b_k, k = 1, 2, 3\}$. Following the same arguments as those for deriving (7.11)–(7.13), we can derive the conditional probability mass function for f_{11+}^* (or f_{11+}^{**}) as given by (7.13) by replacing f_{ijk} with f_{ijk}^* (or f_{ijk}^{**}) and φ_{AC} with φ_{BC} (or φ_{BA}), respectively.

7.1 Testing non-equality of treatments

From equation (7.2), we can see that φ_{AC} represents the square root of the underlying common OR across the three 2×2 tables with cell frequencies $(f_{11k}, f_{12k}, f_{21k}, f_{22k})$ for $k = 1, 2, 3$. We can further see that $\varphi_{AC} = 1$ (i.e., $\eta_{AC} = 0$) if and only if the underlying common OR across these three 2×2 tables equals 1. Similarly, from equations (7.3) and (7.4), we can see that φ_{BC} and φ_{BA} also represent the square root of the underlying common OR across the three 2×2 tables with cell frequencies $\left(f_{11k}^*, f_{12k}^*, f_{21k}^*, f_{22k}^*\right)$ and $\left(f_{11k}^{**}, f_{12k}^{**}, f_{21k}^{**}, f_{22k}^{**}\right)$, respectively. Furthermore, note that $\varphi_{BC} = 1$ (or $\varphi_{BA} = 1$) if and only if the underlying common OR for the corresponding three 2×2 tables equals 1. Thus, we can apply all the summary test procedures and interval estimators for a series of 2×2 tables discussed elsewhere (Fleiss, 1981; Agresti, 1990; Lui, 2004) to do hypothesis testing and interval estimation when studying parameters φ_{AC}, φ_{BC}, or φ_{BA}.

7.1.1 Asymptotic test procedures

Suppose that we want to find out whether there is a difference in effects between treatments A and C. Consider first the WLS test procedure based on $\widehat{OR}_k$ with the logarithmic transformation to test $H_0 : \varphi_{AC} = 1$ versus $H_a : \varphi_{AC} \neq 1$. We will reject $H_0 :$ $\varphi_{AC} = 1$ at the α-level if the following test statistic (Lui, Cumberland, and Chang, 2014)

$$\left(\hat{\eta}_{AC}^{(WLS)}\right)^2 / \widehat{Var}\left(\hat{\eta}_{AC}^{(WLS)}\right) > \chi_\alpha^2(1), \tag{7.14}$$

where $\hat{\eta}_{AC}^{(WLS)} = \sum_k W_k \log\left(\left(\widehat{OR}_k\right)^{1/2}\right)/\sum_k W_k$, $\widehat{OR}_k = (f_{11k}f_{22k})/(f_{12k}f_{21k})$, $W_k = [1/f_{11k} + 1/f_{12k} + 1/f_{21k} + 1/f_{22k}]^{-1}$, $\widehat{Var}\left(\hat{\eta}_{AC}^{(WLS)}\right) = 1/\left(4\sum_k W_k\right)$, and $\chi_\alpha^2(df)$ is the upper $100(\alpha)$th percentile of the central χ^2-distribution with df degree(s) of freedom. Note that if some f_{ijk} equals 0 for any $k (= 1, 2, 3)$, the test statistic (7.14) is undefined. If this should occur, we can apply the ad hoc adjustment procedure for sparse data by adding 0.50 to each cell frequency f_{ijk} in table k when calculating (7.14). To alleviate the concern of using this arbitrary adjustment procedure for sparse data, we can also use the Mantel–Haenszel (MH) summary test procedure (Robins, Breslow, and Greenland, 1986; Agresti, 1990). We will reject $H_0 : \varphi_{AC} = 1$ at the α-level if the following MH test statistic

$$\left(\sum_k f_{11k} - \sum_k f_{1+k}f_{+1k}/f_{++k}\right)^2 / \left\{\sum_k f_{1+k}f_{2+k}f_{+1k}f_{+2k}/\left[f_{++k}^2(f_{++k}-1)\right]\right\} > \chi_\alpha^2(1). \tag{7.15}$$

Similarly, when testing $H_0 : \varphi_{BC} = 1$, we may employ the WLS test procedure based on $\widehat{OR}_k^*$ with the logarithmic transformation. We will reject $H_0 : \varphi_{BC} = 1$ at the α-level if the test statistic

$$\left(\hat{\eta}_{BC}^{(WLS)}\right)^2 / \widehat{Var}\left(\hat{\eta}_{BC}^{(WLS)}\right) > \chi_\alpha^2(1), \tag{7.16}$$

where $\hat{\eta}_{BC}^{(WLS)} = \sum_k W_k^* \log\left(\left(\widehat{OR}_k^*\right)^{1/2}\right)/\sum_k W_k^*$, $\widehat{OR}_k^* = (f_{11k}^* f_{22k}^*)/(f_{12k}^* f_{21k}^*)$, $W_k^* = [1/f_{11k}^* + 1/f_{12k}^* + 1/f_{21k}^* + 1/f_{22k}^*]^{-1}$, and $\widehat{Var}\left(\hat{\eta}_{BC}^{(WLS)}\right) = 1/\left(4\sum_k W_k^*\right)$.

To alleviate the concern of obtaining $f_{ijk}^* = 0$ for some cells in use of (7.16) based on the WLS method, we may apply the arbitrary adjustment procedure for sparse data as described previously or use the following MH summary test procedure to test $H_0 : \varphi_{BC} = 1$. We will reject $H_0 : \varphi_{BC} = 1$ at the α-level if the test statistic

$$\left(\sum_k f_{11k}^* - \sum_k f_{1+k}^* f_{+1k}^*/f_{++k}^*\right)^2 / \left\{\sum_k f_{1+k}^* f_{2+k}^* f_{+1k}^* f_{+2k}^*/\left[\left(f_{++k}^*\right)^2\left(f_{++k}^*-1\right)\right]\right\} > \chi_\alpha^2(1). \tag{7.17}$$

Also, when evaluating whether the effects between treatments A and B are equal (i.e., $\eta_{BC} = \eta_{AC}$), we can apply the WLS summary test procedure based on $\widehat{OR}_k^{**}$ with the logarithmic transformation to test $H_0 : \varphi_{BA}(= \exp(\eta_{BC} - \eta_{AC})) = 1$. We will reject $H_0 : \varphi_{BA} = 1$ at the α-level if the following test statistic

$$\left(\hat{\eta}_{BA}^{(WLS)}\right)^2 / \widehat{Var}\left(\hat{\eta}_{BA}^{(WLS)}\right) > \chi_\alpha^2(1), \tag{7.18}$$

where $\hat{\eta}_{BA}^{(WLS)} = \sum_k W_k^{**} \log\left(\left(\widehat{OR}_k^{**}\right)^{1/2}\right) / \sum_k W_k^{**}$, $\widehat{OR}_k^{**} = \left(f_{11k}^{**} f_{22k}^{**}\right) / \left(f_{12k}^{**} f_{21k}^{**}\right)$,

$W_k^{**} = \left[1/f_{11k}^{**} + 1/f_{12k}^{**} + 1/f_{21k}^{**} + 1/f_{22k}^{**}\right]^{-1}$, and $\widehat{Var}\left(\hat{\eta}_{BA}^{(WLS)}\right) = 1/\left(4\sum_k W_k^{**}\right)$.

When using the MH summary test to alleviate the concern of obtaining $f_{ijk}^{**} = 0$ for some cells in use of (7.18), we will reject $H_0 : \varphi_{BA} = 1$ at the α-level if the test statistic

$$\left(\sum_k f_{11k}^{**} - \sum_k f_{1+k}^{**} f_{+1k}^{**} / f_{++k}^{**}\right)^2 / \left\{\sum_k f_{1+k}^{**} f_{2+k}^{**} f_{+1k}^{**} f_{+2k}^{**} / \left[\left(f_{++k}^{**}\right)^2 \left(f_{++k}^{**} - 1\right)\right]\right\} > \chi_\alpha^2(1).$$
(7.19)

Note that the above test procedures (7.14)–(7.19) can be regarded as an extension of the Mainland–Gart asymptotic test (Mainland, 1963; Gart, 1969; Jones and Kenward, 1989) for testing non-equality of two treatments from an AB/BA crossover trial to a three-treatment three-period crossover trial. Note also that the WLS and MH test procedures are both derived from large-sample theory and are appropriate for use if the observed frequencies f_{ijk} (f_{ijk}^* or f_{ijk}^{**}) for all k are reasonably large. If some of these frequencies are small, we may consider using the exact test procedures, which will be discussed in the next section.

Example 7.1   Consider the data in Table 7.1 taken from a three-period crossover trial comparing the low (treatment A) and high (treatment B) doses of analgesic and placebo (treatment C) for the relief (yes = 1, no = 0) of primary dysmenorrhea. A washout period of one month was applied to separate each treatment period (Jones and Kenward, 1987). When employing test procedures (7.14)–(7.17) for testing non-equality of treatments A and C, and testing non-equality of treatments B and C, we find all p-values to be < 0.0001. These suggest that there will be a difference in the relief rates between treatments A and C, as well as a difference in the relief rates between treatments B and C.

7.1.2   Exact test procedures

Note that under $\varphi_{AC} = 1$, the joint conditional probability mass function (7.12) for the random vector $(f_{111}, f_{112}, f_{113})$, given $f_{-u+} = (f_{u+1}, f_{u+2}, f_{u+3})'$ and $f_{-+v} = (f_{+v1}, f_{+v2}, f_{+v3})'$ fixed (for $u, v = 1, 2$), reduces to

$$P\left(f_{111}, f_{112}, f_{113} \Big| f_{-+1}, f_{-+2}, f_{-1+}, f_{-2+}, \varphi_{AC}^2 = 1\right) = \prod_{k=1}^3 \frac{\binom{f_{+1k}}{f_{11k}}\binom{f_{+2k}}{f_{1+k} - f_{11k}}}{\binom{f_{++k}}{f_{1+k}}}, \quad (7.20)$$

where $a_k \le f_{11k} \le b_k$, $a_k = \max\{0, f_{1+k} - f_{+2k}\}$, and $b_k = \min\{f_{+1k}, f_{1+k}\}$ for $k = 1, 2, 3$.

Given an observed value f_{11+}^0, we can calculate the two tail probabilities as

$$P\left(f_{11+} \le f_{11+}^0 \,|\, f_{+1}, f_{+2}, f_{-1+}, f_{-2+}, \varphi_{AC}^2 = 1\right) = \sum_{f_{11+} \le f_{11+}^0} \prod_{k=1}^{3} \frac{\binom{f_{+1k}}{f_{11k}}\binom{f_{+2k}}{f_{1+k} - f_{11k}}}{\binom{f_{++k}}{f_{1+k}}}, \text{and}$$

$$P\left(f_{11+} \ge f_{11+}^0 \,|\, f_{+1}, f_{+2}, f_{-1+}, f_{-2+}, \varphi_{AC}^2 = 1\right) = \sum_{f_{11+} \ge f_{11+}^0} \prod_{k=1}^{3} \frac{\binom{f_{+1k}}{f_{11k}}\binom{f_{+2k}}{f_{1+k} - f_{11k}}}{\binom{f_{++k}}{f_{1+k}}}.$$

$$(7.21)$$

If $\min\left\{P\left(f_{11+} \le f_{11+}^0 \,|\, f_{+1}, f_{+2}, f_{-1+}, f_{-2+}\right), P\left(f_{11+} \ge f_{11+}^0 \,|\, f_{+1}, f_{+2}, f_{-1+}, f_{-2+}\right)\right\} < \alpha/2$,
then we will reject $H_0 : \varphi_{AC} = 1$ at the α-level. Similarly, when testing $H_0 : \varphi_{BC} = 1$ (or $H_0 : \varphi_{BA} = 1$), we can employ the exact test procedure using the two tailed probabilities as calculated in (7.21) by replacing f_{ijk} with f_{ijk}^* (or f_{ijk}^{**}).

Using Monte Carlo simulations, Lui, Cumberland, and Chang (2014) have found that both the WLS and MH test procedures can generally perform well with respect to Type I error in a variety of situations, while the exact test procedure can be conservative when the number of patients per group n $(= n_1 = n_2 = \cdots = n_6)$ is not large (e.g., 30). They have further noted that the MH test procedure can be slightly preferable to the WLS test procedure and the exact test procedure with respect to power when n is moderate. When the number of patients n per group is so small that all asymptotic test procedures are inappropriate, however, the exact test procedure can still be of use.

7.1.3   Procedures for simultaneously testing non-equality of two experimental treatments versus a placebo

We may sometimes wish to find out whether either of the two experimental treatments A or B is different from treatment C (or a placebo). In other words, we want to test $H_0 : \varphi_{AC} = \varphi_{BC} = 1$ versus $H_a : \varphi_{AC} \ne 1$ or $\varphi_{BC} \ne 1$. To test this H_0, the simplest method is to apply the two WLS procedures (7.14) and (7.16) (or the two MH test procedures (7.15) and (7.17)) and use Bonferroni's inequality to adjust the inflation due to multiple tests in Type I error. Thus, we will reject $H_0 : \varphi_{AC} = \varphi_{BC} = 1$ at the α-level, for example, if either of the following two inequalities holds:

$$\left(\hat{\eta}_{AC}^{(WLS)}\right)^2 / \widehat{Var}\left(\hat{\eta}_{AC}^{(WLS)}\right) > \chi_{\alpha/2}^2(1), \text{ or}$$
$$\left(\hat{\eta}_{BC}^{(WLS)}\right)^2 / \widehat{Var}\left(\hat{\eta}_{BC}^{(WLS)}\right) > \chi_{\alpha/2}^2(1).$$

$$(7.22)$$

Note that the two estimators $\hat{\eta}_{AC}^{(WLS)}$ and $\hat{\eta}_{BC}^{(WLS)}$ are correlated. We can show that the estimated asymptotic covariance between $\hat{\eta}_{AC}^{(WLS)}$ and $\hat{\eta}_{BC}^{(WLS)}$ is given by (Problem 7.4)

$$\widehat{Cov}\left(\hat{\eta}_{AC}^{(WLS)}, \hat{\eta}_{BC}^{(WLS)}\right) = \frac{1}{\left[4\left(\sum_{k=1}^{3} W_k\right)\left(\sum_{k=1}^{3} W_k^*\right)\right]}$$

$$\times \left\{ W_1 W_1^* \widehat{Cov}\left(\log\left(\frac{\hat{\pi}_{01+}^{(1)}}{\hat{\pi}_{10+}^{(1)}}\right), \log\left(\frac{\hat{\pi}_{0+1}^{(1)}}{\hat{\pi}_{1+0}^{(1)}}\right)\right) + W_2 W_2^* \widehat{Cov}\left(\log\left(\frac{\hat{\pi}_{0+1}^{(2)}}{\hat{\pi}_{1+0}^{(2)}}\right), \log\left(\frac{\hat{\pi}_{01+}^{(2)}}{\hat{\pi}_{10+}^{(2)}}\right)\right) \right.$$

$$- W_1 W_3^* \widehat{Cov}\left(\log\left(\frac{\hat{\pi}_{01+}^{(3)}}{\hat{\pi}_{10+}^{(3)}}\right), \log\left(\frac{\hat{\pi}_{+01}^{(3)}}{\hat{\pi}_{+10}^{(3)}}\right)\right) + W_2 W_3^* \widehat{Cov}\left(\log\left(\frac{\hat{\pi}_{0+1}^{(4)}}{\hat{\pi}_{1+0}^{(4)}}\right), \log\left(\frac{\hat{\pi}_{+01}^{(4)}}{\hat{\pi}_{+10}^{(4)}}\right)\right)$$

$$\left. - W_3 W_2^* \widehat{Cov}\left(\log\left(\frac{\hat{\pi}_{01+}^{(5)}}{\hat{\pi}_{10+}^{(5)}}\right), \log\left(\frac{\hat{\pi}_{+01}^{(5)}}{\hat{\pi}_{+10}^{(5)}}\right)\right) + W_3 W_1^* \widehat{Cov}\left(\log\left(\frac{\hat{\pi}_{+01}^{(6)}}{\hat{\pi}_{+10}^{(6)}}\right), \log\left(\frac{\hat{\pi}_{0+1}^{(6)}}{\hat{\pi}_{1+0}^{(6)}}\right)\right) \right\},$$

$$(7.23)$$

where

$$\widehat{Cov}\left(\log\left(\frac{\hat{\pi}_{01+}^{(1)}}{\hat{\pi}_{10+}^{(1)}}\right), \log\left(\frac{\hat{\pi}_{0+1}^{(1)}}{\hat{\pi}_{1+0}^{(1)}}\right)\right) = \hat{\pi}_{011}^{(1)} / \left(n_1 \hat{\pi}_{01+}^{(1)} \hat{\pi}_{0+1}^{(1)}\right) + \hat{\pi}_{100}^{(1)} / \left(n_1 \hat{\pi}_{10+}^{(1)} \hat{\pi}_{1+0}^{(1)}\right),$$

$$\widehat{Cov}\left(\log\left(\frac{\hat{\pi}_{0+1}^{(2)}}{\hat{\pi}_{1+0}^{(2)}}\right), \log\left(\frac{\hat{\pi}_{01+}^{(2)}}{\hat{\pi}_{10+}^{(2)}}\right)\right) = \hat{\pi}_{011}^{(2)} / \left(n_2 \hat{\pi}_{01+}^{(2)} \hat{\pi}_{0+1}^{(2)}\right) + \hat{\pi}_{100}^{(2)} / \left(n_2 \hat{\pi}_{10+}^{(2)} \hat{\pi}_{1+0}^{(2)}\right),$$

$$\widehat{Cov}\left(\log\left(\frac{\hat{\pi}_{01+}^{(3)}}{\hat{\pi}_{10+}^{(3)}}\right), \log\left(\frac{\hat{\pi}_{+01}^{(3)}}{\hat{\pi}_{+10}^{(3)}}\right)\right) = -\left(\hat{\pi}_{010}^{(3)} / \left(n_3 \hat{\pi}_{01+}^{(3)} \hat{\pi}_{+10}^{(3)}\right) + \hat{\pi}_{101}^{(3)} / \left(n_3 \hat{\pi}_{10+}^{(3)} \hat{\pi}_{+01}^{(3)}\right)\right),$$

$$\widehat{Cov}\left(\log\left(\frac{\hat{\pi}_{0+1}^{(4)}}{\hat{\pi}_{1+0}^{(4)}}\right), \log\left(\frac{\hat{\pi}_{+01}^{(4)}}{\hat{\pi}_{+10}^{(4)}}\right)\right) = \hat{\pi}_{001}^{(4)} / \left(n_4 \hat{\pi}_{0+1}^{(4)} \hat{\pi}_{+01}^{(4)}\right) + \hat{\pi}_{110}^{(4)} / \left(n_4 \hat{\pi}_{1+0}^{(4)} \hat{\pi}_{+10}^{(4)}\right),$$

$$\widehat{Cov}\left(\log\left(\frac{\hat{\pi}_{01+}^{(5)}}{\hat{\pi}_{10+}^{(5)}}\right), \log\left(\frac{\hat{\pi}_{+01}^{(5)}}{\hat{\pi}_{+10}^{(5)}}\right)\right) = -\left(\hat{\pi}_{010}^{(5)} / \left(n_5 \hat{\pi}_{01+}^{(5)} \hat{\pi}_{+10}^{(5)}\right) + \hat{\pi}_{101}^{(5)} / \left(n_5 \hat{\pi}_{+01}^{(5)} \hat{\pi}_{10+}^{(5)}\right)\right), \text{ and}$$

$$\widehat{Cov}\left(\log\left(\frac{\hat{\pi}_{+01}^{(6)}}{\hat{\pi}_{+10}^{(6)}}\right), \log\left(\frac{\hat{\pi}_{0+1}^{(6)}}{\hat{\pi}_{1+0}^{(6)}}\right)\right) = \hat{\pi}_{001}^{(6)} / \left(n_6 \hat{\pi}_{0+1}^{(6)} \hat{\pi}_{+01}^{(6)}\right) + \hat{\pi}_{110}^{(6)} / \left(n_6 \hat{\pi}_{1+0}^{(6)} \hat{\pi}_{+10}^{(6)}\right).$$

Note that because the test procedure (7.22) does not account for dependence structure between $\hat{\eta}_{AC}^{(WLS)}$ and $\hat{\eta}_{BC}^{(WLS)}$, we may lose power. Thus, we consider the following bivariate test procedure accounting for $\widehat{Cov}\left(\hat{\eta}_{AC}^{(WLS)}, \hat{\eta}_{BC}^{(WLS)}\right)$ (7.23). We will reject $H_0 : \varphi_{AC} = \varphi_{BC} = 1$ at the α-level if

$$\left(\hat{\eta}_{AC}^{(WLS)}, \hat{\eta}_{BC}^{(WLS)}\right) \hat{\underline{\Sigma}}^{-1} \begin{pmatrix} \hat{\eta}_{AC}^{(WLS)} \\ \hat{\eta}_{BC}^{(WLS)} \end{pmatrix} > \chi_\alpha^2(2), \tag{7.24}$$

where $\hat{\underline{\Sigma}}$ is the estimated covariance matrix with diagonal elements equal to $\widehat{Var}\left(\hat{\eta}_{AC}^{(WLS)}\right)$ and $\widehat{Var}\left(\hat{\eta}_{BC}^{(WLS)}\right)$, and off-diagonal element equal to $\widehat{Cov}\left(\hat{\eta}_{AC}^{(WLS)}, \hat{\eta}_{BC}^{(WLS)}\right)$.

When treatments A and B are known to fall in the same relative direction to treatment C, we may wish to account for this information to improve power and consider the following summary test procedure based on a weighted average of treatment effects $w\hat{\eta}_{AC}^{(WLS)} + (1-w)\hat{\eta}_{BC}^{(WLS)}$, where $0 < w < 1$ is the weight reflecting the relative importance of treatment A to treatment B and can be assigned by clinicians based on their subjective knowledge. This leads us to reject $H_0 : \varphi_{AC} = \varphi_{BC} = 1$ at the α-level if

$$\left(w\hat{\eta}_{AC}^{(WLS)} + (1-w)\hat{\eta}_{BC}^{(WLS)}\right)^2 / Var\left(w\hat{\eta}_{AC}^{(WLS)} + (1-w)\hat{\eta}_{BC}^{(WLS)}\right) > \chi_\alpha^2(1), \qquad (7.25)$$

where $\widehat{Var}\left(w\hat{\eta}_{AC}^{(WLS)} + (1-w)\hat{\eta}_{BC}^{(WLS)}\right) = w^2\widehat{Var}\left(\hat{\eta}_{AC}^{(WLS)}\right) + (1-w)^2\widehat{Var}\left(\hat{\eta}_{BC}^{(WLS)}\right) + 2w(1-w)\widehat{Cov}\left(\hat{\eta}_{AC}^{(WLS)}, \hat{\eta}_{BC}^{(WLS)}\right)$. If we have no prior preference to assign the weight w or feel equally important between the two treatments, we may set w equal to 0.50. Note that the optimal weight w_o to minimize the variance $Var\left(w\hat{\eta}_{AC}^{(WLS)} + (1-w)\hat{\eta}_{BC}^{(WLS)}\right)$ can be approximately given by (Problem 7.5)

$$\hat{w}_o = \left(\widehat{Var}\left(\hat{\eta}_{BC}^{(WLS)}\right) - \widehat{Cov}\left(\hat{\eta}_{AC}^{(WLS)}, \hat{\eta}_{BC}^{(WLS)}\right)\right) / \left[\widehat{Var}\left(\hat{\eta}_{AC}^{(WLS)}\right)\right.$$
$$\left. + \widehat{Var}\left(\hat{\eta}_{BC}^{(WLS)}\right) - 2\widehat{Cov}\left(\hat{\eta}_{AC}^{(WLS)}, \hat{\eta}_{BC}^{(WLS)}\right)\right]. \qquad (7.26)$$

When $Var\left(\hat{\eta}_{BC}^{(WLS)}\right) = Var\left(\hat{\eta}_{AC}^{(WLS)}\right)$, the optimal weight w_o simplifies to 0.50.

7.2   Testing non-inferiority of an experimental treatment to an active control treatment

It is not uncommon to encounter a randomized crossover trial in which we cannot have a placebo arm due to the ethical concern. Instead of testing non-equality between experimental treatments and a placebo, we may wish to test whether either experimental treatment A or B is non-inferior to an active control treatment C, especially when the former has fewer side effects and is easier to administer than the latter.

For assessing the non-inferiority of treatments A or B to an active control treatment C with respect to the efficacy, we consider testing $H_0 : \varphi_{AC} \leq \varphi_l$ and $\varphi_{BC} \leq \varphi_l$ (where $0 < \varphi_l < 1$) versus $H_a : \varphi_{AC} > \varphi_l$ or $\varphi_{BC} > \varphi_l$, where φ_l is the maximum clinically acceptable low margin such that treatment A (or treatment B) can be regarded as non-inferior to treatment C when $\varphi_{AC} > \varphi_l$ (or $\varphi_{BC} > \varphi_l$) holds. As noted in the previous chapters, the determination of the non-inferior margin is usually predetermined by clinicians based on their subjective clinical knowledge. Some good discussions on various choices of the non-inferior margins φ_l can be found elsewhere (Garrett, 2003). Note that because log(x) is an increasing function of x over $(0, \infty)$, both $\varphi_{AC} \leq \varphi_l$ and $\varphi_{BC} \leq \varphi_l$ hold if and only if $\eta_{AC} \leq \log(\varphi_l)$ and $\eta_{BC} \leq \log(\varphi_l)$. Thus, using Bonferroni's inequality to adjust the inflation of Type I error due to multiple tests, we will reject $H_0 : \varphi_{AC} \leq \varphi_l$ and $\varphi_{BC} \leq \varphi_l$ at the α-level if either of the following two inequalities holds:

$$
\begin{aligned}
&\left(\hat{\eta}_{AC}^{(WLS)} - \log(\varphi_l) \right) \Big/ \sqrt{\widehat{Var}\left(\hat{\eta}_{AC}^{(WLS)} \right)} > Z_{\alpha/2}, \text{ or} \\
&\left(\hat{\eta}_{BC}^{(WLS)} - \log(\varphi_l) \right) \Big/ \sqrt{\widehat{Var}\left(\hat{\eta}_{BC}^{(WLS)} \right)} > Z_{\alpha/2},
\end{aligned}
\tag{7.27}
$$

where Z_α is the upper $100(\alpha)$th percentile of the standard normal distribution.

Note that if some of the observed frequencies f_{ijk} or f_{ijk}^* are small, we may consider use of the exact test procedure for testing $H_0 : \varphi_{AC} \leq \varphi_l$ and $\varphi_{BC} \leq \varphi_l$. On the basis of the conditional distribution (7.13) and the corresponding probability mass function for $f_{11+}^* \left(= f_{111}^* + f_{112}^* + f_{113}^* \right)$, we will reject $H_0 : \varphi_{AC} \leq \varphi_l$ and $\varphi_{BC} \leq \varphi_l$ at the α-level if we observe $(f_{11+}^0, f_{11+}^{*0})$ such that

$$
\begin{aligned}
&P\left(f_{11+} \geq f_{11+}^0 \mid f_{\cdot+1}, f_{\cdot+2}, f_{\cdot1+}, f_{\cdot2+}, \varphi_l^2 \right) < \alpha/2, \text{ or} \\
&P\left(f_{11+}^* \geq f_{11+}^{*0} \mid f_{\cdot+1}^*, f_{\cdot+2}^*, f_{\cdot1+}^*, f_{\cdot2+}^*, \varphi_l^2 \right) < \alpha/2.
\end{aligned}
\tag{7.28}
$$

When treatments A and B represent the low (x_L) and high (x_H) doses of an experimental treatment, it can be of interest to find out whether the treatment at a given middle dose x_M (where $x_L < x_M < x_U$) is non-inferior to an active control treatment. If we employ linear interpolation between the relative effects of treatments A and B to treatment C on the log scale, then we want to test $H_0 : w\eta_{AC} + (1-w)\eta_{BC} \leq \log(\varphi_l)$ versus $H_a : w\eta_{AC} + (1-w)\eta_{BC} > \log(\varphi_l)$, where $w = (x_U - x_M)/(x_U - x_L)$. Thus, we will reject H_0 at the α-level if

$$
\left(w\hat{\eta}_{AC}^{(WLS)} + (1-w)\hat{\eta}_{BC}^{(WLS)} - \log(\varphi_l) \right) \Big/ \sqrt{\widehat{Var}\left(w\hat{\eta}_{AC}^{(WLS)} + (1-w)\hat{\eta}_{BC}^{(WLS)} \right)} > Z_\alpha, \quad (7.29)
$$

where $\widehat{Var}\left(w\hat{\eta}_{AC}^{(WLS)} + (1-w)\hat{\eta}_{BC}^{(WLS)} \right) = w^2 \widehat{Var}\left(\hat{\eta}_{AC}^{(WLS)} \right) + (1-w)^2 \widehat{Var}\left(\hat{\eta}_{BC}^{(WLS)} \right) + 2w(1-w)\widehat{Cov}\left(\hat{\eta}_{AC}^{(WLS)}, \hat{\eta}_{BC}^{(WLS)} \right).$

7.3   Testing equivalence between an experimental treatment and an active control treatment

Using the intersection-union test (Casella and Berger, 1990), we can easily modify the procedures for testing non-inferiority to accommodate testing equivalence. When wishing to detect equivalence between either treatment A or B and an active control treatment C with respect to the efficacy, we consider testing $H_0 : (\varphi_{AC} \leq \varphi_l$ or $\varphi_{AC} \geq \varphi_u)$ and $(\varphi_{BC} \leq \varphi_l$ or $\varphi_{BC} \geq \varphi_u)$ versus $H_a : (\varphi_l < \varphi_{AC} < \varphi_u)$ or $(\varphi_l < \varphi_{BC} < \varphi_u)$, where φ_l and φ_u are the maximum clinically acceptable margins such that treatment A (or treatment B) can be regarded as equivalent to an active control treatment C when $\varphi_l < \varphi_{AC} < \varphi_u$ (or $\varphi_l < \varphi_{BC} < \varphi_u$) holds. Thus, when applying $\hat{\eta}_{AC}^{(WLS)}$ and $\hat{\eta}_{BC}^{(WLS)}$ to test equivalence, we will reject $H_0 : (\varphi_{AC} \leq \varphi_l$ or $\varphi_{AC} \geq \varphi_u)$ and $(\varphi_{BC} \leq \varphi_l$ or $\varphi_{BC} \geq \varphi_u)$ at the α-level if either of the following two sets of inequalities holds:

$$\left(\hat{\eta}_{AC}^{(WLS)} - \log(\varphi_l)\right) / \sqrt{\widehat{Var}\left(\hat{\eta}_{AC}^{(WLS)}\right)} > Z_{\alpha/2} \text{ and } \left(\hat{\eta}_{AC}^{(WLS)} - \log(\varphi_u)\right) / \sqrt{\widehat{Var}\left(\hat{\eta}_{AC}^{(WLS)}\right)} < -Z_{\alpha/2};$$

$$\text{or } \left(\hat{\eta}_{BC}^{(WLS)} - \log(\varphi_l)\right) / \sqrt{\widehat{Var}\left(\hat{\eta}_{BC}^{(WLS)}\right)} > Z_{\alpha/2} \text{ and } \left(\hat{\eta}_{BC}^{(WLS)} - \log(\varphi_u)\right) / \sqrt{\widehat{Var}\left(\hat{\eta}_{BC}^{(WLS)}\right)} < -Z_{\alpha/2}.$$

$$(7.30)$$

Note that if some of the observed frequencies f_{ijk} or f_{ijk}^* are small, we may consider the exact test procedure for testing $H_0 : (\varphi_{AC} \leq \varphi_l$ or $\varphi_{AC} \geq \varphi_u)$ and $(\varphi_{BC} \leq \varphi_l$ or $\varphi_{BC} \geq \varphi_u)$. On the basis of the conditional distribution (7.13) and the corresponding probability mass function for f_{11+}^* $(= f_{111}^* + f_{112}^* + f_{113}^*)$, we will reject H_0 at the α-level if we obtain $(f_{11+}^0, f_{11+}^{*0})$ such that

$$P\left(f_{11+} \geq f_{11+}^0 \mid f_{+1}, f_{+2}, f_{-1+}, f_{-2+}, \varphi_l^2\right) < \alpha/2 \text{ and}$$

$$P\left(f_{11+} \leq f_{11+}^0 \mid f_{+1}, f_{+2}, f_{-1+}, f_{-2+}, \varphi_u^2\right) < \alpha/2; \text{ or}$$

$$P\left(f_{11+}^* \geq f_{11+}^{*0} \mid f_{+1}^*, f_{+2}^*, f_{-1+}^*, f_{-2+}^*, \varphi_l^2\right) < \alpha/2 \text{ and}$$

$$P\left(f_{11+}^* \leq f_{11+}^{*0} \mid f_{+1}^*, f_{+2}^*, f_{-1+}^*, f_{-2+}^*, \varphi_u^2\right) < \alpha/2.$$

$$(7.31)$$

Finally, when treatments A and B represent different doses of an experimental treatment, we may be interested in studying whether a weighted average of these doses is equivalent to an active control treatment. Thus, we want to test $H_0 : w\eta_{AC} + (1-w)\eta_{BC} \leq \log(\varphi_l)$ or $w\eta_{AC} + (1-w)\eta_{BC} \geq \log(\varphi_u)$ versus $H_a : \log(\varphi_l) < w\eta_{AC} + (1-w)\eta_{BC} < \log(\varphi_u)$, where $0 < w < 1$. Thus, we will reject H_0 at the α-level if

$$\left(w\hat{\eta}_{AC}^{(WLS)} + (1-w)\hat{\eta}_{BC}^{(WLS)} - \log(\varphi_l)\right) / \sqrt{\widehat{Var}\left(w\hat{\eta}_{AC}^{(WLS)} + (1-w)\hat{\eta}_{BC}^{(WLS)}\right)} > Z_\alpha, \text{ and}$$

$$\left(w\hat{\eta}_{AC}^{(WLS)} + (1-w)\hat{\eta}_{BC}^{(WLS)} - \log(\varphi_u)\right) / \sqrt{\widehat{Var}\left(w\hat{\eta}_{AC}^{(WLS)} + (1-w)\hat{\eta}_{BC}^{(WLS)}\right)} < -Z_\alpha.$$

$$(7.32)$$

7.4 Interval estimation of the odds ratio

To assess the magnitude of the effect for an experimental treatment relative to a placebo is always of importance in an RCT. Because the relative treatment effect measured by φ_{AC} (φ_{BC} or φ_{BA}) is, as shown in (7.2)–(7.4), equal to the square root of the common OR across three 2×2 tables, we can modify all interval estimators for the common OR under stratified sampling developed elsewhere (Fleiss, 1981; Agresti, 1990; Lui, 2004) to produce a confidence interval for the relative treatment effect. For brevity, we consider only interval estimators derived from the WLS method with the logarithmic transformation, the MH type approach, and the exact conditional distribution in the following.

To obtain an interval estimator of φ_{AC}, we first consider use of the WLS estimator with the logarithmic transformation to improve the normal approximation. This leads us to obtain an asymptotic $100(1 - \alpha)\%$ confidence interval for φ_{AC} as given by

$$\left[\exp\left\{ \hat{\eta}_{AC}^{(WLS)} - Z_{\alpha/2} / \left(2\sqrt{\sum_{k=1}^{3} W_k} \right) \right\}, \exp\left\{ \hat{\eta}_{AC}^{(WLS)} + Z_{\alpha/2} / \left(2\sqrt{\sum_{k=1}^{3} W_k} \right) \right\} \right].$$

(7.33)

When estimating φ_{AC}, we can also use the well-known MH point estimator for sparse data as given by

$$\hat{\varphi}_{AC}^{(MH)} = \left(\left(\sum_{k=1}^{3} f_{11k} f_{22k} / f_{++k} \right) / \left(\sum_{k=1}^{3} f_{12k} f_{21k} / f_{++k} \right) \right)^{1/2}.$$

(7.34)

As shown elsewhere (Robins, Breslow, and Greenland, 1986; Agresti, 1990), the asymptotic variance for $\log\left(\hat{\varphi}_{AC}^{(MH)} \right)$ is given by

$$\widehat{Var}\left(\log\left(\hat{\varphi}_{AC}^{(MH)} \right) \right) = \left\{ \frac{\sum_k (f_{11k} + f_{22k})(f_{11k} f_{22k}) / f_{++k}^2}{2 \left(\sum_k f_{11k} f_{22k} / f_{++k} \right)^2} \right.$$

$$+ \frac{\sum_k [(f_{11k} + f_{22k})(f_{12k} f_{21k}) + (f_{12k} + f_{21k})(f_{11k} f_{22k})] / f_{++k}^2}{2 \left(\sum_k f_{11k} f_{22k} / f_{++k} \right) \left(\sum_k f_{12k} f_{21k} / f_{++k} \right)}$$

$$\left. + \frac{\sum_k (f_{12k} + f_{21k})(f_{12k} f_{21k}) / f_{++k}^2}{2 \left(\sum_k f_{12k} f_{21k} / f_{++k} \right)^2} \right\} / 4.$$

(7.35)

From (7.34) and (7.35), we obtain an asymptotic $100(1 - \alpha)\%$ confidence interval for φ_{AC} based on the MH estimator:

$$\left[\hat{\varphi}_{AC}^{(MH)} \exp\left(-Z_{\alpha/2} \sqrt{\widehat{Var}\left(\log\left(\hat{\varphi}_{AC}^{(MH)} \right) \right)} \right), \hat{\varphi}_{AC}^{(MH)} \exp\left(Z_{\alpha/2} \sqrt{\widehat{Var}\left(\log\left(\hat{\varphi}_{AC}^{(MH)} \right) \right)} \right) \right].$$

(7.36)

If some of the observed frequencies f_{ijk} are small, we may consider the interval estimator based on the exact conditional distribution (7.13). For an observed f_{11+}^0, we obtain an exact $100(1-\alpha)\%$ confidence interval for φ_{AC} as given by (Gart, 1970)

$$[\varphi_{ACL}, \varphi_{ACU}], \tag{7.37}$$

where $P\left(f_{11+} \geq f_{11+}^0 \mid f_{-+1}, f_{-+2}, f_{-1+}, f_{-2+}, \varphi_{ACL}^2\right) = \alpha/2$, and $P\left(f_{11+} \leq f_{11+}^0 \mid f_{-+1}, f_{-+2}, f_{-1+}, f_{-2+}, \varphi_{ACU}^2\right) = \alpha/2$.

Similarly, we can obtain asymptotic and exact interval estimators for φ_{BC} (or φ_{BA}) by replacing f_{ijk} with f_{ijk}^* (or f_{ijk}^{**}) in (7.33)–(7.37).

Finally, when treatments A and B represent different doses of an experimental treatment, it can be interesting to obtain an interval estimator for a weighted average of dose effects $w\eta_{AC} + (1-w)\eta_{BC}$ (where $0 < w < 1$). Using the WLS approach with the logarithmic transformation, for example, we obtain an asymptotic $100(1-\alpha)\%$ confidence interval for $w\eta_{AC} + (1-w)\eta_{BC}$ as

$$\left[w\hat{\eta}_{AC}^{(WLS)} + (1-w)\hat{\eta}_{BC}^{(WLS)} - Z_{\alpha/2}\sqrt{\widehat{Var}\left(w\hat{\eta}_{AC}^{(WLS)} + (1-w)\hat{\eta}_{BC}^{(WLS)}\right)}, \right.$$

$$\left. w\hat{\eta}_{AC}^{(WLS)} + (1-w)\hat{\eta}_{BC}^{(WLS)} + Z_{\alpha/2}\sqrt{\widehat{Var}\left(w\hat{\eta}_{AC}^{(WLS)} + (1-w)\hat{\eta}_{BC}^{(WLS)}\right)} \right] \tag{7.38}$$

Note that when $w = 1/2$, we can take the exponential transformation of the confidence limits (7.38) to obtain an asymptotic $100(1-\alpha)\%$ confidence interval for the geometric mean $(\varphi_{AC}\varphi_{BC})^{1/2} = \exp((1/2)\eta_{AC} + (1/2)\eta_{BC})$.

Example 7.2 When applying the WLS and MH methods, we obtain $\hat{\varphi}_{AC}^{(WLS)} = 6.031$ and $\hat{\varphi}_{AC}^{(MH)} = 6.338$ together with their corresponding 95% confidence intervals [2.398, 12.254] and [2.549, 15.755] for φ_{AC}. Similarly, using the WLS and MH methods, we obtain $\hat{\varphi}_{BC}^{(WLS)} = 7.983$ and $\hat{\varphi}_{BC}^{(MH)} = 7.689$ together with their corresponding 95% confidence intervals [3.450, 17.333] and [3.438, 17.195] for φ_{BC}. Because all these resulting lower limits fall above 1, we may claim at the 0.05 level significant evidence that both treatments A and B increase the relief rates of pain as compared with the placebo. Note that the WLS point estimator $\hat{\varphi}_{AC}^{(WLS)}$ (7.6) (or $\hat{\varphi}_{BC}^{(WLS)}$ (7.8)) should not be confused with the point estimator $\exp\left(\hat{\eta}_{AC}^{(WLS)}\right)$ (or $\exp\left(\hat{\eta}_{BC}^{(WLS)}\right)$). Using the WLS and MH methods for assessing φ_{BA} between treatments B and A, we obtain $\hat{\varphi}_{BA}^{(WLS)} = 1.783$ and $\hat{\varphi}_{BA}^{(MH)} = 1.897$ together with their corresponding 95% confidence intervals [0.569, 4.509] and [0.587, 6.134]. Note that these resulting 95% confidence intervals for φ_{BA} do cover $\varphi_{BA} = 1$. Thus, though taking a high dose of the analgesic may increase the relief rate of taking a low dose, there is no evidence that this increase is significant at the 0.05 level.

7.5 Hypothesis testing and estimation for period effects

Under model (7.1), we can show that the OR of a positive response between periods 2 and 1 is equal to (Problem 7.6)

$$
\begin{aligned}
\phi_1 = \exp(\gamma_1) &= \left[\left(\pi_{01+}^{(1)} \pi_{01+}^{(3)} \right) \Big/ \left(\pi_{10+}^{(1)} \pi_{10+}^{(3)} \right) \right]^{1/2} \\
&= \left[\left(\pi_{01+}^{(2)} \pi_{01+}^{(5)} \right) \Big/ \left(\pi_{10+}^{(2)} \pi_{10+}^{(5)} \right) \right]^{1/2} \\
&= \left[\left(\pi_{01+}^{(4)} \pi_{01+}^{(6)} \right) \Big/ \left(\pi_{10+}^{(4)} \pi_{10+}^{(6)} \right) \right]^{1/2}.
\end{aligned}
\tag{7.39}
$$

Similarly, we can show the OR of a positive response between periods 3 and 1 under model (7.1) is equal to (Problem 7.7)

$$
\begin{aligned}
\phi_2 = \exp(\gamma_2) &= \left[\left(\pi_{0+1}^{(1)} \pi_{0+1}^{(6)} \right) \Big/ \left(\pi_{1+0}^{(1)} \pi_{1+0}^{(6)} \right) \right]^{1/2} \\
&= \left[\left(\pi_{0+1}^{(2)} \pi_{0+1}^{(4)} \right) \Big/ \left(\pi_{1+0}^{(2)} \pi_{1+0}^{(4)} \right) \right]^{1/2} \\
&= \left[\left(\pi_{0+1}^{(3)} \pi_{0+1}^{(5)} \right) \Big/ \left(\pi_{1+0}^{(3)} \pi_{1+0}^{(5)} \right) \right]^{1/2}.
\end{aligned}
\tag{7.40}
$$

Furthermore, we can show that the OR, $\phi_{21} (= \exp(\gamma_2 - \gamma_1))$, of a positive response between periods 3 and 2 under model (7.1) is equal to (Problem 7.8)

$$
\begin{aligned}
\phi_{21} &= \left[\left(\pi_{+01}^{(1)} \pi_{+01}^{(2)} \right) \Big/ \left(\pi_{+10}^{(1)} \pi_{+10}^{(2)} \right) \right]^{1/2} \\
&= \left[\left(\pi_{+01}^{(3)} \pi_{+01}^{(4)} \right) \Big/ \left(\pi_{+10}^{(3)} \pi_{+10}^{(4)} \right) \right]^{1/2} \\
&= \left[\left(\pi_{+01}^{(5)} \pi_{+01}^{(6)} \right) \Big/ \left(\pi_{+10}^{(5)} \pi_{+10}^{(6)} \right) \right]^{1/2}.
\end{aligned}
\tag{7.41}
$$

Using the same ideas as those for studying treatment effects, we can do hypothesis testing and interval estimation of the period effect measured by ϕ_1, ϕ_2, and ϕ_{21}. For brevity, we concentrate our attention on the relative effect of period 2 to period 1 here. We define $(g_{11k}, g_{12k}, g_{21k}, g_{22k})$ (for $k = 1, 2, 3$) as the vector of random cell frequencies for the three 2×2 tables corresponding to cells in equation (7.39), each table k ($= 1, 2, 3$) consisting of frequency g_{ijk} in cell (i, j) (for $i, j = 1, 2$):

$$
\begin{aligned}
\left(g_{111} = n_{01+}^{(1)}, g_{121} = n_{10+}^{(3)}, g_{211} = n_{10+}^{(1)}, g_{221} = n_{01+}^{(3)} \right), \\
\left(g_{112} = n_{01+}^{(2)}, g_{122} = n_{10+}^{(5)}, g_{212} = n_{10+}^{(2)}, g_{222} = n_{01+}^{(5)} \right), \text{ and} \\
\left(g_{113} = n_{01+}^{(4)}, g_{123} = n_{10+}^{(6)}, g_{213} = n_{10+}^{(4)}, g_{223} = n_{01+}^{(6)} \right).
\end{aligned}
\tag{7.42}
$$

Suppose that we want to find out whether there is a difference in effects between periods 2 and 1. When employing the WLS test procedure to test $H_0 : \phi_1 = 1$ (or $\gamma_1 = 0$) versus $H_a : \phi_1 \neq 1$, we will reject $H_0 : \phi_1 = 1$ at the α-level if the following test statistic

$$\left(\hat{\gamma}_1^{(WLS)}\right)^2 / \widehat{Var}\left(\hat{\gamma}_1^{(WLS)}\right) > \chi_\alpha^2(1), \tag{7.43}$$

where $\hat{\gamma}_1^{(WLS)} = \sum_k WP_k \log\left(\left(\widehat{ORP}_k\right)^{1/2}\right) / \sum_k WP_k$, $\widehat{ORP}_k = (g_{11k}g_{22k})/(g_{12k}g_{21k})$, $WP_k = [1/g_{11k} + 1/g_{12k} + 1/g_{21k} + 1/g_{22k}]^{-1}$, and $\widehat{Var}\left(\hat{\gamma}_1^{(WLS)}\right) = 1/\left(4\sum_k WP_k\right)$. We can also apply the MH summary test procedure to test $H_0 : \phi_1 = 1$ versus $H_a : \phi_1 \neq 1$. We will reject H_0 at the α-level if the test statistic

$$\left(\sum_k g_{11k} - \sum_k g_{1+k}g_{+1k}/g_{++k}\right)^2 / \left\{\sum_k g_{1+k}g_{2+k}g_{+1k}g_{+2k}/\left[g_{++k}^2(g_{++k}-1)\right]\right\} > \chi_\alpha^2(1). \tag{7.44}$$

Note that the conditional probability distribution of g_{11k}, given $g_{+1k}, g_{+2k}, g_{1+k}$, and g_{2+k} fixed, in table k is given by

$$P\left(g_{11k}|g_{+1k}, g_{+2k}, g_{1+k}, g_{2+k}, \phi_1^2\right) = \frac{\binom{g_{+1k}}{g_{11k}}\binom{g_{+2k}}{g_{1+k}-g_{11k}}(\phi_1^2)^{g_{11k}}}{\sum_{x_k}\binom{g_{+1k}}{x_k}\binom{g_{+2k}}{g_{1+k}-x_k}(\phi_1^2)^{x_k}}, \tag{7.45}$$

where the summation of x_k in the denominator is calculated over $c_k \leq x_k \leq d_k$, $c_k = \max\{0, g_{1+k}-g_{+2k}\}$, and $d_k = \min\{g_{+1k}, g_{1+k}\}$ for $k = 1, 2, 3$. Thus, the joint conditional probability mass function of the random vector $\underline{g}_1 = (g_{111}, g_{112}, g_{113})'$ is given by

$$P\left(g_{111}, g_{112}, g_{113}|\underline{g}_{+1}, \underline{g}_{+2}, \underline{g}_{1+}, \underline{g}_{2+}, \phi_1^2\right) = \prod_{k=1}^{3} \frac{\binom{g_{+1k}}{g_{11k}}\binom{g_{+2k}}{g_{1+k}-g_{11k}}(\phi_1^2)^{g_{11k}}}{\sum_{x_k}\binom{g_{+1k}}{x_k}\binom{g_{+2k}}{g_{1+k}-x_k}(\phi_1^2)^{x_k}}. \tag{7.46}$$

$\underline{g}_{u+} = (g_{u+1}, g_{u+2}, g_{u+3})'$ for $u = 1, 2$, and $\underline{g}_{+v} = (g_{+v1}, g_{+v2}, g_{+v3})'$ for $v = 1, 2$. The probability mass function for $g_{11+}^0 \; (= g_{111}^0 + g_{112}^0 + g_{113}^0)$ based on (7.46) is then given by

$$P\left(g_{11+} = g_{11+}^0|\underline{g}_{+1}, \underline{g}_{+2}, \underline{g}_{1+}, \underline{g}_{2+}, \phi_1^2\right)$$

$$= \sum_{\underline{g}_{11} \in C(g_{11+}^0)} \prod_{k=1}^{3} \frac{\binom{g_{+1k}}{g_{11k}}\binom{g_{+2k}}{g_{1+k}-g_{11k}}(\phi_1^2)^{g_{11k}}}{\sum_{x_k}\binom{g_{+1k}}{x_k}\binom{g_{+2k}}{g_{1+k}-x_k}(\phi_1^2)^{x_k}}, \tag{7.47}$$

where $C\left(g_{11+}^0\right)=\left\{(g_{111},g_{112},g_{113})|g_{111}+g_{112}+g_{113}=g_{11+}^0,c_k\leq g_{11k}\leq d_k,k=1,2,3\right\}$.
On the basis of the conditional distribution (7.47), we can derive, as done previously for treatment effects, an exact test and exact interval estimator for ϕ_1.

7.6   Procedures for testing treatment-by-period interactions

When applying a summary procedure to test non-equality of effects between treatments, we need to assume that there are no treatment-by-period interactions. Otherwise, if the underlying OR of a positive response is > 1 in some tables and is < 1 in other tables, for example, we can easily see that $\hat{\eta}_{AC}^{(WLS)}$ $\left(=\sum_k W_k\log\left(\left(\widehat{OR}_k\right)^{1/2}\right)/\sum_k W_k\right)$ can be small due to cancelation of the positive and negative values $\log\left(\widehat{OR}_k\right)$ between strata. In these cases, a summary test procedure can lack power. Furthermore, if there are treatment-by-period interactions, a summary estimator for the relative treatment effect can be also potentially misleading (Lui, 2004). Thus, it is of interest to test whether there are treatment-by-period interactions.

We can extend model (7.1) to account for treatment-by-period interactions by assuming that the probability of a positive response for patient i in group g at period z is given by the following random effects logistic regression model:

$$P\left(Y_{iz}^{(g)}=1|X_{iz1}^{(g)},X_{iz2}^{(g)},Z_{iz1}^{(g)},Z_{iz2}^{(g)}\right)=$$

$$\frac{\exp\left(\mu_i^{(g)}+\eta_{AC}X_{iz1}^{(g)}+\eta_{BC}X_{iz2}^{(g)}+\gamma_1 Z_{iz1}^{(g)}+\gamma_2 Z_{iz2}^{(g)}+\lambda_{11}X_{iz1}^{(g)}Z_{iz1}^{(g)}+\lambda_{12}X_{iz1}^{(g)}Z_{iz2}^{(g)}+\lambda_{21}X_{iz2}^{(g)}Z_{iz1}^{(g)}+\lambda_{22}X_{iz2}^{(g)}Z_{iz2}^{(g)}\right)}{1+\exp\left(\mu_i^{(g)}+\eta_{AC}X_{iz1}^{(g)}+\eta_{BC}X_{iz2}^{(g)}+\gamma_1 Z_{iz1}^{(g)}+\gamma_2 Z_{iz2}^{(g)}+\lambda_{11}X_{iz1}^{(g)}Z_{iz1}^{(g)}+\lambda_{12}X_{iz1}^{(g)}Z_{iz2}^{(g)}+\lambda_{21}X_{iz2}^{(g)}Z_{iz1}^{(g)}+\lambda_{22}X_{iz2}^{(g)}Z_{iz2}^{(g)}\right)},$$

$$(7.48)$$

where λ_{11} and λ_{12} represent the interactions between treatment A (versus placebo C) and the two periods, as well as λ_{21} and λ_{22} represent the interactions between treatment B (versus placebo C) and the two periods. From model (7.48), we can show that

$$\pi_{10+}^{(1)}=\int\left(\frac{\exp(\mu)}{1+\exp(\mu)}\right)\left(\frac{1}{1+\exp(\mu+\eta_{AC}+\gamma_1+\lambda_{11})}\right)f_1(\mu)d\mu,\text{ and}\qquad(7.49)$$

$$\pi_{01+}^{(1)}=\int\left(\frac{1}{1+\exp(\mu)}\right)\left(\frac{\exp(\mu+\eta_{AC}+\gamma_1+\lambda_{11})}{1+\exp(\mu+\eta_{AC}+\gamma_1+\lambda_{11})}\right)f_1(\mu)d\mu.\qquad(7.50)$$

Hence we obtain the equality

$$\pi_{01+}^{(1)}/\pi_{10+}^{(1)}=\exp(\eta_{AC}+\gamma_1+\lambda_{11}).\qquad(7.51)$$

Similarly, we can show that

$$\pi_{10+}^{(3)} = \int \left(\frac{\exp(\mu+\eta_{AC})}{1+\exp(\mu+\eta_{AC})}\right)\left(\frac{1}{1+\exp(\mu+\gamma_1)}\right)f_3(\mu)d\mu, \text{ and} \tag{7.52}$$

$$\pi_{01+}^{(3)} = \int \left(\frac{1}{1+\exp(\mu+\eta_{AC})}\right)\left(\frac{\exp(\mu+\gamma_1)}{1+\exp(\mu+\gamma_1)}\right)f_3(\mu)d\mu. \tag{7.53}$$

Thus, we obtain the equality

$$\pi_{01+}^{(3)} / \pi_{10+}^{(3)} = \exp(-\eta_{AC}+\gamma_1). \tag{7.54}$$

From (7.51) and (7.54), we obtain

$$\left[\left(\pi_{01+}^{(1)}\pi_{10+}^{(3)}\right) / \left(\pi_{10+}^{(1)}\pi_{01+}^{(3)}\right)\right] = \exp(2\eta_{AC}+\lambda_{11}). \tag{7.55}$$

Following the same arguments as for deriving (7.55), we can show that under model (7.48) (Problem 7.9)

$$\left[\left(\pi_{0+1}^{(2)}\pi_{1+0}^{(4)}\right) / \left(\pi_{1+0}^{(2)}\pi_{0+1}^{(4)}\right)\right] = \exp(2\eta_{AC}+\lambda_{12}) \text{ and} \tag{7.56}$$

$$\left[\left(\pi_{+01}^{(5)}\pi_{+10}^{(6)}\right) / \left(\pi_{+10}^{(5)}\pi_{+01}^{(6)}\right)\right] = \exp(2\eta_{AC}+\lambda_{11}+\lambda_{12}). \tag{7.57}$$

From (7.55) to (7.57), the underlying OR of a positive response for the three 2×2 tables $(f_{11k}, f_{12k}, f_{21k}, f_{22k})$ for $k = 1, 2, 3$ is homogeneous if and only if $\lambda_{11} = \lambda_{12} = 0$. Thus, we may apply the WLS test statistic (Fleiss, 1981) for testing the homogeneity of the OR across strata to detect whether the interactions between treatment A and periods equal 0 (i.e., $\lambda_{11} = \lambda_{12} = 0$). We will reject the null hypothesis $H_0 : \lambda_{11} = \lambda_{12} = 0$ at the α-level if

$$\sum_{k=1}^{3} W_k \left(\log\left(\widehat{OR}_k\right)\right)^2 - \left(\sum_{k=1}^{3} W_k \log\left(\widehat{OR}_k\right)\right)^2 / \sum_{k=1}^{3} W_k > \chi_\alpha^2(2). \tag{7.58}$$

Similarly, we can show that the underlying ORs of a positive response between treatment B and a placebo under model (7.48) for the three 2×2 tables of $\left(f_{11k}^*, f_{12k}^*, f_{21k}^*, f_{22k}^*\right)$ for $k = 1, 2, 3$ are equal to (Problem 7.10)

$$\left[\left(\pi_{0+1}^{(1)}\pi_{1+0}^{(6)}\right) / \left(\pi_{1+0}^{(1)}\pi_{0+1}^{(6)}\right)\right] = \exp(2\eta_{BC}+\lambda_{22}), \tag{7.59}$$

$$\left[\left(\pi_{01+}^{(2)}\pi_{10+}^{(5)}\right) / \left(\pi_{10+}^{(2)}\pi_{01+}^{(5)}\right)\right] = \exp(2\eta_{BC}+\lambda_{21}), \text{ and} \tag{7.60}$$

$$\left[\left(\pi_{+01}^{(3)}\pi_{+10}^{(4)}\right) / \left(\pi_{+10}^{(3)}\pi_{+01}^{(4)}\right)\right] = \exp(2\eta_{BC}+\lambda_{21}+\lambda_{22}). \tag{7.61}$$

Thus, we can apply the WLS procedure for testing the homogeneity of the OR across 2×2 tables of $\left(f_{11k}^*, f_{12k}^*, f_{21k}^*, f_{22k}^*\right)$ for $k = 1, 2, 3$ to test whether the interactions between treatment B and periods equal 0 (i.e., $\lambda_{21} = \lambda_{22} = 0$). We will reject $H_0 : \lambda_{21} = \lambda_{22} = 0$ at the α-level if

$$\sum_{k=1}^{3} W_k^* \left(\log \left(\widehat{OR}_k^* \right) \right)^2 - \left(\sum_{k=1}^{3} W_k^* \log \left(\widehat{OR}_k^* \right) \right)^2 \Big/ \sum_{k=1}^{3} W_k^* > \chi_\alpha^2(2). \quad (7.62)$$

Finally, we can show that the underlying OR of a positive response between treatments B and A under model (7.48) for the three 2×2 tables $\left(f_{11k}^{**}, f_{12k}^{**}, f_{21k}^{**}, f_{22k}^{**} \right)$ for $k = 1, 2, 3$ is equal to (Problem 7.11)

$$\left(\pi_{+01}^{(1)} \pi_{+10}^{(2)} \right) \Big/ \left(\pi_{+10}^{(1)} \pi_{+01}^{(2)} \right) = \exp(2(\eta_{BC} - \eta_{AC}) + (\lambda_{21} - \lambda_{11}) + (\lambda_{22} - \lambda_{12})), \quad (7.63)$$

$$\left(\pi_{0+1}^{(3)} \pi_{1+0}^{(5)} \right) \Big/ \left(\pi_{1+0}^{(3)} \pi_{0+1}^{(5)} \right) = \exp(2(\eta_{BC} - \eta_{AC}) + (\lambda_{22} - \lambda_{12})), \text{ and} \quad (7.64)$$

$$\left(\pi_{01+}^{(4)} \pi_{10+}^{(6)} \right) \Big/ \left(\pi_{10+}^{(4)} \pi_{01+}^{(6)} \right) = \exp(2(\eta_{BC} - \eta_{AC}) + (\lambda_{21} - \lambda_{11})). \quad (7.65)$$

Hence we can use the WLS procedure for testing the homogeneity of the OR across the three observed tables defined by $\left(f_{11k}^{**}, f_{12k}^{**}, f_{21k}^{**}, f_{22k}^{**} \right)$ for $k = 1, 2, 3$ to test whether the interactions between treatment B versus treatment A and periods equal 0 (i.e., $\lambda_{11} = \lambda_{21}$ and $\lambda_{12} = \lambda_{22}$). We will reject $H_0 : \lambda_{11} = \lambda_{21}$ and $\lambda_{12} = \lambda_{22}$ at the α-level if

$$\sum_{k=1}^{3} W_k^{**} \left(\log \left(\widehat{OR}_k^{**} \right) \right)^2 - \left(\sum_{k=1}^{3} W_k^{**} \log \left(\widehat{OR}_k^{**} \right) \right)^2 \Big/ \sum_{k=1}^{3} W_k^{**} > \chi_\alpha^2(2).$$
$$(7.66)$$

Other test procedures (Zelen, 1971; Breslow and Day, 1980; Ejigou and McHugh, 1984) for testing the homogeneity of the OR across tables can also be applied to test whether there are treatment-by-period interactions.

Jones and Kenward (1987) suggested a log-linear model and assumed a specific structural dependence between binary responses within patients for the three-period crossover trial. They proposed the use of nuisance parameters to model this dependence and employing GLIM (Numerical Algorithms Group, Oxford, UK) to obtain parameter estimates under the assumed models. By contrast, we assume a distribution-free random effects logistic regression model and show that our test procedures and estimators can be free from nuisance parameters by using conditional arguments, while accounting for the dependence between responses within patients. Furthermore, since almost all test procedures and estimators derived here can be expressed in closed forms, we can test hypotheses and calculate interval estimators by hand, if necessary. Also, because test statistics and estimators presented here depend on only the marginal frequencies (such as $n_{rs+}^{(g)}$, $n_{r+t}^{(g)}$, and $n_{+st}^{(g)}$) rather than the individual cell frequency $n_{rst}^{(g)}$, use of the approach given here should cause less concern than use of the log-linear model in sparse data. Finally, because the relative treatment effect can be expressed as the square root of the underlying common OR across tables, as shown here, we can use the exact test and exact interval estimators (Gart, 1969,

1970; Agresti, 1990; Lui, 2004) for the common OR under stratified sampling to do hypothesis testing and estimation for a three-treatment three-period crossover trial when the number of patients is small.

Example 7.3   Using the WLS procedures (7.58) and (7.62) to test interactions between treatment A and two periods, as well as interactions between treatment B and two periods, we find the p-values 0.514 and 0.822. Furthermore, using the test procedure (7.66), we obtain the p-value 0.675 for testing the homogeneity of the relative effects between treatment B and treatment A across periods. Thus, there is no significant evidence that there are treatment-by-period interactions, and the summary procedures for testing whether there is a difference between either of the two doses of the analgesic and the placebo should not be illegitimate.

7.7   SAS program codes and results for a logistic regression model with normal random effects

The test procedures discussed in the above do not need to assume any parametric distribution for random effects. On the other hand, if we are willing to assume patient random effects to independently follow a normal distribution, we may apply PROC GLIMMIX in SAS (SAS Institute, 2009) to obtain the pseudo maximum likelihood estimate (PMLE) of parameters and their related tests. We present the SAS codes for using PROC GLIMMIX to analyze the data in Table 7.1 and some outputs for comparison of the results. Because each patient has a treatment response for each of the three periods, we use three data lines to represent these three responses for each patient. The first variable "patid" distinguishes patients from one another; the second and third variables "treat1" and "treat2" represent treatments A and B; the fourth and fifth variables "period1" and "period2" represent periods 1 and 2; the sixth variable "*no*" is the number of responses taken at each period; and the seventh variable "pos" indicates a positive response (or relief) or a negative response (or non-relief).

```
data step1;
input patid treat1 treat2 period1 period2 no pos;
cards;
    1  0  0  0  0  1  1
    1  1  0  1  0  1  1
    1  0  1  0  1  1  1
    2  0  0  0  0  1  1
    2  1  0  1  0  1  1
    2  0  1  0  1  1  0
. . . .
;;;;
```

```
proc glimmix data = step1;
  class patid;
  model pos/no = treat1 treat2 period1 period2/ solution;
  random intercept /subject = patid;
run;
```

We obtain the following main results about the estimates of treatment and period effects:

Effect	Estimate	Error	DF	t Value	Pr > |t|
Intercept	-1.1607	0.3185	85	-3.64	0.0005
treat1	1.9533	0.3431	168	5.69	<.0001
treat2	2.4639	0.3669	168	6.72	<.0001
period1	0.06829	0.3527	168	0.19	0.8467
period2	0.2241	0.3557	168	0.63	0.5295

As shown in the above box, we obtain the PMLE of treatment effects and their estimated SEs as $\hat{\eta}_{AC}^{(PMLE)} = 1.953$ (SE = 0.343) and $\hat{\eta}_{BC}^{(PMLE)} = 2.464$ (SE = 0.367). Using Wald's test procedure, we find that there is strongly significant evidence that both doses can increase the relief rate of pain as compared with the placebo. These results are certainly consistent with the findings based on the WLS or MH test procedures. Also, we obtain $\hat{\varphi}_{AC}^{(PMLE)} = 7.050$ and $\hat{\varphi}_{BC}^{(PMLE)} = 11.752$ together with their corresponding 95% confidence intervals for φ_{AC} and φ_{BC} as given by [3.599, 13.808] and [5.724, 24.127], respectively. Both the point and interval estimates of treatment effects using PROC GLIMMIX seem to shift to the right as compared with those using the WLS or MH method based on the conditional approach. Note that Jones and Kenward (2014) suggested use of "method = quad" when one applies PROC GLIMMIX to binary data. When using "method = quad," we have obtained essentially identical parameter estimates in use of PROC GLIMMIX for data in Table 7.1.

Using Monte Carlo simulation, McCulloch and Neuhaus (2011) noted that the MLE of parameters for "within-cluster" covariates could be insensitive to misspecification of the shape of distribution for random effects. By contrast, test procedures and estimators presented here do not need to assume any parametric distribution for the random effects in model (7.1), and they remain unchanged (conditional upon given data) regardless of any assumed probability density function for random effects. Furthermore, using the conditional arguments, we can easily derive the exact test procedure, which is of use when the number of patients in a crossover trial is small and all asymptotic test procedures are theoretically invalid. Therefore, though the test procedures and estimators using the conditional arguments can be less efficient than the MLE using the likelihood-based approach when the normality assumption is satisfied, we may prefer to use the conditional approaches considered here.

Exercises

Problem 7.1. Show that the OR ($= \varphi_{AC}$) of a positive response between treatment A and C under model (7.1) can be expressed in terms of $\pi_{rst}^{(g)}$'s as those in (7.2) despite the probability density function $f_g(u)$. (Hint: Under model (7.1), the joint probability of patient responses at three periods on a randomly selected subject from group g is

$$P\left(Y_{i1}^{(g)} = y_{i1}^{(g)}, Y_{i2}^{(g)} = y_{i2}^{(g)}, Y_{i3}^{(g)} = y_{i3}^{(g)} \mid X_{iz1}^{(g)}, X_{iz2}^{(g)}, Z_{iz1}^{(g)}, Z_{iz2}^{(g)}\right)$$

$$= \int \prod_{z=1}^{3} \left(\frac{\exp\left(\mu + \eta_{AC}X_{iz1}^{(g)} + \eta_{BC}X_{iz2}^{(g)} + \gamma_1 Z_{iz1}^{(g)} + \gamma_2 Z_{iz2}^{(g)}\right)}{1 + \exp\left(\mu + \eta_{AC}X_{iz1}^{(g)} + \eta_{BC}X_{iz2}^{(g)} + \gamma_1 Z_{iz1}^{(g)} + \gamma_2 Z_{iz2}^{(g)}\right)} \right)^{y_{iz}^{(g)}}$$

$$\times \left(\frac{1}{1 + \exp\left(\mu + \eta_{AC}X_{iz1}^{(g)} + \eta_{BC}X_{iz2}^{(g)} + \gamma_1 Z_{iz1}^{(g)} + \gamma_2 Z_{iz2}^{(g)}\right)} \right)^{1 - y_{iz}^{(g)}} f_g(\mu)d\mu.$$

For simplicity, let $\pi_{rst}^{(g)}$ denote the joint probability of patient responses ($Y_{i1}^{(g)} = r, Y_{i2}^{(g)} = s, Y_{i3}^{(g)} = t$), where $r = 1, 0$, $s = 1, 0$, $t = 1, 0$, for a randomly selected patient from group g. Let "+" represent the summation over that particular subscript. Thus, we can show that $\pi_{10+}^{(1)} = \int \frac{\exp(\mu)}{1 + \exp(\mu)} \left(\frac{1}{1 + \exp(\mu + \eta_{AC} + \gamma_1)} \right) f_1(\mu)d\mu$, and

$\pi_{01+}^{(1)} = \int \frac{1}{1 + \exp(\mu)} \left(\frac{\exp(\mu + \eta_{AC} + \gamma_1)}{1 + \exp(\mu + \eta_{AC} + \gamma_1)} \right) f_1(\mu)d\mu$. These lead to $\pi_{01+}^{(1)} / \pi_{10+}^{(1)} = \exp(\eta_{AC} + \gamma_1)$. Similarly, we can show that $\pi_{10+}^{(3)} = \int \frac{\exp(\mu + \eta_{AC})}{1 + \exp(\mu + \eta_{AC})} \left(\frac{1}{1 + \exp(\mu + \gamma_1)} \right) f_3(\mu)d\mu$, and $\pi_{01+}^{(3)} = \int \frac{1}{1 + \exp(\mu + \eta_{AC})} \times \left(\frac{\exp(\mu + \gamma_1)}{1 + \exp(\mu + \gamma_1)} \right) f_3(\mu)d\mu$. Thus, we obtain $\pi_{01+}^{(3)} / \pi_{10+}^{(3)} = \exp(-\eta_{AC} + \gamma_1)$.)

Problem 7.2. Show that the OR of a positive response between treatments B and C under model (7.1) can be expressed in terms of $\pi_{rst}^{(g)}$'s as those in (7.3).

Problem 7.3. Show that the OR of a positive response between treatments B and A under model (7.1) can be expressed in terms of $\pi_{rst}^{(g)}$'s as those in (7.4).

Problem 7.4. Show that the estimated asymptotic covariance $\widehat{Cov}\left(\hat{\eta}_{AC}^{(WLS)}, \hat{\eta}_{BC}^{(WLS)}\right)$ between $\hat{\eta}_{AC}^{(WLS)}$ and $\hat{\eta}_{BC}^{(WLS)}$ is given by (7.23).

Problem 7.5. Show that the optimal weight to minimize the variance $Var\left(w\hat{\eta}_{AC}^{(WLS)}+(1-w)\hat{\eta}_{BC}^{(WLS)}\right)$ is given by $w_o = \left[Var\left(\hat{\eta}_{BC}^{(WLS)}\right)-Cov\left(\hat{\eta}_{AC}^{(WLS)},\hat{\eta}_{BC}^{(WLS)}\right)\right]/$ $\left[Var\left(\hat{\eta}_{AC}^{(WLS)}\right)+Var\left(\hat{\eta}_{BC}^{(WLS)}\right)-2Cov\left(\hat{\eta}_{AC}^{(WLS)},\hat{\eta}_{BC}^{(WLS)}\right)\right]$.

Problem 7.6. Show that the OR of a positive response between periods 2 and 1 under model (7.1) can be expressed in terms of $\pi_{ijk}^{(g)}$'s as those given in (7.39).

Problem 7.7. Show that the OR of a positive response between periods 3 and 1 under model (7.1) can be expressed in terms of $\pi_{ijk}^{(g)}$'s as those given in (7.40).

Problem 7.8. Show that the OR of a positive response between periods 3 and 2 under model (7.1) can be expressed in terms of $\pi_{ijk}^{(g)}$'s as those given in (7.41).

Problem 7.9. Under model (7.48), derive equations (7.56) and (7.57).

Problem 7.10. Show that the OR of a positive response between treatment B and a placebo for the three corresponding 2×2 tables of $\left(f_{11k}^*,f_{12k}^*,f_{21k}^*,f_{22k}^*\right)$ for $k = 1, 2, 3$ under model (7.48) can be expressed as those in (7.59)–(7.61).

Problem 7.11. Show that the OR of a positive response between treatments B and A under model (7.48) for the three 2×2 tables $\left(f_{11k}^{**},f_{12k}^{**},f_{21k}^{**},f_{22k}^{**}\right)$ for $k = 1, 2, 3$ can be expressed as those in (7.63)–(7.65).

Problem 7.12. Suppose that we decide to employ one of the two 3×3 Latin squares (Senn, 2002, p. 161) to reduce the number of treatment-receipt sequences in a crossover trial. Suppose further that we randomly assign n_g patients to group $g = 1$ with C-A-B treatment-receipt sequence; = 2 with A-B-C treatment-receipt sequence; and = 3 with B-C-A treatment-receipt sequence.

(a) Show that the OR ($=\varphi_{AC}$) of a positive response between treatment A and treatment C under model (7.1) is equal to $\varphi_{AC} = \exp(\eta_{AC}) = \left[\left(\pi_{01+}^{(1)}\pi_{1+0}^{(2)}\pi_{+01}^{(3)}\right)/\left(\pi_{10+}^{(1)}\pi_{0+1}^{(2)}\pi_{+10}^{(3)}\right)\right]^{1/3}$. Thus, we may obtain the following consistent estimator for φ_{AC} as $\hat{\varphi}_{AC} = \left[\left(\hat{\pi}_{01+}^{(1)}\hat{\pi}_{1+0}^{(2)}\hat{\pi}_{+01}^{(3)}\right)/\left(\hat{\pi}_{10+}^{(1)}\hat{\pi}_{0+1}^{(2)}\hat{\pi}_{+10}^{(3)}\right)\right]^{1/3}$.

(b) By use of the delta method, what is the asymptotic variance of $\log(\hat{\varphi}_{AC})$?

Problem 7.13. Suppose that we consider comparing three experimental treatments A, B, and C and one control treatment or placebo D. A crossover design with a complete set of treatment-receipt sequences will consist of 24 groups, which can be too large to be of practical use. If we decide to employ a Latin square ((I, 3) as defined in group I on p. 163 by Senn (2002)). We randomly assign n_g patients to group g = 1 with A-C-B-D treatment-receipt sequence; = 2 with B-D-A-C treatment-receipt sequence; = 3 with C-A-D-B treatment receipt sequence; and = 4 with D-B-C-A treatment-receipt sequence. For patient i ($= 1, 2, \cdots, n_g$) assigned to group g ($= 1, 2, 3,$ 4), let $Y_{iz}^{(g)}$ denote the binary outcome at period z ($= 1, 2, 3, 4$), and $Y_{iz}^{(g)} = 1$ for a positive response, and $= 0$ otherwise. We assume that the probability of a positive response for patient i in group g at period z is given by the following random effects logistic regression model:

$$P\left(Y_{iz}^{(g)} = 1 | X_{iz1}^{(g)}, X_{iz2}^{(g)}, X_{iz3}^{(g)}, Z_{iz1}^{(g)}, Z_{iz2}^{(g)}, Z_{iz3}^{(g)}\right)$$

$$= \frac{\exp\left(\mu_i^{(g)} + \eta_{AD}X_{iz1}^{(g)} + \eta_{BD}X_{iz2}^{(g)} + \eta_{CD}X_{iz3}^{(g)} + \gamma_1 Z_{iz1}^{(g)} + \gamma_2 Z_{iz2}^{(g)} + \gamma_3 Z_{iz3}^{(g)}\right)}{1 + \exp\left(\mu_i^{(g)} + \eta_{AD}X_{iz1}^{(g)} + \eta_{BD}X_{iz2}^{(g)} + \eta_{CD}X_{iz3}^{(g)} + \gamma_1 Z_{iz1}^{(g)} + \gamma_2 Z_{iz2}^{(g)} + \gamma_3 Z_{iz3}^{(g)}\right)},$$

where $X_{iz1}^{(g)}$, $X_{iz2}^{(g)}$, and $X_{iz3}^{(g)}$ denote the indicator functions of treatment-receipt for treatments A, B, and C, and $= 1$ if the patient in group g at period z receives the corresponding treatment, and $= 0$ otherwise; $Z_{iz1}^{(g)}$, $Z_{iz2}^{(g)}$, and $Z_{iz3}^{(g)}$ denote the indicator functions of periods 2, 3, and 4 by setting $Z_{iz1}^{(g)} = 1$ for period $z = 2$, and $= 0$ otherwise; $Z_{iz2}^{(g)} = 1$ for period $z = 3$, and $= 0$ otherwise; $Z_{iz3}^{(g)} = 1$ for period $z = 4$, and $= 0$ otherwise; $\mu_i^{(g)}$ represents the random effect due to the underlying characteristics of the ith patient assigned to group g, and all $\mu_i^{(g)}$'s are assumed to independently follow an unspecified probability density function $f_g(\mu)$; η_{AD}, η_{BD}, and η_{CD} denote the respective effect of treatments A, B, and C relative to treatment (or placebo) D; and γ_1, γ_2, and γ_3 denote the respective effect for periods 2, 3, and 4 versus period 1. Discuss how to apply the conditional approach to derive the consistent estimators for the relative treatment effects η_{AD}, η_{BD}, and η_{CD} based on the WLS method. (Hint: For any given pair of treatments in a given treatment-receipt sequence, we can find that there is another treatment-receipt sequence in which this pair of treatments appears in the reverse order of the same pair of periods.) Note that Kenward and Jones (1992) have provided excellent discussions on the use of Latin square for a 4×4 crossover design in binary data.

8

Three-treatment three-period crossover design in ordinal data

When the underlying patient response is on an ordinal scale, the relative distances between ordinal categories are really incomparable and unsuitable for arithmetic operations. Following Agresti (1980), we propose use of the GOR of patient responses for paired samples or Agresti's α' (Agresti, 1980) to measure the relative treatment effect for comparing two experimental treatments with a placebo (or a control treatment) under a three-period crossover trial (Lui, Chang, and Lin, 2015). For example, consider the data (Table 8.1) taken from a three-period crossover trial comparing an analgesic at low and high doses for the relief of pain in primary dysmenorrhea with a placebo (Kenward and Jones, 1991). Patients were randomly assigned to one of the six groups determined by different treatment-receipt sequences. At the end of each period, each patient rated the treatment as no relief (coded as 1), moderate (coded as 2), and complete (coded as 3). Note that the relative distance between "no relief" and "moderate" is not identical to that between "moderate" and "complete." Thus, taking a difference based on arbitrary scores assigned to these ordinal categories can have no practical meaning or easy interpretation. Although we may often apply the t-test to arbitrary scores (such as 0, 1, 2, $\cdots$) assigned to ordinal categories, it is difficult to provide a meaningful summary index based on these arbitrarily assigned scores to quantify the magnitude of the relative treatment effect. Furthermore, the possibility that one may obtain different test results depending on varying schemes of assigning scores to the same

Crossover Designs: Testing, Estimation, and Sample Size, First Edition. Kung-Jong Lui.
© 2016 John Wiley & Sons, Ltd. Published 2016 by John Wiley & Sons, Ltd.
Companion website: www.wiley.com/go/lui/crossover

Table 8.1   The frequency of patients for the relief of pain in primary dysmenorrhea at the three periods in the six groups with different treatment-receipt sequences in a crossover trial.

Group with treatment-receipt sequence

Group No	$g = 1$	2	3	4	5	6
	P-L-H	P-H-L	L-P-H	L-H-P	H-P-L	H-L-P
Responses						
(1,1,1)	0	2	0	0	3	1
(1,1,2)	1	0	0	1	0	0
(1,1,3)	1	0	1	0	0	0
(1,2,1)	2	0	0	0	0	0
(1,2,2)	3	0	1	0	0	0
(1,2,3)	4	3	1	0	2	0
(1,3,1)	0	0	1	1	0	0
(1,3,2)	0	2	0	0	0	0
(1,3,3)	2	4	1	0	0	1
(2,1,1)	0	1	1	0	0	3
(2,1,2)	0	0	2	0	1	1
(2,1,3)	0	0	1	0	0	0
(2,2,1)	1	0	0	6	1	1
(2,2,2)	0	2	1	0	0	0
(2,2,3)	1	0	0	0	0	0
(2,3,1)	0	0	0	1	0	2
(2,3,2)	0	0	0	0	0	0
(2,3,3)	0	2	0	0	1	0
(3,1,1)	0	0	0	1	0	2
(3,1,2)	0	0	2	0	2	1
(3,1,3)	0	0	3	0	4	1
(3,2,1)	0	0	0	1	0	0
(3,2,2)	0	0	0	1	0	0
(3,2,3)	0	0	0	0	0	0
(3,3,1)	0	0	0	0	0	1
(3,3,2)	0	0	0	0	0	0
(3,3,3)	0	0	0	0	0	0
$n_g =$	15	16	15	12	14	14

1, none or minimal; 2, moderate; 3, complete.
P, placebo; L, low dose; H, high dose.

ordinal data can be undesirable. On the other hand, if we dichotomize ordinal data into binary responses and employ procedures and estimators for dichotomous data, we will probably lose efficiency.

Ezzet and Whitehead (1991) first proposed a normal random effects proportional odds model (Clayton, 1974; Clayton and Cuzick, 1985) to study two treatments under an AB/BA crossover trial. Although we can now use PROC GLIMMIX (SAS Institute, 2009) to obtain the PMLE of model parameters, the implicit assumption of the proportional odds model can be badly violated by many bivariate distributions (Mosteller, 1968; Fleiss, 1981; Agresti, 1980). This may cause concern in use of the random effects proportional odds model, especially when the data are sparse and statistical methods derived from large-sample theory based on the likelihood-based method can be theoretically invalid.

On the basis of the GOR of patient responses, we provide asymptotic and exact test procedures for testing non-equality of treatments in ordinal data (Lui, Chang, and Lin, 2015). We give asymptotic and exact test procedures for testing non-inferiority and equivalence between either of the two experimental treatments and an active control treatment. We address interval estimation of the GOR between treatments. We discuss hypothesis testing and estimation for period effects. We show how one can apply procedures for testing the homogeneity of the OR in stratified analysis to detect whether there are treatment-by-period interactions. For comparison of the test results between the conditional approach using the GOR and the likelihood-based approach assuming the normal random effects proportional odds model, we present the SAS codes and some outputs in use of PROC GLIMMIX (SAS Institute, 2009) to the data in Table 8.1.

Suppose that we compare two experimental treatments A and B with treatment C (that can be a placebo or an active control treatment) in a three-period crossover design. We let U-V-W denote the treatment-receipt sequence of receiving treatments U, V, and W at periods 1, 2, and 3, respectively. We randomly assign n_g patients to group g = 1 with C-A-B treatment-receipt sequence; = 2 with C-B-A treatment-receipt sequence; = 3 with A-C-B treatment-receipt sequence; = 4 with A-B-C treatment-receipt sequence; = 5 with B-C-A treatment-receipt sequence; and = 6 with B-A-C treatment-receipt sequence. For patient i (= 1, 2, $\cdots$, n_g) assigned to group g (= 1, 2, 3, 4, 5, 6), we let $Y_{iz}^{(g)}$ denote the response of the patient at period z (= 1, 2, 3), and take one of the possible ordinal labels C_j, where $C_1 < C_2 < C_3 < \cdots < C_L$. We let $X_{iz1}^{(g)}$ denote the indicator function of treatment-receipt for treatment A, and $X_{iz1}^{(g)} = 1$ if patient i assigned to group g at period z receives treatment A, and = 0 otherwise. Similarly, we let $X_{iz2}^{(g)}$ denote the indicator function of treatment-receipt for treatment B, and $X_{iz2}^{(g)} = 1$ if the corresponding patient at period z receives treatment B, and = 0 otherwise. We further let $Z_{iz1}^{(g)}$ and $Z_{iz2}^{(g)}$ represent the indicator functions of periods with setting $Z_{iz1}^{(g)} = 1$ for period z = 2, and = 0 otherwise; as well as $Z_{iz2}^{(g)} = 1$ for period z = 3, and = 0 otherwise. For patient i (= 1, 2, $\cdots$, n_g) in group g (= 1, 2, 3, 4, 5, 6), we assume that the joint probability of $\left(Y_{iz_1}^{(g)}, Y_{iz_2}^{(g)}\right)$ between periods z_1 and z_2, where $z_1 \neq z_2$, z_1 and $z_2 = 1, 2, 3$, satisfies

$$
P\left(Y_{iz_1}^{(g)} < Y_{iz_2}^{(g)}\right) = \left[1 / \left(1 + \exp\left(\mu_i^{(g)} + \eta_{AC}X_{iz_11}^{(g)} + \eta_{BC}X_{iz_12}^{(g)} + \gamma_1 Z_{iz_11}^{(g)} + \gamma_2 Z_{iz_12}^{(g)}\right)\right)\right]
$$

$$
\times \left[\exp\left(\mu_i^{(g)} + \eta_{AC}X_{iz_21}^{(g)} + \eta_{BC}X_{iz_22}^{(g)} + \gamma_1 Z_{iz_21}^{(g)} + \gamma_2 Z_{iz_22}^{(g)}\right) \right/
$$

$$
\left(1 + \exp\left(\mu_i^{(g)} + \eta_{AC}X_{iz_21}^{(g)} + \eta_{BC}X_{iz_22}^{(g)} + \gamma_1 Z_{iz_21}^{(g)} + \gamma_2 Z_{iz_22}^{(g)}\right)\right)\right],
$$

$$
P\left(Y_{iz_1}^{(g)} > Y_{iz_2}^{(g)}\right) = \left[1 / \left(1 + \exp\left(\mu_i^{(g)} + \eta_{AC}X_{iz_21}^{(g)} + \eta_{BC}X_{iz_22}^{(g)} + \gamma_1 Z_{iz_21}^{(g)} + \gamma_2 Z_{iz_22}^{(g)}\right)\right)\right]
$$

$$
\times \left[\exp\left(\mu_i^{(g)} + \eta_{AC}X_{iz_11}^{(g)} + \eta_{BC}X_{iz_12}^{(g)} + \gamma_1 Z_{iz_11}^{(g)} + \gamma_2 Z_{iz_12}^{(g)}\right) \right/
$$

$$
\left(1 + \exp\left(\mu_i^{(g)} + \eta_{AC}X_{iz_11}^{(g)} + \eta_{BC}X_{iz_12}^{(g)} + \gamma_1 Z_{iz_11}^{(g)} + \gamma_2 Z_{iz_12}^{(g)}\right)\right)\right], \text{ and}
$$

$$
P\left(Y_{iz_1}^{(g)} = Y_{iz_2}^{(g)}\right) = 1 - P\left(Y_{iz_1}^{(g)} > Y_{iz_2}^{(g)}\right) - P\left(Y_{iz_1}^{(g)} < Y_{iz_2}^{(g)}\right), \tag{8.1}
$$

where $\mu_i^{(g)}$ denotes the random effect due to the ith subject in group g, and $\mu_i^{(g)}$'s are assumed to independently follow an unspecified probability density $f_g(\mu)$; η_{AC}, and η_{BC} denote the respective effect of treatments A and B relative to treatment C; and γ_1 and γ_2 denote the respective effect of periods 2 and 3 versus period 1. Based on model (8.1), the GOR of patient responses (Agresti, 1980; Lui, 2002a, 2004) on a given patient i in group g when he/she has covariates $\left(X_{iz_21}^{(g)}, X_{iz_22}^{(g)}, Z_{iz_21}^{(g)}, Z_{iz_22}^{(g)}\right)$ at period z_2 versus when he/she has covariates $\left(X_{iz_11}^{(g)}, X_{iz_12}^{(g)}, Z_{iz_11}^{(g)}, Z_{iz_12}^{(g)}\right)$ at period z_1 is, by definition, equal to

$$
P\left(Y_{iz_1}^{(g)} < Y_{iz_2}^{(g)}\right) \Big/ P\left(Y_{iz_1}^{(g)} > Y_{iz_2}^{(g)}\right) = \exp\left(\eta_{AC}\left(X_{iz_21}^{(g)} - X_{iz_11}^{(g)}\right) + \eta_{BC}\left(X_{iz_22}^{(g)} - X_{iz_12}^{(g)}\right)\right.
$$

$$
\left. + \gamma_1\left(Z_{iz_21}^{(g)} - Z_{iz_11}^{(g)}\right) + \gamma_2\left(Z_{iz_22}^{(g)} - Z_{iz_12}^{(g)}\right)\right). \tag{8.2}
$$

When $\eta_{AC} = 0$, the GOR (8.2) remains unchanged despite receiving treatment A or C. When $\eta_{AC} > 0$, taking treatment A tends to increase the patient response as compared with taking treatment C. When $\eta_{AC} < 0$, taking treatment A tends to decrease the patient response as compared with taking treatment C. Similar interpretations as those for η_{AC} are applicable to parameters η_{BC}, γ_1, and γ_2. We define the GOR of responses for treatment A versus treatment C and that for treatment B versus treatment C as $GOR_{AC} = \exp(\eta_{AC})$ and $GOR_{BC} = \exp(\eta_{BC})$, respectively. Also, we define the GOR of responses for treatment B versus treatment A as $GOR_{BA} = \exp(\eta_{BC} - \eta_{AC})$. On the basis of model (8.1), for a randomly selected patient from group g (= 1, 2) the probability that the patient response $Y_{z_1}^{(g)}$ (of which the non-informative subscript i

has been deleted here for simplicity in notation) at period z_1 is less than his/her response $Y_{z_2}^{(g)}$ at period z_2 is

$$P\left(Y_{z_1}^{(g)} < Y_{z_2}^{(g)}\right) = \int \left[1/\left(1+\exp\left(\mu+\eta_{AC}X_{z_11}^{(g)}+\eta_{BC}X_{z_12}^{(g)}+\gamma_1 Z_{z_11}^{(g)}+\gamma_2 Z_{z_12}^{(g)}\right)\right)\right]$$
$$\times \left[\exp\left(\mu+\eta_{AC}X_{z_21}^{(g)}+\eta_{BC}X_{z_22}^{(g)}+\gamma_1 Z_{z_21}^{(g)}+\gamma_2 Z_{z_22}^{(g)}\right)/\right.$$
$$\left.\left(1+\exp\left(\mu+\eta_{AC}X_{z_21}^{(g)}+\eta_{BC}X_{z_22}^{(g)}+\gamma_1 Z_{z_21}^{(g)}+\gamma_2 Z_{z_22}^{(g)}\right)\right)\right]f_g(\mu)d\mu.$$

$$(8.3)$$

Similarly, for a randomly selected patient from group g ($= 1, 2$) the probability that the patient response $Y_{z_1}^{(g)}$ at period z_1 is larger than his/her response $Y_{z_2}^{(g)}$ at period z_2 is

$$P\left(Y_{z_1}^{(g)} > Y_{z_2}^{(g)}\right) = \int \left[1/\left(1+\exp\left(\mu+\eta_{AC}X_{z_21}^{(g)}+\eta_{BC}X_{z_22}^{(g)}+\gamma_1 Z_{z_21}^{(g)}+\gamma_2 Z_{z_22}^{(g)}\right)\right)\right]$$
$$\times \left[\exp\left(\mu+\eta_{AC}X_{z_11}^{(g)}+\eta_{BC}X_{z_12}^{(g)}+\gamma_1 Z_{z_11}^{(g)}+\gamma_2 Z_{z_12}^{(g)}\right)/\right.$$
$$\left.\left(1+\exp\left(\mu+\eta_{AC}X_{z_11}^{(g)}+\eta_{BC}X_{z_12}^{(g)}+\gamma_1 Z_{z_11}^{(g)}+\gamma_2 Z_{z_12}^{(g)}\right)\right)\right]f_g(\mu)d\mu.$$

$$(8.4)$$

We define $\Pi_C^{(g)}(z_1,z_2) = P\left(Y_{z_1}^{(g)} < Y_{z_2}^{(g)}\right)$ and $\Pi_D^{(g)}(z_1,z_2) = P\left(Y_{z_1}^{(g)} > Y_{z_2}^{(g)}\right)$. From (8.3) and (8.4), we can see that for a randomly selected patient from group g the GOR of patient responses between periods z_2 and z_1 is

$$GOR^{(g)}(z_1,z_2) = \Pi_C^{(g)}(z_1,z_2)/\Pi_D^{(g)}(z_1,z_2)$$
$$= \exp\left(\eta_{AC}\left(X_{z_21}^{(g)}-X_{z_11}^{(g)}\right)+\eta_{BC}\left(X_{z_22}^{(g)}-X_{z_12}^{(g)}\right)+\gamma_1\left(Z_{z_21}^{(g)}-Z_{z_11}^{(g)}\right)+\gamma_2\left(Z_{z_22}^{(g)}-Z_{z_12}^{(g)}\right)\right).$$

$$(8.5)$$

On the basis of model (8.5), we can express the GOR of responses between treatment A and treatment C as (Problem 8.1)

$$GOR_{AC} = \left(GOR^{(1)}(1,2)/GOR^{(3)}(1,2)\right)^{1/2}$$
$$= \left(GOR^{(2)}(1,3)/GOR^{(4)}(1,3)\right)^{1/2} \qquad (8.6)$$
$$= \left(GOR^{(5)}(2,3)/GOR^{(6)}(2,3)\right)^{1/2}.$$

Similarly, we can express the GOR of responses between treatments B and C under model (8.5) as (Problem 8.2)

$$GOR_{BC} = \left(GOR^{(1)}(1,3)/GOR^{(6)}(1,3) \right)^{1/2}$$

$$= \left(GOR^{(2)}(1,2)/GOR^{(5)}(1,2) \right)^{1/2} \tag{8.7}$$

$$= \left(GOR^{(3)}(2,3)/GOR^{(4)}(2,3) \right)^{1/2}.$$

Also, we can show that the GOR of responses between treatments B and A as (Problem 8.3)

$$GOR_{BA} = \exp(\eta_{BC} - \eta_{AC})$$

$$= \left(GOR^{(1)}(2,3)/GOR^{(2)}(2,3) \right)^{1/2}$$

$$= \left(GOR^{(3)}(1,3)/GOR^{(5)}(1,3) \right)^{1/2} \tag{8.8}$$

$$= \left(GOR^{(4)}(1,2)/GOR^{(6)}(1,2) \right)^{1/2}.$$

We let $\pi_{rst}^{(g)}$ denote the joint probability mass function $P\left(Y_1^{(g)} = C_r, Y_2^{(g)} = C_s, Y_3^{(g)} = C_t \right)$, where $r = 1, 2, \cdots, L$, $s = 1, 2, \cdots, L$, and $t = 1, 2, \cdots, L$. We further let the notation "+" denote summation over that particular subscript. For example, the parameter $\pi_{rs+}^{(g)}$ means the marginal probability $P\left(Y_1^{(g)} = C_r, Y_2^{(g)} = C_s \right)$ and equals $\sum_{t=1}^{L} \pi_{rst}^{(g)}$, or the parameter $\pi_{r+t}^{(g)}$ represents $P\left(Y_1^{(g)} = C_r, Y_3^{(g)} = C_t \right)$ and equals $\sum_{s=1}^{L} \pi_{rst}^{(g)}$, and so forth. Thus, for a randomly selected patient from group g (= 1, 2, 3, 4, 5, 6), by definition, we have

$$P\left(Y_1^{(g)} < Y_2^{(g)} \right) = \sum_{r=1}^{L-1} \sum_{s=r+1}^{L} \pi_{rs+}^{(g)}, \text{ and}$$

$$P\left(Y_1^{(g)} > Y_2^{(g)} \right) = \sum_{r=2}^{L} \sum_{s=1}^{r-1} \pi_{rs+}^{(g)}. \tag{8.9}$$

These represent the probability that a randomly selected patient from group g has a response at period 2 higher than his/her response at period 1, and the probability that a randomly selected patient from group g has a response at period 1 higher than his/her response at period 2, respectively. Similarly, when comparing the patient response at period 3 with that at period 1, we can express the above probabilities in terms of $\pi_{rst}^{(g)}$'s as

$$P\left(Y_1^{(g)} < Y_3^{(g)} \right) = \sum_{r=1}^{L-1} \sum_{t=r+1}^{L} \pi_{r+t}^{(g)}, \text{ and}$$

$$P\left(Y_1^{(g)} > Y_3^{(g)} \right) = \sum_{r=2}^{L} \sum_{t=1}^{r-1} \pi_{r+t}^{(g)}. \tag{8.10}$$

Furthermore, when comparing patient responses between periods 3 and 2, we have

$$P\left(Y_2^{(g)} < Y_3^{(g)}\right) = \sum_{s=1}^{L-1}\sum_{t=s+1}^{L}\pi_{+st}^{(g)}, \text{ and}$$
$$P\left(Y_2^{(g)} > Y_3^{(g)}\right) = \sum_{s=2}^{L}\sum_{t=1}^{s-1}\pi_{+st}^{(g)}. \tag{8.11}$$

Let $n_{rst}^{(g)}$ denote the number of patients in group g (= 1, 2, 3, 4, 5, 6) with the vector of responses $P\left(Y_1^{(g)} = C_r, Y_2^{(g)} = C_s, Y_3^{(g)} = C_t\right)$ among n_g patients. The random cell frequencies $\{n_{rst}^{(g)} \mid r = 1, 2, 3, \cdots, L, s = 1, 2, 3, \cdots, L, \text{ and } t = 1, 2, 3, \cdots, L\}$ then follow the multinomial distribution with parameters n_g and $\{\pi_{rst}^{(g)} \mid r = 1, 2, 3, \cdots, L, s = 1, 2, 3, \cdots, L, \text{ and } t = 1, 2, 3, \cdots, L\}$. Note that we can estimate $\pi_{rst}^{(g)}$ by the unbiased consistent sample proportion estimator $\hat{\pi}_{rst}^{(g)} = n_{rst}^{(g)}/n_g$ based on the multinomial distribution. We define $n_C^{(g)}(z_1, z_2)$ as the number of patients with responses at period z_1 lower than their responses at period z_2 in group g. Similarly, we define $n_D^{(g)}(z_1, z_2)$ as the number of patients with responses at period z_1 higher than their responses at period z_2 in group g. For example, $n_C^{(g)}(1,2) = \sum_{r=1}^{L-1}\sum_{s=r+1}^{L}n_{rs+}^{(g)}$ and $n_D^{(g)}(1,2) = \sum_{r=2}^{L}\sum_{s=1}^{r-1}n_{rs+}^{(g)}$. When substituting $\hat{\pi}_{rst}^{(g)}$ for $\pi_{rst}^{(g)}$ in $\Pi_C^{(g)}(z_1, z_2)$ and $\Pi_D^{(g)}(z_1, z_2)$, we obtain $\hat{\Pi}_C^{(g)}(z_1, z_2) = n_C^{(g)}(z_1, z_2)/n_g$ and $\hat{\Pi}_D^{(g)}(z_1, z_2) = n_D^{(g)}(z_1, z_2)/n_g$. Thus, we obtain the consistent estimator for $GOR^{(g)}(z_1, z_2)$ (8.5) as

$$\widehat{GOR}^{(g)}(z_1, z_2) = \hat{\Pi}_C^{(g)}(z_1, z_2)/\hat{\Pi}_D^{(g)}(z_1, z_2). \tag{8.12}$$

Using the delta method, we obtain an estimated asymptotic variance (Problem 8.4) of $\widehat{GOR}^{(g)}(z_1, z_2)$ (8.12) with the logarithmic transformation as given by

$$\widehat{Var}\left(\log\left(\widehat{GOR}^{(g)}(z_1, z_2)\right)\right) = \left(\hat{\Pi}_C^{(g)}(z_1, z_2) + \hat{\Pi}_D^{(g)}(z_1, z_2)\right)/\left(n_g\hat{\Pi}_C^{(g)}(z_1, z_2)\hat{\Pi}_D^{(g)}(z_1, z_2)\right). \tag{8.13}$$

When substituting $\widehat{GOR}^{(g)}(z_1, z_2)$ (8.12) for $GOR^{(g)}(z_1, z_2)$ in (8.6), we obtain the following three consistent estimators for GOR_{AC} as

$$\left(\widehat{GOR}^{(1)}(1,2)/\widehat{GOR}^{(3)}(1,2)\right)^{1/2} = \left[\left(n_C^{(1)}(1,2)n_D^{(3)}(1,2)\right)/\left(n_D^{(1)}(1,2)n_C^{(3)}(1,2)\right)\right]^{1/2},$$
$$\left(\widehat{GOR}^{(2)}(1,3)/\widehat{GOR}^{(4)}(1,3)\right)^{1/2} = \left[\left(n_C^{(2)}(1,3)n_D^{(4)}(1,3)\right)/\left(n_D^{(2)}(1,3)n_C^{(4)}(1,3)\right)\right]^{1/2}, \text{ and}$$
$$\left(\widehat{GOR}^{(5)}(2,3)/\widehat{GOR}^{(6)}(2,3)\right)^{1/2} = \left[\left(n_C^{(5)}(2,3)n_D^{(6)}(2,3)\right)/\left(n_D^{(5)}(2,3)n_C^{(6)}(2,3)\right)\right]^{1/2}. \tag{8.14}$$

For convenience, we define three 2×2 tables, each table k (= 1, 2, 3) consisting of frequency h_{ijk} in cell (i, j) (for $i, j = 1, 2$) with h_{ijk}'s defined by

$$\left(h_{111} = n_C^{(1)}(1,2), h_{121} = n_C^{(3)}(1,2), h_{211} = n_D^{(1)}(1,2), h_{221} = n_D^{(3)}(1,2)\right),$$

$$\left(h_{112} = n_C^{(2)}(1,3), h_{122} = n_C^{(4)}(1,3), h_{212} = n_D^{(2)}(1,3), h_{222} = n_D^{(4)}(1,3)\right), \text{ and} \quad (8.15)$$

$$\left(h_{113} = n_C^{(5)}(2,3), h_{123} = n_C^{(6)}(2,3), h_{213} = n_D^{(5)}(2,3), h_{223} = n_D^{(6)}(2,3)\right).$$

On the basis of (8.12)–(8.15), we may obtain the commonly used WLS estimator for GOR_{AC} as given by (Fleiss, 1981)

$$\widehat{GOR}_{AC}^{(WLS)} = \sum_k W_k \left(\widehat{OR}_k\right)^{1/2} \Big/ \left(\sum_k W_k\right), \quad (8.16)$$

where $\widehat{OR}_k = (h_{11k}h_{22k})/(h_{12k}h_{21k})$, and $W_k = 1/\widehat{Var}\left(\log\left(\widehat{OR}_k\right)\right) = [1/h_{11k} + 1/h_{12k} + 1/h_{21k} + 1/h_{22k}]^{-1}$.

Similarly, we define three 2×2 tables, each table k (= 1, 2, 3) consisting of frequency h_{ijk}^* in cell (i, j) (for $i, j = 1, 2$) with h_{ijk}^*'s defined by

$$\left(h_{111}^* = n_C^{(1)}(1,3), h_{121}^* = n_C^{(6)}(1,3), h_{211}^* = n_D^{(1)}(1,3), h_{221}^* = n_D^{(6)}(1,3)\right),$$

$$\left(h_{112}^* = n_C^{(2)}(1,2), h_{122}^* = n_C^{(5)}(1,2), h_{212}^* = n_D^{(2)}(1,2), h_{222}^* = n_D^{(5)}(1,2)\right), \text{ and} \quad (8.17)$$

$$\left(h_{113}^* = n_C^{(3)}(2,3), h_{123}^* = n_C^{(4)}(2,3), h_{213}^* = n_D^{(3)}(2,3), h_{223}^* = n_D^{(4)}(2,3)\right).$$

Thus, on the basis of (8.7) and (8.17), we obtain the WLS estimator for GOR_{BC} as

$$\widehat{GOR}_{BC}^{(WLS)} = \sum_k W_k^* \left(\widehat{OR}_k^*\right)^{1/2} \Big/ \left(\sum_k W_k^*\right), \quad (8.18)$$

where $\widehat{OR}_k^* = (h_{11k}^* h_{22k}^*)/(h_{12k}^* h_{21k}^*)$, and $W_k^* = 1/\widehat{Var}\left(\log\left(\widehat{OR}_k^*\right)\right) = [1/h_{11k}^* + 1/h_{12k}^* + 1/h_{21k}^* + 1/h_{22k}^*]^{-1}$.

Also, we define three 2×2 tables, each table k (= 1, 2, 3) consisting of frequency h_{ijk}^{**} in cell (i, j) (for $i, j = 1, 2$) with h_{ijk}^{**}'s defined by

$$\left(h_{111}^{**} = n_C^{(1)}(2,3), h_{121}^{**} = n_C^{(2)}(2,3), h_{211}^{**} = n_D^{(1)}(2,3), h_{221}^{**} = n_D^{(2)}(2,3)\right),$$

$$\left(h_{112}^{**} = n_C^{(3)}(1,3), h_{122}^{**} = n_C^{(5)}(1,3), h_{212}^{**} = n_D^{(3)}(1,3), h_{222}^{**} = n_D^{(5)}(1,3)\right), \text{ and} \quad (8.19)$$

$$\left(h_{113}^{**} = n_C^{(4)}(1,2), h_{123}^{**} = n_C^{(6)}(1,2), h_{213}^{**} = n_D^{(4)}(1,2), h_{223}^{**} = n_D^{(6)}(1,2)\right).$$

On the basis of (8.8) and (8.19), we obtain the WLS estimator for GOR_{BA} as

$$\widehat{GOR}_{BA}^{(WLS)} = \sum_k W_k^{**} \left(\widehat{OR}_k^{**} \right)^{1/2} \Big/ \left(\sum_k W_k^{**} \right), \tag{8.20}$$

where $\widehat{OR}_k^{**} = \left(h_{11k}^{**} h_{22k}^{**} \right) / \left(h_{12k}^{**} h_{21k}^{**} \right)$, and $W_k^{**} = 1 / \widehat{Var} \left(\log \left(\widehat{OR}_k^{**} \right) \right) = \left[1 / h_{11k}^{**} + 1 / h_{12k}^{**} + 1 / h_{21k}^{**} + 1 / h_{22k}^{**} \right]^{-1}$. Note that if $h_{ijk} = 0$ for some cells in a 2×2 table k, we cannot calculate $\widehat{GOR}_{AC}^{(WLS)}$ (8.16). We may apply the commonly used ad hoc arbitrary adjustment procedure for sparse data by adding 0.50 to each observed frequency h_{ijk} in this particular table k. Similarly, we may apply this ad hoc adjustment procedure for sparse data if $h_{ijk}^* = 0$ (or $h_{ijk}^{**} = 0$) for some cells when using $\widehat{GOR}_{BC}^{(WLS)}$ (8.18) [or $\widehat{GOR}_{BA}^{(WLS)}$ (8.20)].

Define $n_{dis}^{(g)}(z_1, z_2) = n_C^{(g)}(z_1, z_2) + n_D^{(g)}(z_1, z_2)$ as the total number of patients with responses falling in different ordinal categories between periods z_1 and z_2 in group g. Given $n_{dis}^{(g)}(z_1, z_2)$ fixed, we can show that $n_C^{(g)}(z_1, z_2)$ follows the binomial distribution with parameters $n_{dis}^{(g)}(z_1, z_2)$ and $\Pi_C^{(g)}(z_1, z_2) / \left(\Pi_C^{(g)}(z_1, z_2) + \Pi_D^{(g)}(z_1, z_2) \right)$ $\left(= GOR^{(g)}(z_1, z_2) / (1 + GOR^{(g)}(z_1, z_2)) \right)$. Thus, we can show that the conditional probability distribution of h_{11k}, given $h_{+1k}, h_{+2k}, h_{1+k}$ and h_{2+k} fixed, is given by (see Problem 3.4)

$$P\left(h_{11k} | h_{+1k}, h_{+2k}, h_{1+k}, h_{2+k}, GOR_{AC}^2 \right) = \frac{\binom{h_{+1k}}{h_{11k}} \binom{h_{+2k}}{h_{1+k} - h_{11k}} \left(GOR_{AC}^2 \right)^{h_{11k}}}{\sum_{x_k} \binom{h_{+1k}}{x_k} \binom{h_{+2k}}{h_{1+k} - x_k} \left(GOR_{AC}^2 \right)^{x_k}}, \tag{8.21}$$

where the summation of x_k in the denominator is calculated over $a_k \leq x_k \leq b_k$, $a_k = \max\{0, h_{1+k} - h_{+2k}\}$, and $b_k = \min\{h_{+1k}, h_{1+k}\}$ for $k = 1, 2, 3$. Thus, the joint conditional probability distribution of $\underline{h}_{11} = (h_{111}, h_{112}, h_{113})'$ is simply

$$P\left(h_{111}, h_{112}, h_{113} | \underline{h}_{+1}, \underline{h}_{+2}, \underline{h}_{1+}, \underline{h}_{2+}, GOR_{AC}^2 \right)$$

$$= \prod_{k=1}^3 \frac{\binom{h_{+1k}}{h_{11k}} \binom{h_{+2k}}{h_{1+k} - h_{11k}} \left(GOR_{AC}^2 \right)^{h_{11k}}}{\sum_{x_k} \binom{h_{+1k}}{x_k} \binom{h_{+2k}}{h_{1+k} - x_k} \left(GOR_{AC}^2 \right)^{x_k}}, \tag{8.22}$$

where $\underline{h}_{u+} = (h_{u+1}, h_{u+2}, h_{u+3})'$ for $u = 1, 2$, and $\underline{h}_{+v} = (h_{+v1}, h_{+v2}, h_{+v3})'$ for $v = 1, 2$. The probability mass function for a given value h_{11+}^0 $(= h_{111}^0 + h_{112}^0 + h_{113}^0)$ based on (8.22) is then given by

$$P\left(h_{11+} = h_{11+}^0 \mid \underline{h}_{+1}, \underline{h}_{+2}, \underline{h}_{1+}, \underline{h}_{2+}, GOR_{AC}^2\right)$$

$$= \sum_{\underline{h}_{11} \in C\left(h_{11+}^0\right)} \prod_{k=1}^3 \frac{\binom{h_{+1k}}{h_{11k}} \binom{h_{+2k}}{h_{1+k}-h_{11k}} \left(GOR_{AC}^2\right)^{h_{11k}}}{\sum_{x_k} \binom{h_{+1k}}{x_k} \binom{h_{+2k}}{h_{1+k}-x_k} \left(GOR_{AC}^2\right)^{x_k}}, \tag{8.23}$$

where $C\left(h_{11+}^0\right) = \left\{\left(h_{111}, h_{112}, h_{113}\right)' \mid h_{111} + h_{112} + h_{113} = h_{11+}^0, a_k \le h_{11k} \le b_k, k = 1, 2, 3\right\}$.
Following the same arguments as for deriving (8.21)–(8.23), we can derive the conditional probability mass function for h_{11+}^* (or h_{11+}^{**}) as given by (8.23) with replacing h_{ijk} by h_{ijk}^* (or h_{ijk}^{**}) and GOR_{AC} by GOR_{BC} (or GOR_{BA}).

8.1   Testing non-equality of treatments

From (8.6), (8.14), and (8.15), GOR_{AC} represents the square root of the underlying common OR of responses across the three 2×2 tables consisting of observed cell frequencies $(h_{11k}, h_{12k}, h_{21k}, h_{22k})$ for $k = 1$, 2, 3. Thus, $GOR_{AC} = 1$ if and only if the underlying common OR equals 1. Furthermore, we can see from equations (8.7), (8.8), (8.17), and (8.19) that GOR_{BC} and GOR_{BA} represent the square roots of the underlying common OR across the three 2×2 tables consisting of observed cell frequencies $\left(h_{11k}^*, h_{12k}^*, h_{21k}^*, h_{22k}^*\right)$ and $\left(h_{11k}^{**}, h_{12k}^{**}, h_{21k}^{**}, h_{22k}^{**}\right)$, respectively. Therefore, we have $GOR_{BC} = 1$ or $GOR_{BA} = 1$ if and only if the underlying common OR of the corresponding three 2×2 tables equals 1. These results suggest that we should be able to apply all summary test procedures and interval estimators for a series of 2×2 tables discussed elsewhere (Fleiss, 1981; Agresti, 1990; Lui, 2004) to do hypothesis testing and interval estimation when studying GOR_{AC}, GOR_{BC}, or GOR_{BA}.

8.1.1   Asymptotic test procedures

When testing the null hypothesis $H_0 : GOR_{AC} = 1$ (or equivalently, $\eta_{AC} = 0$) versus the alternative hypothesis $H_a : GOR_{AC} \ne 1$, we may consider using the WLS summary test procedure. We will reject $H_0 : GOR_{AC} = 1$ at the α-level if

$$\hat{\eta}_{AC}^2 / \widehat{Var}(\hat{\eta}_{AC}) > Z_{\alpha/2}^2, \tag{8.24}$$

where $\hat{\eta}_{AC} = \sum_{k=1}^3 W_k \log\left(\widehat{OR}_k\right) / \left(2 \sum_{k=1}^3 W_k\right)$, $W_k = (1/h_{11k} + 1/h_{12k} + 1/h_{21k} +$
$1/h_{22k})^{-1}$, $\widehat{OR}_k = (h_{11k} h_{22k})/(h_{12k} h_{21k})$, $\widehat{Var}(\hat{\eta}_{AC}) = 1/\left(4 \sum_{k=1}^3 W_k\right)$, and Z_α is the upper $100(\alpha)$th percentile of the standard normal distribution.

When applying the WLS summary procedure to test $H_0 : GOR_{BC} = 1$ versus $H_a : GOR_{BC} \neq 1$, we will reject H_0 at the α-level if

$$(\hat{\eta}_{BC}^2)/\widehat{Var}(\hat{\eta}_{BC}) > Z_{\alpha/2}^2, \tag{8.25}$$

where $\hat{\eta}_{BC} = \sum_{k=1}^{3} W_k^* \log\left(\widehat{OR}_k^*\right)/\left(2\sum_{k=1}^{3} W_k^*\right)$, $W_k^* = \left(1/h_{11k}^* + 1/h_{12k}^* + 1/h_{21k}^* + 1/h_{22k}^*\right)^{-1}$, $\widehat{OR}_k^* = \left(h_{11k}^* h_{22k}^*\right)/\left(h_{12k}^* h_{21k}^*\right)$, and $\widehat{Var}(\hat{\eta}_{BC}) = 1/\left(4\sum_{k=1}^{3} W_k^*\right)$.

Similarly, when testing $H_0 : GOR_{BA} = 1$ versus $H_a : GOR_{BA} \neq 1$, we will reject H_0 at the α-level if

$$(\hat{\eta}_{BA}^2)/\widehat{Var}(\hat{\eta}_{BA}) > Z_{\alpha/2}^2, \tag{8.26}$$

where $\hat{\eta}_{BA} = \sum_{k=1}^{3} W_k^{**} \log\left(\widehat{OR}_k^{**}\right)/\left(2\sum_{k=1}^{3} W_k^{**}\right)$, $W_k^{**} = \left(1/h_{11k}^{**} + 1/h_{12k}^{**} + 1/h_{21k}^{**} + 1/h_{22k}^{**}\right)^{-1}$, $\widehat{OR}_k^{**} = \left(h_{11k}^{**} h_{22k}^{**}\right)/\left(h_{12k}^{**} h_{21k}^{**}\right)$, and $\widehat{Var}(\hat{\eta}_{BA}) = 1/\left(4\sum_{k=1}^{3} W_k^{**}\right)$.

Note that if any h_{ijk} (h_{ijk}^* or h_{ijk}^{**}) for some cells is 0, then we cannot apply the WLS test procedure (8.24) ((8.25) or (8.26)). To alleviate this concern, we may apply either the ad hoc adjustment procedure for sparse data as described previously or the following MH summary test procedure (Fleiss, 1981; Agresti, 1990; Lui, 2004). Note that $GOR_{AC} = 1$ if and only if $GOR_{AC}^2 = 1$. Based on (8.6) and (8.15), we will reject $H_0 : GOR_{AC} = 1$ at the α-level if the following MH test statistic

$$\left(\sum_k h_{11k} - \sum_k h_{1+k}h_{+1k}/h_{++k}\right)^2 / \left\{\sum_k h_{1+k}h_{2+k}h_{+1k}h_{+2k}/[h_{++}k2(h_{++k}-1)]\right\} > Z_{\alpha/2}^2. \tag{8.27}$$

When using the MH procedure to test $H_0 : GOR_{BC} = 1$ versus $H_a : GOR_{BC} \neq 1$, we will reject H_0 at the α-level if the following MH test statistic

$$\left(\sum_k h_{11k}^* - \sum_k h_{1+k}^* h_{+1k}^* / h_{++k}^*\right)^2 / \left\{\sum_k h_{1+k}^* h_{2+k}^* h_{+1k}^* h_{+2k}^* / \left[\left(h_{++k}^*\right)^2\left(h_{++k}^*-1\right)\right]\right\} > Z_{\alpha/2}^2. \tag{8.28}$$

Similarly, when using the MH procedure to test $H_0 : GOR_{BA} = 1$ versus $H_a : GOR_{BA} \neq 1$, we will reject H_0 at the α-level if the following MH test statistic

$$\left(\sum_k h_{11k}^{**} - \sum_k h_{1+k}^{**} h_{+1k}^{**} / h_{++k}^{**}\right)^2 / \left\{\sum_k h_{1+k}^{**} h_{2+k}^{**} h_{+1k}^{**} h_{+2k}^{**} / \left[\left(h_{++k}^{**}\right)^2\left(h_{++k}^{**}-1\right)\right]\right\} > Z_{\alpha/2}^2. \tag{8.29}$$

8.1.2   Exact test procedure

When the number $n_C^{(g)}(z_1, z_2)$ or $n_D^{(g)}(z_1, z_2)$ for some pairs (z_1, z_2) in group g is small, we may consider use of the test procedure based on the exact conditional distribution (8.23). Note that the conditional probability distribution of h_{11+}^0 $(= h_{111}^0 + h_{112}^0 + h_{113}^0)$ when $GOR_{AC} = 1$ simplifies to

$$P\left(h_{11+} = h_{11+}^0 \mid \underline{h}_{+1}, \underline{h}_{+2}, \underline{h}_{1+}, \underline{h}_{2+}, GOR_{AC}^2 = 1\right)$$

$$= \sum_{\underline{h}_{11} \in C\left(h_{11+}^0\right)} \prod_{k=1}^{3} \frac{\binom{h_{+1k}}{h_{11k}} \binom{h_{+2k}}{h_{1+k} - h_{11k}}}{\binom{h_{++k}}{h_{1+k}}}, \qquad (8.30)$$

where $C\left(h_{11+}^0\right) = \left\{ (h_{111}, h_{112}, h_{113})' \mid h_{111} + h_{112} + h_{113} = h_{11+}^0, a_k \le h_{11k} \le b_k \right\}$. On the basis of (8.30), we will reject $H_0 : GOR_{BC} = 1$ at the α-level if we obtain h_{11+}^0 such that

$$\min\left\{ P\left(h_{11+} \le h_{11+}^0 \mid \underline{h}_{+1}, \underline{h}_{+2}, \underline{h}_{1+}, \underline{h}_{2+}, GOR_{AC}^2 = 1\right) \right.$$
$$\left. P\left(h_{11+} \ge h_{11+}^0 \mid \underline{h}_{+1}, \underline{h}_{+2}, \underline{h}_{1+}, \underline{h}_{2+}, GOR_{AC}^2 = 1\right) \right\} \le \alpha/2. \qquad (8.31)$$

Similarly, when testing $H_0 : GOR_{BC} = 1$ (or $H_0 : GOR_{BA} = 1$), we can employ the exact test procedure based on the critical region (8.31) with substituting h_{ijk}^* (or h_{ijk}^{**}) for h_{ijk}.

Example 8.1   Consider the data in Table 8.1 taken from a crossover trial comparing an analgesic at low (L) and high (H) doses with a placebo (P) for relief of pain in primary dysmenorrhea patients (Kenward and Jones, 1991, p. 1608). Here, we regard the low and high doses as treatments A and B, as well as placebo as treatment C. There were 86 patients randomly assigned to one of six groups distinguished by treatment-receipt sequences: P-L-H ($g = 1$); P-H-L ($g = 2$); L-P-H ($g = 3$); L-H-P ($g = 4$); H-P-L ($g = 5$); and H-L-P ($g = 6$). At the end of each treatment period, each patient was assessed the extent of relief on the ordinal scale: none, moderate, and complete. We code these as 1, 2, and 3, respectively. When applying the WLS procedures (8.24) and (8.25), the MH procedures (8.27) and (8.28), as well as the corresponding exact test procedure to test $H_0 : GOR_{AC} = 1$ (or $H_0 : \eta_{AC} = 0$) and $H_0 : GOR_{BC} = 1$ (or $H_0 : \eta_{BC} = 0$), we obtain all the p-values < 0.0001. These suggest that there may be strong evidence that taking either the low or high dose of the analgesic versus the placebo can affect the relief of pain in primary dysmenorrhea. Furthermore, to study the effect on the relief extent of pain between the high and low doses, we apply the WLS and MH procedures (8.26) and (8.29), as well as the exact procedure to test $H_0 : GOR_{BA} = 1$. We obtain the p-values 0.433, 0.447, and 0.649, respectively. Thus, we have no significant evidence that there is a difference in the relief extent of pain between the high and low doses.

8.2 Testing non-inferiority of an experimental treatment to an active control treatment

When treatment C represents an active control treatment, we may sometimes want to assess whether either treatment A or treatment B is non-inferior (rather than equal) to treatment C. This leads us to test $H_0 : GOR_{AC} \leq GOR_l$ and $GOR_{BC} \leq GOR_l$ (where $0 < GOR_l < 1$) versus $H_a : GOR_{AC} > GOR_l$ or $GOR_{BC} > GOR_l$, where GOR_l is the maximum clinically acceptable low margin such that treatment A (or treatment B) can be regarded as non-inferior to treatment C when $GOR_{AC} > GOR_l$ (or $GOR_{BC} > GOR_l$) holds. Some discussions on how to determine the non-inferior margin based on the GOR can be found in Chapter 4. When testing $H_0 : GOR_{AC} \leq GOR_l$ and $GOR_{BC} \leq GOR_l$ we will reject H_0 at the α-level if either of the following two inequalities holds:

$$
\begin{aligned}
(\hat{\eta}_{AC} - \log(GOR_l)) / \sqrt{\widehat{Var}(\hat{\eta}_{AC})} > Z_{\alpha/2}, \text{ or} \\
(\hat{\eta}_{BC} - \log(GOR_l)) / \sqrt{\widehat{Var}(\hat{\eta}_{BC})} > Z_{\alpha/2}.
\end{aligned}
\tag{8.32}
$$

Note that if some of observed frequencies h_{ijk} or h_{ijk}^* are small, we may consider use of the exact test procedure for testing $H_0 : GOR_{AC} \leq GOR_l$ and $GOR_{BC} \leq GOR_l$. On the basis of the conditional distribution (8.23) and its corresponding probability mass function for the random variable h_{11+}^* $(= h_{111}^* + h_{112}^* + h_{113}^*)$, we will reject $H_0 :$ $GOR_{AC} \leq GOR_l$ and $GOR_{BC} \leq GOR_l$ at the α-level if we observe $(h_{11+}^0, h_{11+}^{*0})$ such that

$$
\begin{aligned}
P\left(h_{11+} \geq h_{11+}^0 \mid \underline{h}_{+1}, \underline{h}_{+2}, \underline{h}_{1+}, \underline{h}_{2+}, GOR_l^2\right) < \alpha/2, \text{ or} \\
P\left(h_{11+}^* \geq h_{11+}^{*0} \mid \underline{h}_{+1}^*, \underline{h}_{+2}^*, \underline{h}_{1+}^*, \underline{h}_{2+}^*, GOR_l^2\right) < \alpha/2.
\end{aligned}
\tag{8.33}
$$

We claim that treatment A (or treatment B) is non-inferior to treatment C when $P\left(h_{11+} \geq h_{11+}^0 \mid \underline{h}_{+1}, \underline{h}_{+2}, \underline{h}_{1+}, \underline{h}_{2+}, GOR_l^2\right)$ (or $P\left(h_{11+}^* \geq h_{11+}^{*0} \mid \underline{h}_{+1}^*, \underline{h}_{+2}^*, \underline{h}_{1+}^*, \underline{h}_{2+}^*, GOR_l^2\right)) < \alpha/2$.

8.3 Testing equivalence between an experimental treatment and an active control treatment

Using the intersection-union test (Casella and Berger, 1990), we can modify procedures for testing non-inferiority to accommodate testing equivalence. When testing equivalence between either treatment A or B and an active control treatment C with respect to the GOR, we want to test $H_0 : (GOR_{AC} \leq GOR_l$ or $GOR_{AC} \geq GOR_u)$ and $(GOR_{BC} \leq GOR_l$ or $GOR_{BC} \geq GOR_u)$ versus $H_a : (GOR_l < GOR_{AC} < GOR_u)$ or $(GOR_l < GOR_{BC} < GOR_u)$, where GOR_l and GOR_u are the maximum clinically acceptable margins such that treatment A (or treatment B) can be regarded as equivalent to an active control treatment C when $GOR_l < GOR_{AC} < GOR_u$

(or $GOR_l < GOR_{BC} < GOR_u$) holds. Thus, when applying $\hat{\eta}_{AC}$ and $\hat{\eta}_{BC}$ to test equivalence, we will reject H_0 at the α-level if either of the following two sets of inequalities holds:

$$(\hat{\eta}_{AC} - \log(GOR_l))/\sqrt{\widehat{Var}(\hat{\eta}_{AC})} > Z_{\alpha/2} \text{ and}$$

$$(\hat{\eta}_{AC} - \log(GOR_u))/\sqrt{\widehat{Var}(\hat{\eta}_{AC})} < -Z_{\alpha/2}; \text{ or}$$

$$(\hat{\eta}_{BC} - \log(GOR_l))/\sqrt{\widehat{Var}(\hat{\eta}_{BC})} > Z_{\alpha/2} \text{ and}$$

$$(\hat{\eta}_{BC} - \log(GOR_u))/\sqrt{\widehat{Var}(\hat{\eta}_{BC})} < -Z_{\alpha/2}. \tag{8.34}$$

Note that if some of observed frequencies h_{ijk} or h_{ijk}^* are small, we may apply the exact test procedure to test $H_0 : (GOR_{AC} \le GOR_l \text{ or } GOR_{AC} \ge GOR_u)$ and $(GOR_{BC} \le GOR_l \text{ or } GOR_{BC} \ge GOR_u)$. On the basis of the conditional distribution (8.23) and its corresponding probability mass function for the random variable h_{11+}^*, we will reject H_0 at the α-level if we obtain $(h_{11+}^0, h_{11+}^{*0})$ such that

$$P\left(h_{11+} \ge h_{11+}^0 \mid \underline{h}_{+1}, \underline{h}_{+2}, \underline{h}_{1+}, \underline{h}_{2+}, GOR_l^2\right) < \alpha/2 \text{ and}$$

$$P\left(h_{11+} \le h_{11+}^0 \mid \underline{h}_{+1}, \underline{h}_{+2}, \underline{h}_{1+}, \underline{h}_{2+}, GOR_u^2\right) < \alpha/2; \text{ or}$$

$$P\left(h_{11+}^* \ge h_{11+}^{*0} \mid \underline{h}_{+1}^*, \underline{h}_{+2}^*, \underline{h}_{1+}^*, \underline{h}_{2+}^*, GOR_l^2\right) < \alpha/2 \text{ and}$$

$$P\left(h_{11+}^* \le h_{11+}^{*0} \mid \underline{h}_{+1}^*, \underline{h}_{+2}^*, \underline{h}_{1+}^*, \underline{h}_{2+}^*, GOR_u^2\right) < \alpha/2. \tag{8.35}$$

8.4   Interval estimation of the GOR

It is always of importance to obtain an interval estimator of the relative effect between treatments in a crossover trial. When all observed frequencies h_{ijk} are large, we employ the WLS method to obtain an asymptotic $100(1 - \alpha)\%$ confidence interval for GOR_{AC} as given by

$$\left[\exp\left\{\hat{\eta}_{AC} - Z_{\alpha/2}\Big/\sqrt{\left(4\sum_{k=1}^{3} W_k\right)}\right\}, \exp\left\{\hat{\eta}_{AC} + Z_{\alpha/2}\Big/\sqrt{\left(4\sum_{k=1}^{3} W_k\right)}\right\}\right]. \tag{8.36}$$

When some of the observed frequencies h_{ijk} are not large, the weights used in the WLS method can be subject to a large variation, and hence the interval estimator based on the WLS method can lose accuracy. This may lead us to consider use of the MH point estimator as given by

$$\widehat{GOR}_{AC}^{(MH)} = \left(\left(\sum_{k=1}^{3} h_{11k}h_{22k}/h_{++k}\right)\Big/\left(\sum_{k=1}^{3} h_{12k}h_{21k}/h_{++k}\right)\right)^{1/2}. \tag{8.37}$$

As given elsewhere (Robins, Breslow, and Greenland, 1986; Agresti, 1990), the asymptotic variance for $\log\left(\widehat{GOR}_{AC}^{(MH)}\right)$ is given by

$$\widehat{Var}\left(\log\left(\widehat{GOR}_{AC}^{(MH)}\right)\right) = \left\{ \frac{\sum_k (h_{11k}+h_{22k})(h_{11k}h_{22k})/h_{++k}^2}{2\left(\sum_k h_{11k}h_{22k}/h_{++k}\right)^2} \right.$$

$$+ \frac{\sum_k [(h_{11k}+h_{22k})(h_{12k}h_{21k}) + (h_{12k}+h_{21k})(h_{11k}h_{22k})]/h_{++k}^2}{2\left(\sum_k h_{11k}h_{22k}/h_{++k}\right)\left(\sum_k h_{12k}h_{21k}/h_{++k}\right)}$$

$$\left. + \frac{\sum_k (h_{12k}+h_{21k})(h_{12k}h_{21k})/h_{++k}^2}{2\left(\sum_k h_{12k}h_{21k}/h_{++k}\right)^2} \right\} /4. \tag{8.38}$$

On the basis of (8.37) and (8.38), we obtain an asymptotic $100(1-\alpha)\%$ confidence interval for GOR_{AC} based on the MH estimator as given by

$$\left[\widehat{GOR}_{AC}^{(MH)} \exp\left(-Z_{\alpha/2}\sqrt{\widehat{Var}\left(\log\left(\widehat{GOR}_{AC}^{(MH)}\right)\right)} \right) \right.$$
$$\left. \widehat{GOR}_{AC}^{(MH)} \exp\left(Z_{\alpha/2}\sqrt{\widehat{Var}\left(\log\left(\widehat{GOR}_{AC}^{(MH)}\right)\right)} \right) \right]. \tag{8.39}$$

When the observed frequencies h_{ijk} are small, we can derive an exact interval estimator based on the conditional distribution (8.23) for GOR_{AC} (Gart, 1970; Zelen, 1971; Breslow and Day, 1980).

Given an observed value h_{11+}^0 $(= h_{111}^0 + h_{112}^0 + h_{113}^0)$, we obtain an exact $100(1-\alpha)\%$ confidence interval for GOR_{AC} as given by (Gart, 1970)

$$[GOR_{ACL}, GOR_{ACU}], \tag{8.40}$$

where GOR_{ACL} and GOR_{ACU} are the solutions of the following two equations: $P\left(h_{11+} \geq h_{11+}^0 \mid \underline{h}_{+1}, \underline{h}_{+2}, \underline{h}_{1+}, \underline{h}_{2+}, GOR_{ACL}^2\right) = \alpha/2$, and $P\left(h_{11+} \leq h_{11+}^0 \mid \underline{h}_{+1}, \underline{h}_{+2}, \underline{h}_{1+}, \underline{h}_{2+}, GOR_{ACU}^2\right) = \alpha/2$. We may obtain the corresponding asymptotic and exact $100(1-\alpha)\%$ confidence intervals for GOR_{BC} (or GOR_{BA}) by replacing h_{ijk} with h_{ijk}^* (or h_{ijk}^{**}) in (8.36)–(8.40).

Example 8.2   When using $\widehat{GOR}_{AC}^{(WLS)}$ (8.16) and $\widehat{GOR}_{AC}^{(MH)}$ (8.37), we obtain estimates of GOR_{AC} as 6.652 and 7.080, respectively. These translate to the probability that a patient taking the low dose of analgesic has better outcomes than a patient taking the placebo approximately 6.5 to 7 times the probability that the former has worse outcomes than the latter. When employing asymptotic interval estimators (8.36),

(8.39), and the exact interval estimator (8.40), we obtain 95% confidence intervals for GOR_{AC} as [2.654, 13.431], [2.833, 17.691], and [2.784, 22.997], respectively. Because all these lower limits fall above 1, we may conclude that there is evidence that taking the low dose of the analgesic affects the patient response with respect to the relief extent of pain in primary dysmenorrhea. This is consistent with the previous findings based on hypothesis testing. Similarly, when employing $\widehat{GOR}_{BC}^{(WLS)}$ (8.18) and $\widehat{GOR}_{BC}^{(MH)}$ (obtained by substituting h_{ijk}^* for h_{ijk} in (8.37)) to assess the effect of the high dose relative to the placebo, we obtain 8.099 and 7.527, respectively. Furthermore, when using the WLS and MH interval estimators with the logarithmic transformation as well as the exact interval estimator, we obtain the 95% confidence intervals for the GOR_{BC} as [3.478, 16.802], [3.430, 16.521], and [3.141, 17.953], respectively. To assess the dose effect between the high and low doses, we obtain $\widehat{GOR}_{BA}^{(WLS)} = 1.291$ and $\widehat{GOR}_{BA}^{(MH)} = 1.290$, as well as the asymptotic WLS, MH, and exact 95% confidence intervals as given by [0.683, 2.438], [0.683, 2.438], and [0.622, 2.570]. On the basis of these results, we may conclude that though taking the high dose of the analgesic slightly increases the extent of relief in pain as compared with taking the low dose, this increase is not significant at the 5% level.

8.5   Hypothesis testing and estimation for period effects

In a crossover trial, we may wish to study whether there are period effects. Note that under model (8.5), we can easily see that the GOR of patient responses between periods 2 and 1 is (Problem 8.5)

$$GOR_{21} = \exp(\gamma_1) = \left(GOR^{(1)}(1,2)GOR^{(3)}(1,2) \right)^{1/2}$$

$$= \left(GOR^{(2)}(1,2)GOR^{(5)}(1,2) \right)^{1/2} \qquad (8.41)$$

$$= \left(GOR^{(4)}(1,2)GOR^{(6)}(1,2) \right)^{1/2}.$$

Furthermore, we can show that the GOR of patient responses between periods 3 and 1 is (Problem 8.6)

$$GOR_{31} = \exp(\gamma_2) = \left(GOR^{(1)}(1,3)GOR^{(6)}(1,3) \right)^{1/2}$$

$$= \left(GOR^{(2)}(1,3)GOR^{(4)}(1,3) \right)^{1/2} \qquad (8.42)$$

$$= \left(GOR^{(3)}(1,3)GOR^{(5)}(1,3) \right)^{1/2}.$$

Thus, when substituting $\widehat{GOR}^{(g)}(z_1, z_2)$ for $GOR^{(g)}(z_1, z_2)$ in (8.41), we obtain the following consistent estimators for GOR_{21} as

$$\widehat{ORP}_1 = \left(\widehat{GOR}^{(1)}(1,2)\widehat{GOR}^{(3)}(1,2) \right)^{1/2},$$

$$\widehat{ORP}_2 = \left(\widehat{GOR}^{(2)}(1,2)\widehat{GOR}^{(5)}(1,2) \right)^{1/2}, \text{ and} \qquad (8.43)$$

$$\widehat{ORP}_3 = \left(\widehat{GOR}^{(4)}(1,2)\widehat{GOR}^{(6)}(1,2) \right)^{1/2}.$$

For convenience, we define $(l_{11k}, l_{12k}, l_{21k}, l_{22k})$ (for $k = 1, 2, 3$) as the vector of random frequencies corresponding to the three 2×2 tables, each table k ($= 1, 2, 3$) consisting of frequency l_{ijk} in cell (i,j) (for $i, j = 1, 2$) with l_{ijk}'s defined by

$$\left(l_{111} = n_C^{(1)}(1,2), l_{121} = n_D^{(3)}(1,2), l_{211} = n_D^{(1)}(1,2), l_{221} = n_C^{(3)}(1,2) \right),$$

$$\left(l_{112} = n_C^{(2)}(1,2), l_{122} = n_D^{(5)}(1,2), l_{212} = n_D^{(2)}(1,2), l_{222} = n_C^{(5)}(1,2) \right), \text{ and} \qquad (8.44)$$

$$\left(l_{113} = n_C^{(4)}(1,2), l_{123} = n_D^{(6)}(1,2), l_{213} = n_D^{(4)}(1,2), l_{223} = n_C^{(6)}(1,2) \right).$$

On the basis of (8.41), (8.43), and (8.44), we obtain the WLS estimator for γ_1 as

$$\hat{\gamma}_1 = \sum_k WP_k \log\left(\widehat{ORP}_k \right) / \left(2\sum_k WP_k \right), \qquad (8.45)$$

where $\widehat{ORP}_k = (l_{11k}l_{22k})/(l_{12k}l_{21k})$ and $WP_k = [1/l_{11k} + 1/l_{12k} + 1/l_{21k} + 1/l_{22k}]^{-1}$. The asymptotic variance for $\hat{\gamma}_1$ (8.45) is

$$\widehat{Var}(\hat{\gamma}_1) = 1/\left(4\sum_k WP_k \right). \qquad (8.46)$$

On the basis of (8.45) and (8.46), we will reject $H_0 : GOR_{21} = 1$ at the α-level if

$$(\hat{\gamma}_1)^2 / \widehat{Var}(\hat{\gamma}_1) > Z_{\alpha/2}^2. \qquad (8.47)$$

We may also obtain an asymptotic $100(1 - \alpha)\%$ confidence interval for GOR_{21} based on (8.45) and (8.46) as given by

$$\left[\exp\left\{ \hat{\gamma}_1 - Z_{\alpha/2} / \sqrt{\left(4\sum_{k=1}^3 WP_k \right)} \right\}, \exp\left\{ \hat{\gamma}_1 + Z_{\alpha/2} / \sqrt{\left(4\sum_{k=1}^3 WP_k \right)} \right\} \right]. \qquad (8.48)$$

Following the same idea as that for studying treatment effects, we can derive the MH test procedure and estimator for studying the relative effect between periods 2 and 1 as well. Note that the conditional probability distribution of l_{11k}, given $l_{+1k}, l_{+2k}, l_{1+k}$ and l_{2+k} fixed, is given by

$$P\left(l_{11k}|l_{+1k},l_{+2k},l_{1+k},l_{2+k},GOR_{21}^2\right) = \frac{\binom{l_{+1k}}{l_{11k}}\binom{l_{+2k}}{l_{1+k}-l_{11k}}\left(GOR_{21}^2\right)^{l_{11k}}}{\sum_{x_k}\binom{l_{+1k}}{x_k}\binom{l_{+2k}}{l_{1+k}-x_k}\left(GOR_{21}^2\right)^{x_k}}, \quad (8.49)$$

where the summation of x_k in the denominator is calculated over $ap_k \le x_k \le bp_k$, $ap_k = \max\{0, l_{1+k}-l_{+2k}\}$, and $bp_k = \min\{l_{+1k}, l_{1+k}\}$ for $k = 1, 2, 3$. Thus, the joint conditional probability distribution of $\underline{l}_{11} = (l_{111}, l_{112}, l_{113})'$ is simply

$$P\left(l_{111},l_{112},l_{113}|\underline{l}_{+1},\underline{l}_{+2},\underline{l}_{1+},\underline{l}_{2+},GOR_{21}^2\right)$$
$$= \prod_{k=1}^{3} \frac{\binom{l_{+1k}}{l_{11k}}\binom{l_{+2k}}{l_{1+k}-l_{11k}}\left(GOR_{21}^2\right)^{l_{11k}}}{\sum_{x_k}\binom{l_{+1k}}{x_k}\binom{l_{+2k}}{l_{1+k}-x_k}\left(GOR_{21}^2\right)^{x_k}}, \quad (8.50)$$

where $\underline{l}_{u+} = (l_{u+1}, l_{u+2}, l_{u+3})'$ for $u = 1, 2$, and $\underline{l}_{+v} = (l_{+v1}, l_{+v2}, l_{+v3})'$ for $v = 1, 2$. The probability mass function for a given value l_{11+}^0 based on (8.50) is then given by

$$P\left(l_{11+} = l_{11+}^0|\underline{l}_{+1},\underline{l}_{+2},\underline{l}_{1+},\underline{l}_{2+},GOR_{21}^2\right)$$
$$= \sum_{\underline{l}_{11} \in C\left(l_{11+}^0\right)} \prod_{k=1}^{3} \frac{\binom{l_{+1k}}{l_{11k}}\binom{l_{+2k}}{l_{1+k}-l_{11k}}\left(GOR_{21}^2\right)^{l_{11k}}}{\sum_{x_k}\binom{l_{+1k}}{x_k}\binom{l_{+2k}}{l_{1+k}-x_k}\left(GOR_{21}^2\right)^{x_k}}, \quad (8.51)$$

where $C\left(l_{11+}^0\right) = \left\{(l_{111}, l_{112}, l_{113})'|l_{111}+l_{112}+l_{113} = l_{11+}^0, ap_k \le l_{11k} \le bp_k\right\}$.

Given an observed l_{11+}^0, we obtain an exact $100(1-\alpha)\%$ confidence interval for GOR_{21} as given by (Gart, 1970)

$$[GOR_{21L}, GOR_{21U}], \quad (8.52)$$

where GOR_{21L} and GOR_{21U} are the solutions of the following two equations:

$$P\left(l_{11+} \ge l_{11+}^0|\underline{l}_{+1},\underline{l}_{+2},\underline{l}_{1+},\underline{l}_{2+},GOR_{21L}^2\right) = \alpha/2, \quad \text{and}$$
$$P\left(l_{11+} \le l_{11+}^0|\underline{l}_{+1},\underline{l}_{+2},\underline{l}_{1+},\underline{l}_{2+},GOR_{21U}^2\right) = \alpha/2.$$

Following the same idea as above, we can derive test procedures and interval estimators for GOR_{31} or $GOR_{32}(= \exp(\gamma_2 - \gamma_1))$.

8.6 Procedures for testing treatment-by-period interactions

When employing summary test procedures (8.24)–(8.29) and (8.31), as well as summary interval estimators (8.36), (8.39), and (8.40), we implicitly assume that there is no treatment-by-period interaction. To account for treatment-by-period interactions, we can extend model (8.1) to include the interaction terms between treatments and periods. Following the same idea as for deriving (8.5), we can show that the GOR of responses between periods z_2 and z_1 is

$$
\begin{aligned}
GOR^{(g)}(z_1, z_2) &= P\left(Y_{z_1}^{(g)} < Y_{z_2}^{(g)}\right) / P\left(Y_{z_1}^{(g)} > Y_{z_2}^{(g)}\right) \\
&= \exp\Big(\eta_{AC}\left(X_{z_2 1}^{(g)} - X_{z_1 1}^{(g)}\right) + \eta_{BC}\left(X_{z_2 2}^{(g)} - X_{z_1 2}^{(g)}\right) \\
&\quad + \gamma_1\left(Z_{z_2 1}^{(g)} - Z_{z_1 1}^{(g)}\right) + \gamma_2\left(Z_{z_2 2}^{(g)} - Z_{z_1 2}^{(g)}\right) \\
&\quad + \tau_{11}\left(X_{z_2 1}^{(g)} Z_{z_2 1}^{(g)} - X_{z_1 1}^{(g)} Z_{z_1 1}^{(g)}\right) + \tau_{12}\left(X_{z_2 1}^{(g)} Z_{z_2 2}^{(g)} - X_{z_1 1}^{(g)} Z_{z_1 2}^{(g)}\right) \\
&\quad + \tau_{21}\left(X_{z_2 2}^{(g)} Z_{z_2 1}^{(g)} - X_{z_1 2}^{(g)} Z_{z_1 1}^{(g)}\right) + \tau_{22}\left(X_{z_2 2}^{(g)} Z_{z_2 2}^{(g)} - X_{z_1 2}^{(g)} Z_{z_1 2}^{(g)}\right)\Big),
\end{aligned}
\tag{8.53}
$$

where τ_{11} and τ_{12} denote the interactions between treatment A (versus placebo C) and period effects, and τ_{21} and τ_{22} denote the interactions between treatment B (versus placebo C) and period effects. On the basis of model (8.53), we can show that (Problem 8.7)

$$
\begin{aligned}
OR_1 &= \left(GOR^{(1)}(1,2)/GOR^{(3)}(1,2)\right) = \exp(2\eta_{AC} + \tau_{11}), \\
OR_2 &= \left(GOR^{(2)}(1,3)/GOR^{(4)}(1,3)\right) = \exp(2\eta_{AC} + \tau_{12}), \text{ and} \\
OR_3 &= \left(GOR^{(5)}(2,3)/GOR^{(6)}(2,3)\right) = \exp(2\eta_{AC} + \tau_{11} + \tau_{12}).
\end{aligned}
\tag{8.54}
$$

Note that $OR_1 = OR_2 = OR_3$ if and only if $\tau_{11} = \tau_{12} = 0$. Thus, we can test $H_0 : \tau_{11} = \tau_{12} = 0$ by employing the WLS procedure for testing the homogeneity of OR (Fleiss, 1981). We will reject $H_0 : \tau_{11} = \tau_{12} = 0$ at the α-level if

$$
\sum_{k=1}^{3} W_k \left(\log\left(\widehat{OR}_k\right)\right)^2 - \left(\sum_{k=1}^{3} W_k \log\left(\widehat{OR}_k\right)\right)^2 / \left(\sum_{k=1}^{3} W_k\right) > \chi_\alpha^2(2),
\tag{8.55}
$$

where $\chi_\alpha^2(2)$ stands for the upper $100(\alpha)$th percentile of the chi-squared distribution with two degrees of freedom. Furthermore, we can show that (Problem 8.8)

$$
\begin{aligned}
OR_1^* &= \left(GOR^{(1)}(1,3)/GOR^{(6)}(1,3)\right) = \exp(2\eta_{BC} + \tau_{22}), \\
OR_2^* &= \left(GOR^{(2)}(1,2)/GOR^{(5)}(1,2)\right) = \exp(2\eta_{BC} + \tau_{21}), \text{ and} \\
OR_3^* &= \left(GOR^{(3)}(2,3)/GOR^{(4)}(2,3)\right) = \exp(2\eta_{BC} + \tau_{21} + \tau_{22}).
\end{aligned}
\tag{8.56}
$$

On the basis of (8.56), we will reject $H_0 : \tau_{21} = \tau_{22} = 0$ at the α-level if

$$\sum_{k=1}^{3} W_k^* \left(\log\left(\widehat{OR}_k^* \right) \right)^2 - \left(\sum_{k=1}^{3} W_k^* \log\left(\widehat{OR}_k^* \right) \right)^2 / \left(\sum_{k=1}^{3} W_k^* \right) > \chi_\alpha^2(2). \quad (8.57)$$

Other test procedures (Zelen, 1971; Breslow and Day, 1980; Ejigou and McHugh, 1984) for testing the homogeneity of the OR across table can also be applied to test whether there is a treatment-by-period interaction.

Example 8.3   To illustrate the use of procedures (8.55) (or (8.57)), we consider the data given in Table 8.1. We obtain the p-value 0.517 (or 0.686) for testing whether there are no interactions between treatment A (or treatment B) and two periods. Thus, we may reasonably assume that both effects for the low dose and high dose of the analgesic relative to the placebo on the patient response remain constant across periods.

Note that when there are four treatments, including three experimental treatments A, B, and C, and one placebo D, there are 24 groups in a crossover design with a complete set of different treatment-receipt sequences. This number of groups is likely too large to be of use in practice. We may consider using a Latin square to reduce the number of groups. We summarize the details in Problem 8.9.

8.7   SAS program codes and results for the proportional odds model with normal random effects

When assuming the proportional odds model with normal random effects (Ezzet and Whitehead, 1991), we may apply PROC GLIMMIX (SAS Institute, 2009) to analyze the data in Table 8.1. We present the SAS codes in the following box, in which placebo (coded as 1), low dose (coded as 2), and high dose (coded as 3) are used for the variable "treat."

```
data step1;
input patient treat period response;
datalines;
         1   1   1   1
         1   2   2   1
         1   3   3   2
         2   1   1   1
         2   2   2   1
         2   3   3   3
.... .
```

```
                86  3  1  3
                86  2  2  3
                86  1  3  1
;;;;
proc glimmix;
  class treat period;
    model response= treat period/ solution dist=multinomial
                                  link=cumlogit;
    random intercept /subject=patient;
    estimate 'treatment 3 versus treatment 1' treat -1 0 1;
    estimate 'treatment 2 versus treatment 1' treat -1 1 0;
    estimate 'treatment 3 versus treatment 2' treat 0 -1 1;
    run;
```

For brevity, we present only the partial output regarding the estimates of the relative treatment effects in the following box.

Label	Estimate	Standard Error	DF	t Value	Pr > |t|
	The GLIMMIX Procedure				
treatment 3 versus treatment 1	-2.4156	0.3331	167	-7.25	<.0001
treatment 2 versus treatment 1	-2.0413	0.3265	167	-6.25	<.0001
treatment 3 versus treatment 2	-0.3743	0.2842	167	-1.32	0.1896

On the basis of these estimates (of which the signs are all < 0), we may conclude that both the low dose and high dose can significantly improve, as compared with the placebo, the relief extent of pain at the 5% level; both p-values are < 0.0001. Furthermore, though the high dose can improve the outcome of patients as compared with the low dose, this improvement is not significant at the 5% level. All these test results are the same as those reported previously for using test procedures based on the GOR. For reader's information, we have used "method = quad" (Jones and Kenward, 2014) in the use of PROC GLIMMIX and obtained essentially identical parameter estimates and p-values (to the third decimal places).

The GOR has simple interpretations and is well defined for continuous variables (Agresti, 1980). A few publications discussing estimation of the GOR and its applications under various situations can be found elsewhere (Edwardes and Baltzan, 2000; Lui, 2002a, 2002b, 2004; Lui and Chang, 2013a, 2013b). When using the GOR to summarize the relative effect between treatments, we show that one can apply the WLS and MH summary test procedures or estimators to study the relative effect between treatments in crossover trials. All these asymptotic test procedures or estimators are in closed forms and are valid for use despite the distribution for patient random effects. In practice, we may often encounter sparse data, in which the cell frequencies are, as shown in Table 8.1, small or zero. The likelihood-based methods, such as Wald's tests or Wald's interval estimators derived from large-sample theory, can be inappropriate. By contrast, test procedures and estimators presented here are functions of marginal total frequencies $n_C^{(g)}(z_1, z_2)$ and $n_D^{(g)}(z_1, z_2)$. Thus, use of the proposed conditional approach may have less concern than use of the likelihood-based approach in trials of a small size. Furthermore, the exact test procedures and exact interval estimators derived here are of use when the number of patients in our trials is small and all asymptotic methods are theoretically invalid. Using similar ideas as presented here, we can easily extend all the results, including the exact procedures and interval estimators, to a four-treatment four-period crossover design with use of a Latin square (Problem 8.9).

Exercises

Problem 8.1. Under model (8.5), show that the GOR of treatment A versus treatment C can be expressed as given by equations in (8.6).

Problem 8.2. Under model (8.5), show that the GOR of treatment B versus treatment C can be expressed as given by equations in (8.7).

Problem 8.3. Under model (8.5), show that the GOR of treatment B versus treatment A can be expressed as given by equations in (8.8).

Problem 8.4. Using the delta method, show that an estimated asymptotic variance of $\widehat{GOR}^{(g)}(z_1, z_2)$ (8.12) with the logarithmic transformation is given in (8.13).

Problem 8.5. Under model (8.5), show that the GOR of patient responses between periods 2 and 1 can be expressed as given by equations in (8.41).

Problem 8.6. Under model (8.5), show that the GOR of patient responses between periods 3 and 1 can be expressed as given by equations in (8.42).

Problem 8.7. Under model (8.53), derive equations in (8.54).

Problem 8.8. Under model (8.53), derive equations in (8.56).

Problem 8.9. Suppose that we employ one of the Latin squares (e.g,, the one in the cell (I, 3) on p. 163 in Senn (2002)) for comparing three experimental treatments A, B, and C with a placebo (P). Suppose further that we randomly assign n_g patients to group $g = 1$ with A-C-B-P treatment-receipt sequence; $= 2$ with B-P-A-C treatment-receipt sequence; $= 3$ with C-A-P-B treatment receipt sequence; and $= 4$ with P-B-C-A treatment-receipt sequence. For patient i ($= 1, 2, \cdots, n_g$) assigned to group g ($= 1, 2, 3, 4$), let $Y_{iz}^{(g)}$ denote the patient response at period z ($= 1, 2, 3, 4$), where $Y_{iz}^{(g)}$ takes one of the possible ordinal labels C_j (where $C_1 < C_2 < C_3 < \cdots < C_L$). We let $X_{z1}^{(g)}$, $X_{z2}^{(g)}$, and $X_{z3}^{(g)}$ denote the indicator functions of treatment-receipt for treatments A, B, and C, respectively. We further let $1_{z1}^{(g)}$, $1_{z2}^{(g)}$, and $1_{z3}^{(g)}$ be the indicator functions of period covariate for periods 2, 3, and 4.

(a) Describe what model assumptions for the patient responses $(Y_{iz_1}^{(g)}, Y_{iz_2}^{(g)})$ are so that the GOR for a randomly selected patient from group g can be given by $GOR^{(g)}(z_1, z_2) = P\left(Y_{z_1}^{(g)} < Y_{z_2}^{(g)}\right) / P\left(Y_{z_1}^{(g)} > Y_{z_2}^{(g)}\right) = \exp\left(\eta_{AP}\left(X_{z_2 1}^{(g)} - X_{z_1 1}^{(g)}\right) + \eta_{BP}\left(X_{z_2 2}^{(g)} - X_{z_1 2}^{(g)}\right) + \eta_{CP}\left(X_{z_2 3}^{(g)} - X_{z_1 3}^{(g)}\right) + \gamma_1\left(1_{z_2 1}^{(g)} - 1_{z_1 1}^{(g)}\right) + \gamma_2\left(1_{z_2 2}^{(g)} - 1_{z_1 2}^{(g)}\right) + \gamma_3\left(1_{z_2 3}^{(g)} - 1_{z_1 3}^{(g)}\right)\right)$, where η_{AP}, η_{BP}, and η_{CP} denote the relative effects of treatments A, B, and C versus placebo, and γ_1, γ_2, and γ_3 denote the relative effects of periods 2, 3, and 4 versus period 1.

(b) Under the above model, show that the GOR of responses for treatment A versus placebo is $GOR_{AP} = \exp(\eta_{AP}) = (GOR^{(4)}(1, 4)/GOR^{(1)}(1, 4))^{1/2} = (GOR^{(2)}(2, 3)/GOR^{(3)}(2, 3))^{1/2}$.

(c) Show that the GOR of responses for treatment B versus placebo is $GOR_{BP} = \exp(\eta_{BP}) = (GOR^{(3)}(3, 4)/GOR^{(1)}(3, 4))^{1/2} = (GOR^{(4)}(1, 2)/GOR^{(2)}(1, 2))^{1/2}$.

(d) Show that the GOR of responses for treatment C versus placebo is $GOR_{CP} = \exp(\eta_{CP}) = \left(GOR^{(2)}(2,4)/GOR^{(1)}(2,4)\right)^{1/2} = (GOR^{(4)}(1, 3)/GOR^{(3)}(1, 3))^{1/2}$.

(e) Discuss how to use the above results to derive the WLS, MH, and exact test procedures and interval estimators (Lui, Chang, and Lin, 2015).

9

Three-treatment three-period crossover design in frequency data

When studying treatments for epilepsy, angina pectoris, and asthma, we often come across count data, such as the number of seizures in epilepsy, the count of episodes in angina pectoris, or the frequency of exacerbations in asthma (Hills and Armitage, 1979; Fleiss, 1986a; Nicholson *et al.*, 1998; Taylor *et al.*, 1998; Senn, 2002; Lemanske *et al.*, 2010). Because we may want to compare two or more experimental treatments with a placebo for reducing the number of patients assigned to receive inert placebo or studying nonlinear dose responses, the extension of results in frequency data from the AB/BA design to a three-treatment three-period crossover design is of use. Since the number of event occurrences is either 0 or a positive integer on a discrete scale and is often skewed to the right, test procedures and estimators derived under the normality assumption are probably not adequate for use in count data. Note that, not like the ordinal data, the frequency data are suitable for arithmetic operations and the mean frequency is meaningful and easily understood.

We focus our attention on count data in situations in which there are three treatments in a three-period crossover trial. For example, consider the trial comprising a 4-week run-in period and three treatment periods of 24 weeks, each of which was followed by a 4-week washout interval (Taylor *et al.*, 1998, 2000). There was a total of 165 patients randomly assigned to six groups with different treatment-receipt sequences. There were five patients ($\approx 3\%$) with incomplete information on the number of exacerbations. We summarize in Table 9.1 the data (kindly provided by Profs. Herbison and Taylor at the University of Otago) regarding the subtotal frequencies of

Crossover Designs: Testing, Estimation, and Sample Size, First Edition. Kung-Jong Lui.
© 2016 John Wiley & Sons, Ltd. Published 2016 by John Wiley & Sons, Ltd.
Companion website: www.wiley.com/go/lui/crossover

Table 9.1   The frequencies $\left(Y^{(g)}_{+1}, Y^{(g)}_{+2}, Y^{(g)}_{+3}\right)'$ of exacerbations at the three periods over n_g patients with complete information on the number of exacerbations in group g (= 1, 2, 3, 4, 5, 6) distinguished with different treatment-receipt sequences.

Group	$\left(Y^{(g)}_{+1}, Y^{(g)}_{+2}, Y^{(g)}_{+3}\right)'$	n_g
P–A–B (g = 1)	(5,4,4)'	27
P–B–A (g = 2)	(26,12,34)'	26
A–P–B (g = 3)	(23,24,3)'	27
A–B–P (g = 4)	(12,1,4)'	26
B–P–A (g = 5)	(9,14,4)'	28
B–A–P (g = 6)	(3,13,19)'	26

P, placebo; A, salbutamol; B, salmeterol.

exacerbations based on the rest of the 160 patients for the three periods in each of the six groups. We want to study whether taking salbutamol (400 ug four times daily) or salmeterol (50 ug twice daily) can reduce, as compared with taking the placebo, the mean frequency of exacerbations in asthma patients.

On the basis of a random effects exponential multiplicative risk model, we assume that the frequency of event occurrences follows a Poisson distribution. We provide asymptotic and exact test procedures for testing non-equality of treatments. We give procedures for testing non-inferiority and equivalence between either of the two experimental treatments and an active control treatment. We address interval estimation of the ratio of mean frequencies between treatments. We discuss hypothesis testing and estimation for period effects. Finally, we show procedures for testing treatment-by-period interactions.

Suppose that we compare two experimental treatments A and B with treatment C (that can be a placebo or an active control treatment) in a three-period crossover trial. We use the treatment-receipt sequence U-V-W to denote that a patient receives treatments U, V, and W at periods 1, 2, and 3, respectively. Suppose that we randomly assign n_g patients to group $g = 1$ with C-A-B treatment-receipt sequence; = 2 with C-B-A treatment-receipt sequence; = 3 with A-C-B treatment-receipt sequence; = 4 with A-B-C treatment-receipt sequence; = 5 with B-C-A treatment-receipt sequence; and = 6 with B-A-C treatment-receipt sequence. For patient i (= 1, 2, $\cdots$, n_g) assigned to group g (= 1, 2, 3, 4, 5, 6), let $Y^{(g)}_{iz}$ denote the frequency of event occurrences at period z (= 1, 2, 3). Let $X^{(g)}_{iz1}$ denote the indicator function of treatment-receipt for treatment A, and $X^{(g)}_{iz1} = 1$ if the corresponding patient at period z receives treatment A, and = 0 otherwise. Similarly, let $X^{(g)}_{iz2}$ denote the indicator function of treatment-receipt for treatment B, and $X^{(g)}_{iz2} = 1$ if the corresponding patient at period

z receives treatment B, and $= 0$ otherwise. Furthermore, we let $Z_{iz1}^{(g)}$ and $Z_{iz2}^{(g)}$ denote the indicator functions of periods 2 and 3 with setting $Z_{iz1}^{(g)} = 1$ for period $z = 2$, and $= 0$ otherwise; and $Z_{iz2}^{(g)} = 1$ for period $z = 3$, and $= 0$ otherwise. As commonly assumed for a crossover design, we assume with an adequate washout period that there is no carry-over effect due to the treatment administered at an earlier period on the patient response. We assume that the frequency $Y_{iz}^{(g)}$ of event occurrences on patient i ($= 1, 2, \cdots, n_g$) assigned to group g ($= 1, 2, \cdots, 6$) at period z ($= 1, 2, 3$) follows the Poisson distribution with mean that can be modeled as

$$E\left(Y_{iz}^{(g)}\right) = \exp\left(\mu_i^{(g)} + \eta_{AC}X_{iz1}^{(g)} + \eta_{BC}X_{iz2}^{(g)} + \gamma_1 Z_{iz1}^{(g)} + \gamma_2 Z_{iz2}^{(g)}\right), \tag{9.1}$$

where $\mu_i^{(g)}$ represents the random effect due to the ith patient assigned to group g and all $\mu_i^{(g)}$'s are assumed to independently follow an unspecified probability density function $f_g(\mu)$; η_{AC} and η_{BC} denote the respective effect of treatments A and B relative to treatment C; and γ_1 and γ_2 denote the respective effect for periods 2 and 3 versus period 1. At a fixed period, the ratio of mean frequencies for a given patient between treatments A and C under model (9.1) is equal to $RM_{AC} = \exp(\eta_{AC})$. If there is no difference in effects between treatments A and C, the ratio of mean frequencies $RM_{AC} = 1$ (or equivalently, $\eta_{AC} = 0$). If treatment A tends to increase (or decrease) the frequency of event occurrences as compared with treatment C, $RM_{AC} > 1$ (or $RM_{AC} < 1$). Similarly, the ratio of mean frequencies between treatments B and C at a fixed period on a given patient is $RM_{BC} = \exp(\eta_{BC})$. Similar interpretations as for RM_{AC} are applicable to RM_{BC}, γ_1, and γ_2. Note that the ratio of mean frequencies between treatments B and A is equal to $RM_{BA} = \exp(\eta_{BC} - \eta_{AC})$.

Conditional upon patient i in group g ($= 1, 2, \cdots, 6$), we can show that the random vector of occurrence frequencies $\left(Y_{i1}^{(g)}, Y_{i2}^{(g)}, Y_{i3}^{(g)}\right)'$ at the three periods, given the sum $Y_{i+}^{(g)} = Y_{i1}^{(g)} + Y_{i2}^{(g)} + Y_{i3}^{(g)} = y_{i+}^{(g)}$ fixed, follows the conditional trinomial distribution with parameters $y_{i+}^{(g)}$ and $\left(p_1^{(g)}, p_2^{(g)}, p_3^{(g)}\right)'$, where $\left(p_1^{(g)}, p_2^{(g)}, p_3^{(g)}\right)'$ are defined in Problem 9.1. Define $Y_{+z}^{(g)} = \sum_{i=1}^{n_g} Y_{iz}^{(g)}$ as the total frequency of event occurrences over n_g patients in group g at period z ($= 1, 2, 3$). Because the vector of cell probabilities $\left(p_1^{(g)}, p_2^{(g)}, p_3^{(g)}\right)'$ does not depend on random effects $\mu_i^{(g)}$, the random vector $\left(Y_{+1}^{(g)}, Y_{+2}^{(g)}, Y_{+3}^{(g)}\right)'$, given $\underline{y}_{-+}^{(g)} = \left(y_{1+}^{(g)}, y_{2+}^{(g)}, \cdots, y_{n_g+}^{(g)}\right)'$ fixed, follows the conditional trinomial distribution with parameters $y_{++}^{(g)}$ ($= \sum_{i=1}^{n_g} y_{i+}^{(g)}$) and $\left(p_1^{(g)}, p_2^{(g)}, p_3^{(g)}\right)'$. Thus, we can estimate $p_z^{(g)}$ by the consistent sample proportion estimator $\hat{p}_z^{(g)} = Y_{+z}^{(g)} / Y_{++}^{(g)}$ for $z = 1, 2, 3$. We will base the following arguments on the above conditional trinomial distributions for the six groups distinguished with different treatment-receipt sequences.

Under model (9.1), we can show that the ratio of mean frequencies $RM_{AC} = \exp(\eta_{AC})$ between treatments A and C is equal to the following three ORs (Problem 9.2) in the corresponding 2×2 contingency tables:

$$OR_1 = \left[\left(p_2^{(1)}p_1^{(3)}\right)/\left(p_1^{(1)}p_2^{(3)}\right)\right]^{1/2},$$

$$OR_2 = \left[\left(p_3^{(2)}p_1^{(4)}\right)/\left(p_1^{(2)}p_3^{(4)}\right)\right]^{1/2}, \text{ and} \qquad (9.2)$$

$$OR_3 = \left[\left(p_3^{(5)}p_2^{(6)}\right)/\left(p_2^{(5)}p_3^{(6)}\right)\right]^{1/2}.$$

Thus, we can apply the WLS method (Fleiss, 1981) to estimate $\eta_{AC}(= \log(RM_{AC}))$ and obtain

$$\hat{\eta}_{AC}^{(WLS)} = \sum_{k=1}^{3} W_k \log\left(\widehat{OR}_k\right)/\left(2\sum_{i=1}^{3} W_k\right), \qquad (9.3)$$

where $\widehat{OR}_1 = \left(\hat{p}_2^{(1)}\hat{p}_1^{(3)}\right)/\left(\hat{p}_1^{(1)}\hat{p}_2^{(3)}\right)$, $\widehat{OR}_2 = \left(\hat{p}_3^{(2)}\hat{p}_1^{(4)}\right)/\left(\hat{p}_1^{(2)}\hat{p}_3^{(4)}\right)$, $\widehat{OR}_3 = \left(\hat{p}_3^{(5)}\hat{p}_2^{(6)}\right)/$ $\left(\hat{p}_2^{(5)}\hat{p}_3^{(6)}\right)$, $W_1 = 1/\widehat{Var}\left(\log\left(\widehat{OR}_1\right)\right) = \left(1/Y_{+2}^{(1)}+1/Y_{+1}^{(3)}+1/Y_{+1}^{(1)}+1/Y_{+2}^{(3)}\right)^{-1}$, $W_2 =$ $1/\widehat{Var}\left(\log\left(\widehat{OR}_2\right)\right) = \left(1/Y_{+3}^{(2)}+1/Y_{+1}^{(4)}+1/Y_{+1}^{(2)}+1/Y_{+3}^{(4)}\right)^{-1}$, and $W_3 = 1/\widehat{Var}\left(\log\left(\widehat{OR}_3\right)\right) =$ $\left(1/Y_{+3}^{(5)}+1/Y_{+2}^{(6)}+1/Y_{+2}^{(5)}+1/Y_{+3}^{(6)}\right)^{-1}$. We can further show that an estimated asymptotic variance for $\hat{\eta}_{AC}^{(WLS)}$ (9.3) is (Problem 9.3)

$$\widehat{Var}\left(\hat{\eta}_{AC}^{(WLS)}\right) = 1/\left(4\sum_{k=1}^{3} W_k\right). \qquad (9.4)$$

Similarly, we can show that the ratio of mean frequencies $RM_{BC} = \exp(\eta_{BC})$ between treatments B and C under model (9.1) is equal to the following three ORs (Problem 9.4):

$$OR_1^* = \left[\left(p_3^{(1)}p_1^{(6)}\right)/\left(p_1^{(1)}p_3^{(6)}\right)\right]^{1/2},$$

$$OR_2^* = \left[\left(p_2^{(2)}p_1^{(5)}\right)/\left(p_1^{(2)}p_2^{(5)}\right)\right]^{1/2}, \text{ and} \qquad (9.5)$$

$$OR_3^* = \left[\left(p_3^{(3)}p_2^{(4)}\right)/\left(p_2^{(3)}p_3^{(4)}\right)\right]^{1/2}.$$

To estimate η_{BC} (= $\log(RM_{BC})$), we may also consider the WLS estimator as given by

$$\hat{\eta}_{BC}^{(WLS)} = \sum_{k=1}^{3} W_k^* \log\left(\widehat{OR}_k^*\right)/\left(2\sum_{i=1}^{3} W_k^*\right), \qquad (9.6)$$

where $\widehat{OR}_1^* = \left(\hat{p}_3^{(1)}\hat{p}_1^{(6)}\right)/\left(\hat{p}_1^{(1)}\hat{p}_3^{(6)}\right)$, $\widehat{OR}_2^* = \left(\hat{p}_2^{(2)}\hat{p}_1^{(5)}\right)/\left(\hat{p}_1^{(2)}\hat{p}_2^{(5)}\right)$, $\widehat{OR}_3^* = \left(\hat{p}_3^{(3)}\hat{p}_2^{(4)}\right)/$

$\left(\hat{p}_2^{(3)}\hat{p}_3^{(4)}\right)$, $W_1^* = 1/\widehat{Var}\left(\log\left(\widehat{OR}_1^*\right)\right) = \left(1/Y_{+3}^{(1)}+1/Y_{+1}^{(6)}+1/Y_{+1}^{(1)}+1/Y_{+3}^{(6)}\right)^{-1}$, $W_2^* =$

$1/\widehat{Var}\left(\log\left(\widehat{OR}_2^*\right)\right) = \left(1/Y_{+2}^{(2)}+1/Y_{+1}^{(5)}+1/Y_{+1}^{(2)}+1/Y_{+2}^{(5)}\right)^{-1}$, and $W_3^* = 1/\widehat{Var}\left(\log\left(\widehat{OR}_3^*\right)\right)$

$= \left(1/Y_{+3}^{(3)}+1/Y_{+2}^{(4)}+1/Y_{+2}^{(3)}+1/Y_{+3}^{(4)}\right)^{-1}$. An estimated asymptotic variance estima-

tor for $\hat{\eta}_{BC}^{(WLS)}$ (9.6) is

$$\widehat{Var}\left(\hat{\eta}_{BC}^{(WLS)}\right) = 1/\left(4\sum_{k=1}^{3}W_k^*\right). \tag{9.7}$$

Also, we can show that the ratio of mean frequencies $RM_{BA} = \exp(\eta_{BC}-\eta_{AC})$ between treatments B and A under model (9.1) is equal to the following three ORs (Problem 9.5):

$$OR_1^{**} = \left[\left(p_3^{(1)}p_2^{(2)}\right)/\left(p_2^{(1)}p_3^{(2)}\right)\right]^{1/2},$$

$$OR_2^{**} = \left[\left(p_3^{(3)}p_1^{(5)}\right)/\left(p_1^{(3)}p_3^{(5)}\right)\right]^{1/2}, \text{and} \tag{9.8}$$

$$OR_3^{**} = \left[\left(p_2^{(4)}p_1^{(6)}\right)/\left(p_1^{(4)}p_2^{(6)}\right)\right]^{1/2}.$$

To estimate η_{BA} (= $\log(RM_{BA})$), we may again use the WLS estimator as given by

$$\hat{\eta}_{BA}^{(WLS)} = \sum_{k=1}^{3}W_k^{**}\log\left(\widehat{OR}_k^{**}\right)/\left(2\sum_{i=1}^{3}W_k^{**}\right), \tag{9.9}$$

where $\widehat{OR}_1^{**} = \left(\hat{p}_3^{(1)}\hat{p}_2^{(2)}\right)/\left(\hat{p}_2^{(1)}\hat{p}_3^{(2)}\right)$, $\widehat{OR}_2^{**} = \left(\hat{p}_3^{(3)}\hat{p}_1^{(5)}\right)/\left(\hat{p}_1^{(3)}\hat{p}_3^{(5)}\right)$, $\widehat{OR}_3^{**} = \left(\hat{p}_2^{(4)}\hat{p}_1^{(6)}\right)/$

$\left(\hat{p}_1^{(4)}\hat{p}_2^{(6)}\right)$, $W_1^{**} = 1/\widehat{Var}\left(\log\left(\widehat{OR}_1^{**}\right)\right) = \left(1/Y_{+3}^{(1)}+1/Y_{+3}^{(2)}+1/Y_{+2}^{(1)}+1/Y_{+2}^{(2)}\right)^{-1}$,

$W_2^{**} = 1/\widehat{Var}\left(\log\left(\widehat{OR}_2^{**}\right)\right) = \left(1/Y_{+3}^{(3)}+1/Y_{+3}^{(5)}+1/Y_{+1}^{(3)}+1/Y_{+1}^{(5)}\right)^{-1}$, and $W_3^{**} = 1/$

$\widehat{Var}\left(\log\left(\widehat{OR}_3^{**}\right)\right) = \left(1/Y_{+2}^{(4)}+1/Y_{+2}^{(6)}+1/Y_{+1}^{(4)}+1/Y_{+1}^{(6)}\right)^{-1}$. Furthermore, we obtain

an estimated asymptotic variance estimator for $\hat{\eta}_{BA}$ (9.9) as

$$\widehat{Var}\left(\hat{\eta}_{BA}^{(WLS)}\right) = 1/\left(4\sum_{k=1}^{3}W_k^{**}\right). \tag{9.10}$$

For simplicity in notation, we will let "+" denote the summation over that subscript for all notation in the following. We define $(o_{11k}, o_{12k}, o_{21k}, o_{22k})$ (for $k = 1, 2, 3$) as the vector of random frequencies for the three 2×2 tables, each table k (= 1, 2, 3) consisting of frequency o_{ij} in cell (i, j) (for $i, j = 1, 2$) corresponding to equations in (9.2):

$$\left(o_{111} = Y_{+2}^{(1)}, o_{121} = Y_{+2}^{(3)}, o_{211} = Y_{+1}^{(1)}, o_{221} = Y_{+1}^{(3)}\right),$$

$$\left(o_{112} = Y_{+3}^{(2)}, o_{122} = Y_{+3}^{(4)}, o_{212} = Y_{+1}^{(2)}, o_{222} = Y_{+1}^{(4)}\right), \text{ and} \qquad (9.11)$$

$$\left(o_{113} = Y_{+3}^{(5)}, o_{123} = Y_{+3}^{(6)}, o_{213} = Y_{+2}^{(5)}, o_{223} = Y_{+2}^{(6)}\right).$$

Similarly, we define $\left(o_{11k}^{*}, o_{12k}^{*}, o_{21k}^{*}, o_{22k}^{*}\right)$ (for $k = 1, 2, 3$) as the vector of random frequencies for the three 2×2 tables, each table k $(= 1, 2, 3)$ consisting of frequency o_{ijk}^{*} in cell (i, j) (for $i, j = 1, 2$) corresponding to equations in (9.5):

$$\left(o_{111}^{*} = Y_{+3}^{(1)}, o_{121}^{*} = Y_{+3}^{(6)}, o_{211}^{*} = Y_{+1}^{(1)}, o_{221}^{*} = Y_{+1}^{(6)}\right),$$

$$\left(o_{112}^{*} = Y_{+2}^{(2)}, o_{122}^{*} = Y_{+2}^{(5)}, o_{212}^{*} = Y_{+1}^{(2)}, o_{222}^{*} = Y_{+1}^{(5)}\right), \text{ and} \qquad (9.12)$$

$$\left(o_{113}^{*} = Y_{+3}^{(3)}, o_{123}^{*} = Y_{+3}^{(4)}, o_{213}^{*} = Y_{+2}^{(3)}, o_{223}^{*} = Y_{+2}^{(4)}\right).$$

Furthermore, we define $\left(o_{11k}^{**}, o_{12k}^{**}, o_{21k}^{**}, o_{22k}^{**}\right)$ (for $k = 1, 2, 3$) as the vector of random frequencies for the three 2×2 tables, each table k $(= 1, 2, 3)$ consisting of frequency o_{ijk}^{**} in cell (i, j) (for $i, j = 1, 2$) corresponding to equations in (9.8):

$$\left(o_{111}^{**} = Y_{+3}^{(1)}, o_{121}^{**} = Y_{+3}^{(2)}, o_{211}^{**} = Y_{+2}^{(1)}, o_{221}^{**} = Y_{+2}^{(2)}\right),$$

$$\left(o_{112}^{**} = Y_{+3}^{(3)}, o_{122}^{**} = Y_{+3}^{(5)}, o_{212}^{**} = Y_{+1}^{(3)}, o_{222}^{**} = Y_{+1}^{(5)}\right), \text{ and} \qquad (9.13)$$

$$\left(o_{113}^{**} = Y_{+2}^{(4)}, o_{123}^{**} = Y_{+2}^{(6)}, o_{213}^{**} = Y_{+1}^{(4)}, o_{223}^{**} = Y_{+1}^{(6)}\right).$$

On the basis of (9.2) and (9.11), we can show that the conditional probability distribution of o_{11k}, given $o_{+1k}, o_{+2k}, o_{1+k}$, and o_{2+k} fixed, is given by

$$P\left(o_{11k} | o_{+1k}, o_{+2k}, o_{1+k}, o_{2+k}, RM_{AC}^{2}\right) = \frac{\binom{o_{+1k}}{o_{11k}} \binom{o_{+2k}}{o_{1+k} - o_{11k}} \left(RM_{AC}^{2}\right)^{o_{11k}}}{\sum_{x_k} \binom{o_{+1k}}{x_k} \binom{o_{+2k}}{o_{1+k} - x_k} \left(RM_{AC}^{2}\right)^{x_k}},$$

$$(9.14)$$

where the summation of x_k in the denominator is calculated over $a_k \le x_k \le b_k$, $a_k = \max\{0, o_{1+k} - o_{+2k}\}$, and $b_k = \min\{o_{+1k}, o_{1+k}\}$ for $k = 1, 2, 3$. Thus, the joint conditional probability distribution of $\underline{o}_{11} = (o_{111}, o_{112}, o_{113})'$ is

$$P\left(o_{111}, o_{112}, o_{113} | \underline{o}_{+1}, \underline{o}_{+2}, \underline{o}_{1+}, \underline{o}_{2+}, RM_{AC}^2\right)$$

$$= \prod_{k=1}^{3} \frac{\binom{o_{+1k}}{o_{11k}} \binom{o_{+2k}}{o_{1+k}-o_{11k}} \left(RM_{AC}^2\right)^{o_{11k}}}{\sum_{x_k} \binom{o_{+1k}}{x_k} \binom{o_{+2k}}{o_{1+k}-x_k} \left(RM_{AC}^2\right)^{x_k}}, \qquad (9.15)$$

where $\underline{o}_{w+} = (o_{w+1}, o_{w+2}, o_{w+3})'$ for $w = 1, 2$, and $\underline{o}_{+v} = (o_{+v1}, o_{+v2}, o_{+v3})'$ for $v = 1$, 2. The probability mass function for a given value o_{11+}^0 $(= o_{111}^0 + o_{112}^0 + o_{113}^0)$ based on (9.15) is then

$$P\left(o_{11+} = o_{11+}^0 | \underline{o}_{+1}, \underline{o}_{+2}, \underline{o}_{1+}, \underline{o}_{2+}, RM_{AC}^2\right)$$

$$= \sum_{\underline{o}_{11} \in C\left(o_{11+}^0\right)} \prod_{k=1}^{3} \frac{\binom{o_{+1k}}{o_{11k}} \binom{o_{+2k}}{o_{1+k}-o_{11k}} \left(RM_{AC}^2\right)^{o_{11k}}}{\sum_{x_k} \binom{o_{+1k}}{x_k} \binom{o_{+2k}}{o_{1+k}-x_k} \left(RM_{AC}^2\right)^{x_k}}, \qquad (9.16)$$

where $C\left(o_{11+}^0\right) = \left\{(o_{111}, o_{112}, o_{113})' | o_{111} + o_{112} + o_{113} = o_{11+}^0, a_k \le o_{11k} \le b_k\right\}$. Following the same arguments as for deriving (9.14)–(9.16), we can derive the conditional probability mass function for o_{11+}^* (or o_{11+}^{**}) as given by (9.16) by replacing o_{ijk} with o_{ijk}^* (or o_{ijk}^{**}) and RM_{AC} with RM_{BC} (or RM_{BA}).

9.1   Testing non-equality between treatments and placebo

When treatments A and B represent two experimental treatments, and treatment C represents a placebo (or a control group), as noted by Dunnett (1964, p. 484), we are often interested in studying whether either of two experimental treatments differs from the placebo (or the control group), while whether there is a difference between the two experimental treatments is not of our concern. In other words, we want to study whether $\eta_{AC} \ne 0$ or $\eta_{BC} \ne 0$. Thus, we consider testing the null hypothesis $H_0 : RM_{AC} = RM_{BC} = 1$ (or equivalently, $\eta_{AC} = \eta_{BC} = 0$) versus the alternative hypothesis $H_a : RM_{AC} \ne 1$ or $RM_{BC} \ne 1$ (i.e., $\eta_{AC} \ne 0$ or $\eta_{BC} \ne 0$). Note that the equality $RM_{AC} = RM_{BC} = 1$ implies that $\left(p_1^{(1)}, p_2^{(1)}, p_3^{(1)}\right)' = \left(p_1^{(2)}, p_2^{(2)}, p_3^{(2)}\right)' = \cdots = \left(p_1^{(6)}, p_2^{(6)}, p_3^{(6)}\right)'$. When testing $H_0 : RM_{AC} = RM_{BC} = 1$, one can apply Pearson's chi-squared goodness-of-fit test to study whether the distributions of cell frequencies are identical among the six groups (Fleiss, 1981; Agresti, 1990). We will reject $H_0 : RM_{AC} = RM_{BC} = 1$ at the α-level if

$$\sum_{g=1}^{6}\sum_{z=1}^{3}\left[Y_{+z}^{(g)}-\left(Y_{+z}^{(+)}y_{++}^{(g)}\right)/y_{++}^{(+)}\right]^{2}/\left[\left(Y_{+z}^{(+)}y_{++}^{(g)}\right)/y_{++}^{(+)}\right]>\chi_{\alpha}^{2}(10),\quad(9.17)$$

where $y_{+z}^{(+)}=\sum_{g=1}^{6}y_{+z}^{(g)}$, $y_{++}^{(+)}=\sum_{g=1}^{6}y_{++}^{(g)}$, and $\chi_{\alpha}^{2}(df)$ is the upper $100(\alpha)$th percentile of the central chi-squared distribution with df degree(s) of freedom. To test $H_{0}:RM_{AC}=RM_{BC}=1$, we may also apply the asymptotic likelihood ratio test based on the above conditional trinomial distribution of $\left(Y_{+1}^{(g)},Y_{+2}^{(g)},Y_{+3}^{(g)}\right)'$ (Agresti, 1990).

We let $\left(p_{1}^{(0)},p_{2}^{(0)},p_{3}^{(0)}\right)'$ denote the common value of $\left(p_{1}^{(g)},p_{2}^{(g)},p_{3}^{(g)}\right)'$ (for $g=1,2,3,$ 4, 5, 6) under $H_{0}:\eta_{AC}=\eta_{BC}=0$. Thus, we will reject $H_{0}:RM_{AC}=RM_{BC}=1$ at the α-level if

$$2\left[\sum_{g=1}^{6}\sum_{z=1}^{3}Y_{+z}^{(g)}\log\left(\hat{p}_{z}^{(g)}\right)-\sum_{z=1}^{3}Y_{+z}^{(+)}\log\left(\hat{p}_{z}^{(0)}\right)\right]>\chi_{\alpha}^{2}(10),\qquad(9.18)$$

where $\hat{p}_{z}^{(g)}=Y_{+z}^{(g)}/y_{++}^{(g)}$ and $\hat{p}_{z}^{(0)}=Y_{+z}^{(+)}/y_{++}^{(+)}$ for $z=1,2,3$.

When n_{g} is large, we may test $H_{0}:RM_{AC}=RM_{BC}=1$ by use of asymptotic test procedures based on (9.3), (9.4), (9.6), and (9.7), and Bonferroni's inequality to adjust the inflation due to multiple tests in Type I error. We will reject $H_{0}:RM_{AC}=RM_{BC}=1$ at the α-level if either of the following two inequalities holds:

$$|\hat{\eta}_{AC}^{(WLS)}|/\sqrt{\widehat{\text{var}}\left(\hat{\eta}_{AC}^{(WLS)}\right)}>Z_{\alpha/4}\,\text{or}\,|\hat{\eta}_{BC}^{(WLS)}|/\sqrt{\widehat{\text{var}}\left(\hat{\eta}_{BC}^{(WLS)}\right)}>Z_{\alpha/4},\qquad(9.19)$$

where Z_{α} is the upper $100(\alpha)$th percentile of the standard normal distribution.

Note that the two WLS estimators $\hat{\eta}_{AC}^{(WLS)}$ (9.3) and $\hat{\eta}_{BC}^{(WLS)}$ (9.6) are correlated. Using the delta method (Agresti, 1990), we can show that an estimated covariance between $\hat{\eta}_{AC}$ and $\hat{\eta}_{BC}$ is (Problem 9.6)

$$\widehat{Cov}\left(\hat{\eta}_{AC}^{(WLS)},\hat{\eta}_{BC}^{(WLS)}\right)$$

$$=\frac{1}{\left[4\left(\sum_{k=1}^{3}W_{k}\right)\left(\sum_{k=1}^{3}W_{k}^{*}\right)\right]}\left\{W_{1}W_{1}^{*}\widehat{Cov}\left(\log\left(\frac{\hat{p}_{2}^{(1)}}{\hat{p}_{1}^{(1)}}\right),\log\left(\frac{\hat{p}_{3}^{(1)}}{\hat{p}_{1}^{(1)}}\right)\right)\right.$$

$$+W_{2}W_{2}^{*}\widehat{Cov}\left(\log\left(\frac{\hat{p}_{3}^{(2)}}{\hat{p}_{1}^{(2)}}\right),\log\left(\frac{\hat{p}_{2}^{(2)}}{\hat{p}_{1}^{(2)}}\right)\right)-W_{1}W_{3}^{*}\widehat{Cov}\left(\log\left(\frac{\hat{p}_{2}^{(3)}}{\hat{p}_{1}^{(3)}}\right),\log\left(\frac{\hat{p}_{3}^{(3)}}{\hat{p}_{2}^{(3)}}\right)\right)$$

$$+W_{2}W_{3}^{*}\widehat{Cov}\left(\log\left(\frac{\hat{p}_{3}^{(4)}}{\hat{p}_{1}^{(4)}}\right),\log\left(\frac{\hat{p}_{3}^{(4)}}{\hat{p}_{2}^{(4)}}\right)\right)-W_{3}W_{2}^{*}\widehat{Cov}\left(\log\left(\frac{\hat{p}_{3}^{(5)}}{\hat{p}_{2}^{(5)}}\right),\log\left(\frac{\hat{p}_{2}^{(5)}}{\hat{p}_{1}^{(5)}}\right)\right)$$

$$\left.+W_{3}W_{1}^{*}\widehat{Cov}\left(\log\left(\frac{\hat{p}_{3}^{(6)}}{\hat{p}_{2}^{(6)}}\right),\log\left(\frac{\hat{p}_{3}^{(6)}}{\hat{p}_{1}^{(6)}}\right)\right)\right\},\qquad(9.20)$$

where $\widehat{Cov}\left(\log\left(\frac{\hat{p}_2^{(1)}}{\hat{p}_1^{(1)}}\right),\log\left(\frac{\hat{p}_3^{(1)}}{\hat{p}_1^{(1)}}\right)\right)=1/Y_{+1}^{(1)}$, $\widehat{Cov}\left(\log\left(\frac{\hat{p}_3^{(2)}}{\hat{p}_1^{(2)}}\right),\log\left(\frac{\hat{p}_2^{(2)}}{\hat{p}_1^{(2)}}\right)\right)=1/Y_{+1}^{(2)}$,

$\widehat{Cov}\left(\log\left(\frac{\hat{p}_2^{(3)}}{\hat{p}_3^{(3)}}\right),\log\left(\frac{\hat{p}_3^{(3)}}{\hat{p}_2^{(3)}}\right)\right)=-\left(1/Y_{+2}^{(3)}\right)$, $\widehat{Cov}\left(\log\left(\frac{\hat{p}_3^{(4)}}{\hat{p}_1^{(4)}}\right),\log\left(\frac{\hat{p}_3^{(4)}}{\hat{p}_2^{(4)}}\right)\right)=1/Y_{+3}^{(4)}$,

$\widehat{Cov}\left(\log\left(\frac{\hat{p}_2^{(5)}}{\hat{p}_3^{(5)}}\right),\log\left(\frac{\hat{p}_2^{(5)}}{\hat{p}_1^{(5)}}\right)\right)=-\left(1/Y_{+2}^{(5)}\right)$, and $\widehat{Cov}\left(\log\left(\frac{\hat{p}_3^{(6)}}{\hat{p}_2^{(6)}}\right),\log\left(\frac{\hat{p}_3^{(6)}}{\hat{p}_1^{(6)}}\right)\right)=1/Y_{+3}^{(6)}$.

Because the test procedure (9.19) does not account for dependence structure between $\hat{\eta}_{AC}^{(WLS)}$ (9.3) and $\hat{\eta}_{BC}^{(WLS)}$ (9.6), we may lose power. Thus, we consider the following bivariate test procedure accounting for $\widehat{Cov}\left(\hat{\eta}_{AC}^{(WLS)},\hat{\eta}_{BC}^{(WLS)}\right)$ (9.20). We will reject H_0 : $RM_{AC}=RM_{BC}=1$ at the α-level if

$$\left(\hat{\eta}_{AC}^{(WLS)},\hat{\eta}_{BC}^{(WLS)}\right)\hat{\underline{\Sigma}}^{-1}\begin{pmatrix}\hat{\eta}_{AC}^{(WLS)}\\\hat{\eta}_{BC}^{(WLS)}\end{pmatrix}>\chi_\alpha^2(2), \qquad (9.21)$$

where $\hat{\underline{\Sigma}}$ is the estimated covariance matrix with diagonal elements equal to $\widehat{Var}\left(\hat{\eta}_{AC}^{(WLS)}\right)$ (9.4) and $\widehat{Var}\left(\hat{\eta}_{BC}^{(WLS)}\right)$ (9.7), and off-diagonal element equal to $\widehat{Cov}\left(\hat{\eta}_{AC}^{(WLS)},\hat{\eta}_{BC}^{(WLS)}\right)$ (9.20).

When treatments A and B are known to fall in the same relative direction as compared with the placebo, we may wish to account for this information to improve power and consider the following summary test procedure based on a weighted average of treatment effects $w\hat{\eta}_{AC}^{(WLS)}+(1-w)\hat{\eta}_{BC}^{(WLS)}$, where $0<w<1$ is the weight reflecting the relative importance of treatment A to that of treatment B and can be assigned by clinicians based on their subjective knowledge. This leads us to reject $H_0:RM_{AC}=RM_{BC}=1$ at the α-level if

$$\left|w\hat{\eta}_{AC}^{(WLS)}+(1-w)\hat{\eta}_{BC}^{(WLS)}\right|/\sqrt{\widehat{Var}\left(w\hat{\eta}_{AC}^{(WLS)}+(1-w)\hat{\eta}_{BC}^{(WLS)}\right)}>Z_{\alpha/2}, \qquad (9.22)$$

where $\widehat{Var}\left(w\hat{\eta}_{AC}^{(WLS)}+(1-w)\hat{\eta}_{BC}^{(WLS)}\right)=w^2\widehat{Var}\left(\hat{\eta}_{AC}^{(WLS)}\right)+(1-w)^2\widehat{Var}\left(\hat{\eta}_{BC}^{(WLS)}\right)+2w(1-w)\widehat{Cov}\left(\hat{\eta}_{AC}^{(WLS)},\hat{\eta}_{BC}^{(WLS)}\right)$. If we have no prior preference to assign the weight w or feel equally important between the two treatments, we may set w equal to 0.50. Note that the optimal weight w_o to minimize the variance $Var\left(w\hat{\eta}_{AC}^{(WLS)}+(1-w)\hat{\eta}_{BC}^{(WLS)}\right)$ is approximately given by

$$\hat{w}_o=\left(\widehat{Var}\left(\hat{\eta}_{BC}^{(WLS)}\right)-\widehat{Cov}\left(\hat{\eta}_{AC}^{(WLS)},\hat{\eta}_{BC}^{(WLS)}\right)\right)/ \\ \left[\widehat{Var}\left(\hat{\eta}_{AC}^{(WLS)}\right)+\widehat{Var}\left(\hat{\eta}_{BC}^{(WLS)}\right)-2\widehat{Cov}\left(\hat{\eta}_{AC}^{(WLS)},\hat{\eta}_{BC}^{(WLS)}\right)\right]. \qquad (9.23)$$

When $Var\left(\hat{\eta}_{BC}^{(WLS)}\right)=Var\left(\hat{\eta}_{AC}^{(WLS)}\right)$, the optimal weight w_o simplifies to 0.50.

Using Monte Carlo simulations, Lui and Chang (2014) found that all the above asymptotic test procedures can perform well with respect to Type I error when the mean size $(E(n_g) =) n$ of patients per group is even moderate. Lui and Chang (2014) noted that the powers of the two most commonly used test procedures (9.17) and (9.18) for the contingency table are generally less than those of the WLS test procedures (9.19) and (9.21). When there is only one of the two experimental treatments with a nonzero effect as compared with the placebo, the bivariate test procedure (9.21) seems to be preferable to the others with respect to power. When two experimental treatments have the same magnitude of nonnegligible effects in the same direction, the summary test procedure (with $w = 0.50$) (9.22) can be the best with respect to power among all test procedures considered here. When one of two experimental treatments has an effect relatively large to placebo, the test procedure (9.19) based on the univariate test procedure with Bonferroni's equality can still be of use.

Example 9.1   Consider the data (Table 9.1) taken from a double-blind three-period crossover trial comparing salbutamol (400 ug four times daily) (treatment A), salmeterol (50 ug twice daily) (treatment B), and placebo (treatment C) in asthma patients (Taylor *et al.*, 1998, 2000). For illustration purpose only, we consider the data on only 160 patients with complete information on the vector $\left(Y_{+1}^{(g)}, Y_{+2}^{(g)}, Y_{+3}^{(g)}\right)$ of total frequencies of exacerbations at the three periods in group g (= 1, 2, 3, 4, 5, 6) and the number n_g of patients assigned to each group. When applying test procedures (9.17)–(9.19), (9.21), and (9.22) to test $H_0 : \eta_{AC} = \eta_{BC} = 0$, we obtain the corresponding p-values to be 0.000, 0.000, 0.000, 0.000, and 0.008, respectively. All these small values suggest that there should be strong evidence that the mean numbers of exacerbations are different between either of the two experimental treatments and placebo. The average numbers of exacerbations per patient for taking placebo, salbutamol, and salmeterol based on the data in Table 9.1 are 0.575, 0.563, and 0.200, respectively. It seems obvious that the mean number of exacerbations for salmeterol is less than those for the other two treatments.

9.2   Testing non-inferiority of an experimental treatment to an active control treatment

Since it is sometimes unethical to have a placebo arm, we may need to use an active control treatment. Instead of testing non-equality between treatments, we may wish to test whether either experimental treatment A or B is non-inferior to an active control treatment C, especially when the former has fewer side effects and less cost or is easier to administer than the latter.

Suppose that the higher the mean frequency of responses, the better is the treatment. Thus, to detect the non-inferiority of treatment A or B to treatment C, we want to test $H_0 : RM_{AC} \leq RM_l$ and $RM_{BC} \leq RM_l$ (where $0 < RM_l < 1$) versus $H_a : RM_{AC} > RM_l$ or $RM_{BC} > RM_l$, where RM_l is the maximum clinically acceptable low margin such that treatment A (or treatment B) can be regarded as non-inferior to treatment C when $RM_{AC} > RM_l$ (or $RM_{BC} > RM_l$). When the observed frequencies $Y^{(g)}_{+z}$ for $z = 1, 2, 3$ are reasonably large for all groups, we may apply statistics $\hat{\eta}^{(WLS)}_{AC}$ (9.3) and $\hat{\eta}^{(WLS)}_{BC}$ (9.6) as well as their estimated asymptotic variances $\widehat{Var}\left(\hat{\eta}^{(WLS)}_{AC}\right)$ (9.4) and $\widehat{Var}\left(\hat{\eta}^{(WLS)}_{BC}\right)$ (9.7) to test $H_0 : RM_{AC} \leq RM_l$ and $RM_{BC} \leq RM_l$. We will reject H_0 at the α-level and claim that treatment A or treatment B is non-inferior to treatment C if

$$\left(\hat{\eta}^{(WLS)}_{AC} - \log(RM_l)\right) \Big/ \sqrt{\widehat{var}\left(\hat{\eta}^{(WLS)}_{AC}\right)} > Z_{\alpha/2}, \text{ or}$$

$$\left(\hat{\eta}^{(WLS)}_{BC} - \log(RM_l)\right) \Big/ \sqrt{\widehat{var}\left(\hat{\eta}^{(WLS)}_{BC}\right)} > Z_{\alpha/2}. \tag{9.24}$$

When some of the observed frequencies $Y^{(g)}_{+z}$ are not large, the weights used in the WLS estimators $\hat{\eta}^{(WLS)}_{AC}$ (9.3) and $\hat{\eta}^{(WLS)}_{BC}$ (9.6) can be subject to a large variation, and thereby the test procedures (9.24) can lose accuracy. In this case, we may consider use of the test procedure based on the exact conditional probability mass function (9.16). We will reject H_0 at the α-level and claim that treatment A or B is non-inferior to treatment C if we obtain the vector of observed frequencies $(o^0_{11+}, o^{*0}_{11+})'$ such that the tail probabilities

$$P\left(o_{11+} \geq o^0_{11+} | \underline{o}_{+1}, \underline{o}_{+2}, \underline{o}_{1+}, \underline{o}_{2+}, RM^2_l\right) < \alpha/2, \text{ or}$$

$$P\left(o^*_{11+} \geq o^{*0}_{11+} | \underline{o}^*_{+1}, \underline{o}^*_{+2}, \underline{o}^*_{1+}, \underline{o}^*_{2+}, RM^2_l\right) < \alpha/2. \tag{9.25}$$

9.3 Testing equivalence between an experimental treatment and an active control treatment

Using the intersection-union test (Casella and Berger, 1990), we can easily modify procedures for testing non-inferiority to accommodate testing equivalence. When testing equivalence between either treatment A or B and an active control treatment C, we want to test $H_0 : (RM_{AC} \leq RM_l$ or $RM_{AC} \geq RM_u)$ and $(RM_{BC} \leq RM_l$ or $RM_{BC} \geq RM_u)$ versus $H_a : (RM_l < RM_{AC} < RM_u)$ or $(RM_l < RM_{BC} < RM_u)$, where RM_l and RM_u are the maximum clinically acceptable margins such that treatment A (or treatment B) can be regarded as equivalent to an active control treatment C when $RM_l < RM_{AC} < RM_u$ (or $RM_l < RM_{BC} < RM_u$) holds. Thus, using $\hat{\eta}^{(WLS)}_{AC}$ (9.3) and $\hat{\eta}^{(WLS)}_{BC}$ (9.6), we will reject H_0 at the α-level if either of the following two sets of inequalities holds:

$$\left(\hat{\eta}_{AC}^{(WLS)}-\log(RM_l)\right)\Big/\sqrt{\widehat{Var}\left(\hat{\eta}_{AC}^{(WLS)}\right)}>Z_{\alpha/2} \text{ and}$$

$$\left(\hat{\eta}_{AC}^{(WLS)}-\log(RM_u)\right)\Big/\sqrt{\widehat{Var}\left(\hat{\eta}_{AC}^{(WLS)}\right)}<-Z_{\alpha/2}; \text{or}$$

$$\left(\hat{\eta}_{BC}^{(WLS)}-\log(RM_l)\right)\Big/\sqrt{\widehat{Var}\left(\hat{\eta}_{BC}^{(WLS)}\right)}>Z_{\alpha/2} \text{ and} \qquad (9.26)$$

$$\left(\hat{\eta}_{BC}^{(WLS)}-\log(RM_u)\right)\Big/\sqrt{\widehat{Var}\left(\hat{\eta}_{BC}^{(WLS)}\right)}<-Z_{\alpha/2}.$$

Note that if some of the observed frequencies o_{ijk} or o_{ijk}^* are small, we may use the exact test procedure to test $H_0: (RM_{AC} \le RM_l$ or $RM_{AC} \ge RM_u)$ and $(RM_{BC} \le RM_l$ or $RM_{BC} \ge RM_u)$. On the basis of the conditional distribution (9.16) and the corresponding conditional probability mass function for the random vector $(o_{111}^*, o_{112}^*, o_{113}^*)$, we will reject H_0 at the α-level if we obtain $(o_{11+}^0, o_{11+}^{*0})$ such that

$$P\left(o_{11+} \ge o_{11+}^0 \mid o_{+1}, o_{+2}, o_{1+}, o_{2+}, RM_l^2\right) < \alpha/2 \text{ and}$$
$$P\left(o_{11+} \le o_{11+}^0 \mid o_{+1}, o_{+2}, o_{1+}, o_{2+}, RM_u^2\right) < \alpha/2; \text{ or} \qquad (9.27)$$
$$P\left(o_{11+}^* \ge o_{11+}^{*0} \mid o_{+1}^*, o_{+2}^*, o_{1+}^*, o_{2+}^*, RM_l^2\right) < \alpha/2 \text{ and}$$
$$P\left(o_{11+}^* \le o_{11+}^{*0} \mid o_{+1}^*, o_{+2}^*, o_{1+}^*, o_{2+}^*, RM_u^2\right) < \alpha/2.$$

9.4   Interval estimation of the ratio of mean frequencies

To quantify the magnitude of the relative treatment effect, we want to obtain an interval estimator of the ratio of mean frequencies. For brevity, we focus our attention on interval estimation of RM_{AC} and RM_{BC}. All results presented here can be easily modified to estimate RM_{BA}.

On the basis of $\hat{\eta}_{AC}^{(WLS)}$ (9.3) and $\widehat{Var}\left(\hat{\eta}_{AC}^{(WLS)}\right)$ (9.4), we obtain an asymptotic $100(1 - \alpha)\%$ confidence interval for RM_{AC} as

$$\left[\exp\left(\hat{\eta}_{AC}^{(WLS)}-Z_{\alpha/2}\sqrt{\widehat{Var}\left(\hat{\eta}_{AC}^{(WLS)}\right)}\right), \exp\left(\hat{\eta}_{AC}^{(WLS)}+Z_{\alpha/2}\sqrt{\widehat{Var}\left(\hat{\eta}_{AC}^{(WLS)}\right)}\right)\right]. \quad (9.28)$$

When some of the observed frequencies $Y_{+z}^{(g)}$ are not large, the weights used in the WLS estimator (9.28) can be subject to a large variation, and hence interval estimator (9.28) can lose accuracy. This may lead us to consider use of the MH estimator (Agresti, 1990) for RM_{AC} as given by

$$\widehat{RM}_{AC}^{(MH)} = \left(\left(\sum_{k=1}^{3} o_{11k}o_{22k}/o_{++k}\right)\Big/\left(\sum_{k=1}^{3} o_{12k}o_{21k}/o_{++k}\right)\right)^{1/2}. \quad (9.29)$$

As given elsewhere (Robins, Breslow, and Greenland, 1986; Agresti, 1990), we obtain an estimated asymptotic variance for $\log\left(\widehat{RM}_{AC}^{(MH)}\right)$ as

$$
\widehat{Var}\left(\log\left(\widehat{RM}_{AC}^{(MH)}\right)\right) = \left\{ \frac{\sum_k (o_{11k} + o_{22k})(o_{11k}o_{22k})/o_{++k}^2}{2\left(\sum_k o_{11k}o_{22k}/o_{++k}\right)^2} \right.
$$

$$
+ \frac{\sum_k [(o_{11k} + o_{22k})(o_{12k}o_{21k}) + (o_{12k} + o_{21k})(o_{11k}o_{22k})]/o_{++k}^2}{2\left(\sum_k o_{11k}o_{22k}/o_{++k}\right)\left(\sum_k o_{12k}o_{21k}/o_{++k}\right)}
$$

$$
\left. + \frac{\sum_k (o_{12k} + o_{21k})(o_{12k}o_{21k})/o_{++k}^2}{2\left(\sum_k o_{12k}o_{21k}/o_{++k}\right)^2} \right\} /4.
$$

(9.30)

On the basis of (9.29) and (9.30), we obtain an asymptotic $100(1 - \alpha)\%$ confidence interval for RM_{AC} based on the MH estimator (9.29) as

$$
\left[\widehat{RM}_{AC}^{(MH)} \exp\left(-Z_{\alpha/2}\sqrt{\widehat{Var}\left(\log\left(\widehat{RM}_{AC}^{(MH)}\right)\right)} \right), \right.
$$

$$
\left. \widehat{RM}_{AC}^{(MH)} \exp\left(Z_{\alpha/2}\sqrt{\widehat{Var}\left(\log\left(\widehat{RM}_{AC}^{(MH)}\right)\right)} \right) \right].
$$

(9.31)

Similarly, based on $\hat{\eta}_{BC}^{(WLS)}$ (9.6) and $\widehat{Var}\left(\hat{\eta}_{BC}^{(WLS)}\right)$ (9.7), we obtain an asymptotic $100(1 - \alpha)\%$ confidence interval for RM_{BC} as

$$
\left[\exp\left(\hat{\eta}_{BC}^{(WLS)} - Z_{\alpha/2}\sqrt{\widehat{Var}\left(\hat{\eta}_{BC}^{(WLS)}\right)} \right), \exp\left(\hat{\eta}_{BC}^{(WLS)} + Z_{\alpha/2}\sqrt{\widehat{Var}\left(\hat{\eta}_{BC}^{(WLS)}\right)} \right) \right]. \quad (9.32)
$$

Furthermore, we may consider use of the MH estimator (Agresti, 1990) for RM_{BC} as given by

$$
\widehat{RM}_{BC}^{(MH)} = \left(\left(\sum_{k=1}^3 o_{11k}^* o_{22k}^* / o_{++k}^* \right) \Big/ \left(\sum_{k=1}^3 o_{12k}^* o_{21k}^* / o_{++k}^* \right) \right)^{1/2}, \quad (9.33)
$$

with its estimated asymptotic variance $\widehat{Var}\left(\log\left(\widehat{RM}_{BC}^{(MH)}\right)\right)$ given by (9.30) by replacing o_{ijk} with o_{ijk}^*. Thus, we obtain an asymptotic $100(1 - \alpha)\%$ confidence interval for RM_{BC} based on the MH estimator as

$$\left[\widehat{RM}_{BC}^{(MH)}\exp\left(-Z_{\alpha/2}\sqrt{\widehat{Var}\left(\log\left(\widehat{RM}_{BC}^{(MH)}\right)\right)}\right),\right.$$

$$\left.\widehat{RM}_{BC}^{(MH)}\exp\left(Z_{\alpha/2}\sqrt{\widehat{Var}\left(\log\left(\widehat{RM}_{BC}^{(MH)}\right)\right)}\right)\right].$$

$$(9.34)$$

When treatments A and B represent different doses of an experimental treatment, it can be of interest to obtain an interval estimator for a weighted average of dose effects $w\eta_{AC}+(1-w)\eta_{BC}$ (where $0<w<1$). For example, suppose that parameters η_{AC} and η_{BC} represent the effects corresponding to the low dose x_L and the high dose x_H of a treatment, respectively. If we wish to estimate the effect at dose x_M falling between these two doses (i.e., $x_L<x_M<x_U$) by use of the linear interpolation method, we can then set w equal to $(x_U-x_M)/(x_U-x_L)$. Using the WLS method, we may obtain an asymptotic $100(1-\alpha)\%$ confidence interval for $w\eta_{AC}+(1-w)\eta_{BC}$ at dose x_M as

$$\left[w\hat{\eta}_{AC}^{(WLS)}+(1-w)\hat{\eta}_{BC}^{(WLS)}-Z_{\alpha/2}\sqrt{\widehat{Var}\left(w\hat{\eta}_{AC}^{(WLS)}+(1-w)\hat{\eta}_{BC}^{(WLS)}\right)},\right.$$

$$\left.w\hat{\eta}_{AC}^{(WLS)}+(1-w)\hat{\eta}_{BC}^{(WLS)}+Z_{\alpha/2}\sqrt{\widehat{Var}\left(w\hat{\eta}_{AC}^{(WLS)}+(1-w)\hat{\eta}_{BC}^{(WLS)}\right)}\right].$$

$$(9.35)$$

Note that when $w=1/2$, we can take the exponential transformation of the confidence limits (9.35) to obtain an asymptotic $100(1-\alpha)\%$ confidence interval for the geometric mean $(RM_{AC}RM_{BC})^{1/2}$ $(=\exp((1/2)\eta_{AC}+(1/2)\eta_{BC}))$.

Example 9.2   When assessing the magnitude of the relative treatment effects between salbutamol and placebo, we obtain the WLS and MH point estimators $\widehat{RM}_{AC}\left(=\exp\left(\hat{\eta}_{AC}^{(WLS)}\right)\right)=0.948$ and $\widehat{RM}_{AC}^{(MH)}=0.955$, as well as the corresponding 95% confidence intervals using interval estimators (9.28) and (9.31) as [0.647, 1.388] and [0.681, 1.338]. Although taking salbutamol can slightly reduce the mean number of exacerbations as compared with the placebo, we have no evidence that this decrease is significant at the 0.05 level, because the above resulting confidence intervals cover 1. When comparing salmeterol with placebo, we obtain $\widehat{RM}_{BC}\left(=\exp\left(\hat{\eta}_{BC}^{(WLS)}\right)\right)=0.430$ and $\widehat{RM}_{BC}^{(MH)}=0.433$, as well as the corresponding 95% confidence intervals using interval estimators (9.32) and (9.34) as [0.279, 0.664] and [0.283, 0.661]. Both of these point estimates suggest that taking salmeterol reduces the mean number of exacerbations by more than 50% as compared with the placebo. Furthermore, because the above resulting upper confidence limits fall below 1, there is significant evidence that taking salmeterol can reduce the mean number of exacerbations as compared with the placebo at the 5% level.

When the observed frequencies o_{ijk} are small, note that the exact interval estimator for the common OR across strata under stratified sampling published elsewhere

(Gart, 1970; Zelen, 1971; Breslow and Day, 1980) based on the conditional distribution (9.16) can be used to derive the confidence interval for RM_{AC} (RM_{BC} or RM_{BA}). Given an observed value o_{11+}^0 ($= o_{111}^0 + o_{112}^0 + o_{113}^0$), for example, we obtain an exact $100(1 - \alpha)\%$ confidence interval for RM_{AC} as given by (Gart, 1970)

$$[RM_{ACL}, RM_{ACU}], \tag{9.36}$$

where RM_{ACL} and RM_{ACU} are the solutions of the following two equations: $P\left(o_{11+} \geq o_{11+}^0 \mid \underline{o}_{+1}, \underline{o}_{+2}, \underline{o}_{1+}, \underline{o}_{2+}, RM_{ACL}^2\right) = \alpha/2$ and $P\left(o_{11+} \leq o_{11+}^0 \mid \underline{o}_{+1}, \underline{o}_{+2}, \underline{o}_{1+}, \underline{o}_{2+}, RM_{ACU}^2\right) = \alpha/2$.

The exact $100(1 - \alpha)\%$ confidence intervals for RM_{BC} (or RM_{BA}) can be obtained by substituting o_{ijk}^* (or o_{ijk}^{**}) for o_{ijk} in (9.36) and solving the corresponding equations.

9.5   Hypothesis testing and estimation for period effects

When studying the period effect measured by the ratio of mean frequencies $RM_{21}(= \exp(\gamma_1))$ between periods 2 and 1, we can show that (Problem 9.7)

$$
\begin{aligned}
RM_{21} &= \left[\left(p_2^{(1)} p_2^{(3)}\right) / \left(p_1^{(1)} p_1^{(3)}\right)\right]^{1/2} \\
&= \left[\left(p_2^{(2)} p_2^{(5)}\right) / \left(p_1^{(2)} p_1^{(5)}\right)\right]^{1/2} \\
&= \left[\left(p_2^{(4)} p_2^{(6)}\right) / \left(p_1^{(4)} p_1^{(6)}\right)\right]^{1/2}.
\end{aligned}
\tag{9.37}
$$

Similarly, we can show that the ratio of mean frequencies $RM_{31}(= \exp(\gamma_2))$ between periods 3 and 1 is given by (Problem 9.8)

$$
\begin{aligned}
RM_{31} &= \left[\left(p_3^{(1)} p_3^{(6)}\right) / \left(p_1^{(1)} p_1^{(6)}\right)\right]^{1/2} \\
&= \left[\left(p_3^{(2)} p_3^{(4)}\right) / \left(p_1^{(2)} p_1^{(4)}\right)\right]^{1/2} \\
&= \left[\left(p_3^{(3)} p_3^{(5)}\right) / \left(p_1^{(3)} p_1^{(5)}\right)\right]^{1/2}.
\end{aligned}
\tag{9.38}
$$

On the basis of (9.37), we obtain the WLS estimator for γ_1 as

$$\hat{\gamma}_1^{(WLS)} = \sum_{k=1}^{3} WP_k \log\left(\widehat{ORP}_k\right) / \left(2\sum_{i=1}^{3} WP_k\right), \tag{9.39}$$

where $\widehat{ORP}_1 = \left(\hat{p}_2^{(1)} \hat{p}_2^{(3)}\right) / \left(\hat{p}_1^{(1)} \hat{p}_1^{(3)}\right)$, $\widehat{ORP}_2 = \left(\hat{p}_2^{(2)} \hat{p}_2^{(5)}\right) / \left(\hat{p}_1^{(2)} \hat{p}_1^{(5)}\right)$, $\widehat{ORP}_3 = \left(\hat{p}_2^{(4)} \hat{p}_2^{(6)}\right) / \left(\hat{p}_1^{(4)} \hat{p}_1^{(6)}\right)$, $WP_1 = 1/\widehat{Var}\left(\log\left(\widehat{ORP}_1\right)\right) = \left(1/Y_{+2}^{(1)} + 1/Y_{+1}^{(3)} + 1/Y_{+1}^{(1)} + \right.$

$1/Y_{+2}^{(3)})^{-1}$, $WP_2 = 1/\widehat{Var}\left(\log\left(\widehat{ORP}_2\right)\right) = \left(1/Y_{+2}^{(2)} + 1/Y_{+1}^{(5)} + 1/Y_{+1}^{(2)} + 1/Y_{+2}^{(5)}\right)^{-1}$,

and $WP_3 = 1/\widehat{Var}\left(\log\left(\widehat{ORP}_3\right)\right) = \left(1/Y_{+2}^{(4)} + 1/Y_{+1}^{(6)} + 1/Y_{+1}^{(4)} + 1/Y_{+2}^{(6)}\right)^{-1}$. We can

further show that an asymptotic variance for $\hat{\gamma}_1^{(WLS)}$ (9.39) is

$$\widehat{Var}\left(\hat{\gamma}_1^{(WLS)}\right) = 1\bigg/\left(4\sum_{k=1}^{3} WP_k\right). \tag{9.40}$$

On the basis of (9.38), we obtain the WLS estimator for $RM_{31}(=\exp(\gamma_2))$ as

$$\hat{\gamma}_2^{(WLS)} = \sum_{k=1}^{3} WP_k^* \log\left(\widehat{ORP}_k^*\right)\bigg/\left(2\sum_{i=1}^{3} WP_k^*\right), \tag{9.41}$$

where $\widehat{ORP}_1^* = \left(\hat{p}_3^{(1)}\hat{p}_3^{(6)}\right)\big/\left(\hat{p}_1^{(1)}\hat{p}_1^{(6)}\right)$, $\widehat{ORP}_2^* = \left(\hat{p}_3^{(2)}\hat{p}_3^{(4)}\right)\big/\left(\hat{p}_1^{(2)}\hat{p}_1^{(4)}\right)$, $\widehat{ORP}_3^* = \left(\hat{p}_3^{(3)}\hat{p}_3^{(5)}\right)\big/\left(\hat{p}_1^{(3)}\hat{p}_1^{(5)}\right)$, $WP_1^* = 1/\widehat{Var}\left(\log\left(\widehat{ORP}_1^*\right)\right) = \left(1/Y_{+3}^{(1)} + 1/Y_{+1}^{(6)} + 1/Y_{+1}^{(1)} + 1/Y_{+3}^{(6)}\right)^{-1}$, $WP_2^* = 1/\widehat{Var}\left(\log\left(\widehat{ORP}_2^*\right)\right) = \left(1/Y_{+3}^{(2)} + 1/Y_{+1}^{(4)} + 1/Y_{+1}^{(2)} + 1/Y_{+3}^{(4)}\right)^{-1}$,

and $WP_3^* = 1/\widehat{Var}\left(\log\left(\widehat{ORP}_3^*\right)\right) = \left(1/Y_{+3}^{(3)} + 1/Y_{+1}^{(5)} + 1/Y_{+1}^{(3)} + 1/Y_{+3}^{(5)}\right)^{-1}$. Further-

more, we obtain an estimated asymptotic variance estimator for $\hat{\gamma}_2^{(WLS)}$ (9.41) as

$$\widehat{Var}\left(\hat{\gamma}_2^{(WLS)}\right) = 1\bigg/\left(4\sum_{k=1}^{3} WP_k^*\right). \tag{9.42}$$

When n_g is large, we may test $H_0 : \gamma_1 = \gamma_2 = 0$ by use of asymptotic test procedures (9.39)–(9.42) and Bonferroni's inequality to adjust the inflation due to multiple tests in Type I error. We will reject $H_0 : \gamma_1 = \gamma_2 = 0$ at the α-level if either of the following two inequalities holds:

$$|\hat{\gamma}_1^{(WLS)}|\bigg/\sqrt{\widehat{var}\left(\hat{\gamma}_1^{(WLS)}\right)} > Z_{\alpha/4}, \text{ or}$$
$$|\hat{\gamma}_2^{(WLS)}|\bigg/\sqrt{\widehat{var}\left(\hat{\gamma}_2^{(WLS)}\right)} > Z_{\alpha/4}. \tag{9.43}$$

Following the same ideas as those presented previously for assessing the treatment effect, we can derive other test procedures as well as interval estimators for γ_1 and γ_2 on the basis of the MH and exact methods.

9.6   Procedures for testing treatment-by-period interactions

To examine whether there are interactions between treatments and periods, we extend model (9.1) to include the interaction terms by assuming that the frequency $Y_{iz}^{(g)}$ of event occurrences on patient i ($= 1, 2, \cdots, n_g$) assigned to group g ($= 1, 2, 3, 4, 5, 6$) at period z ($= 1, 2, 3$) follows the Poisson distribution with mean given by

$$
\begin{aligned}
E\left(Y_{iz}^{(g)}\right) = \exp\big(\mu_i^{(g)} &+ \eta_{AC}X_{iz1}^{(g)} + \eta_{BC}X_{iz2}^{(g)} + \gamma_1 Z_{iz1}^{(g)} + \gamma_2 Z_{iz2}^{(g)} \\
&+ \nu_{11}X_{iz1}^{(g)}Z_{iz1}^{(g)} + \nu_{12}X_{iz1}^{(g)}Z_{iz2}^{(g)} + \nu_{21}X_{iz2}^{(g)}Z_{iz1}^{(g)} + \nu_{22}X_{iz2}^{(g)}Z_{iz2}^{(g)}\big),
\end{aligned}
\tag{9.44}
$$

where ν_{11} and ν_{12} represent the interaction terms between treatment A (versus placebo C) and periods 1 and 2, and ν_{21} and ν_{22} represent the interaction terms between treatment B (versus placebo C) and periods 1 and 2. On the basis of model (9.44), we can show that (Problem 9.9)

$$
\begin{aligned}
OR_1 &= \left[\left(p_2^{(1)}p_1^{(3)}\right) \big/ \left(p_1^{(1)}p_2^{(3)}\right)\right] = \exp(2\eta_{AC} + \nu_{11}), \\
OR_2 &= \left[\left(p_3^{(2)}p_1^{(4)}\right) \big/ \left(p_1^{(2)}p_3^{(4)}\right)\right] = \exp(2\eta_{AC} + \nu_{12}), \text{ and} \\
OR_3 &= \left[\left(p_3^{(5)}p_2^{(6)}\right) \big/ \left(p_2^{(5)}p_3^{(6)}\right)\right] = \exp(2\eta_{AC} + \nu_{11} + \nu_{12}).
\end{aligned}
\tag{9.45}
$$

Note that we can see from (9.45) that $OR_1 = OR_2 = OR_3$ if and only if $\nu_{11} = \nu_{12} = 0$. Thus, we can test the null hypothesis $H_0: \nu_{11} = \nu_{12} = 0$ by employing the WLS procedure for testing the homogeneity of OR across a series of 2×2 tables (Fleiss, 1981). We will reject $H_0: \nu_{11} = \nu_{12} = 0$ at the α-level if

$$
\sum_{k=1}^{3} W_k\left(\log\left(\widehat{OR}_k\right)\right)^2 - \left(\sum_{k=1}^{3} W_k\log\left(\widehat{OR}_k\right)\right)^2 \big/ \left(\sum_{k=1}^{3} W_k\right) > \chi_\alpha^2(2). \tag{9.46}
$$

Furthermore, we can show that under model (9.44) (Problem 9.10)

$$
\begin{aligned}
OR_1^* &= \left[\left(p_3^{(1)}p_1^{(6)}\right) \big/ \left(p_1^{(1)}p_3^{(6)}\right)\right] = \exp(2\eta_{BC} + \nu_{22}), \\
OR_2^* &= \left[\left(p_2^{(2)}p_1^{(5)}\right) \big/ \left(p_1^{(2)}p_2^{(5)}\right)\right] = \exp(2\eta_{BC} + \nu_{21}), \text{ and} \\
OR_3^* &= \left[\left(p_3^{(3)}p_2^{(4)}\right) \big/ \left(p_2^{(3)}p_3^{(4)}\right)\right] = \exp(2\eta_{BC} + \nu_{21} + \nu_{22}).
\end{aligned}
\tag{9.47}
$$

On the basis of (9.47), we will reject $H_0: \nu_{21} = \nu_{22} = 0$ at the α-level if

$$
\sum_{k=1}^{3} W_k^*\left(\log\left(\widehat{OR}_k^*\right)\right)^2 - \left(\sum_{k=1}^{3} W_k^*\log\left(\widehat{OR}_k^*\right)\right)^2 \big/ \left(\sum_{k=1}^{3} W_k^*\right) > \chi_\alpha^2(2). \tag{9.48}
$$

Other test procedures published elsewhere (Zelen, 1971; Breslow and Day, 1980; Ejigou and McHugh, 1984; Lui, 2004) for testing the homogeneity of the OR across 2×2 tables can be also applied to test whether there are treatment-by-period interactions.

Example 9.3 When applying test procedures (9.46) and (9.48), we obtain the p-values 0.005 and 0.240, respectively. Thus, there seems to evidence that the relative effects of treatment A (salbutamol) to the placebo vary between periods. When calculating OR_i (9.45) by substituting $\hat{p}_z^{(g)}$ for $p_z^{(g)}$, we obtain $\widehat{OR}_1 = 0.767$, $\widehat{OR}_2 = 3.923$, and $\widehat{OR}_3 = 0.195$. Because $\widehat{OR}_2$ is larger than $\widehat{OR}_1$, the relative effect of salbutamol to placebo seems to deteriorate at period 2 versus period 1. This result is consistent with the observation that the asthma score for salbutamol might deteriorate over time noted elsewhere (Taylor *et al.*, 1998).

Exercises

Problem 9.1. Show that conditional upon patient i in group g (= 1, 2, $\cdots$, 6), the random vector of frequencies $\left(Y_{i1}^{(g)}, Y_{i2}^{(g)}, Y_{i3}^{(g)}\right)'$, given $Y_{i+}^{(g)} = Y_{i1}^{(g)} + Y_{i2}^{(g)} + Y_{i3}^{(g)} = y_{i+}^{(g)}$ fixed, follows the multinomial distribution with parameters $y_{i+}^{(g)}$ and $\left(p_1^{(g)}, p_2^{(g)}, p_3^{(g)}\right)'$, where

for $g = 1$:

$$p_1^{(1)} = 1/(1 + \exp(\eta_{AC} + \gamma_1) + \exp(\eta_{BC} + \gamma_2)),$$

$$p_2^{(1)} = \exp(\eta_{AC} + \gamma_1)/(1 + \exp(\eta_{AC} + \gamma_1) + \exp(\eta_{BC} + \gamma_2)),$$

$$p_3^{(1)} = \exp(\eta_{BC} + \gamma_2)/(1 + \exp(\eta_{AC} + \gamma_1) + \exp(\eta_{BC} + \gamma_2));$$

for $g = 2$:

$$p_1^{(2)} = 1/(1 + \exp(\eta_{BC} + \gamma_1) + \exp(\eta_{AC} + \gamma_2)),$$

$$p_2^{(2)} = \exp(\eta_{BC} + \gamma_1)/(1 + \exp(\eta_{BC} + \gamma_1) + \exp(\eta_{AC} + \gamma_2)),$$

$$p_3^{(2)} = \exp(\eta_{AC} + \gamma_2)/(1 + \exp(\eta_{BC} + \gamma_1) + \exp(\eta_{AC} + \gamma_2));$$

for $g = 3$:

$$p_1^{(3)} = \exp(\eta_{AC})/(\exp(\eta_{AC}) + \exp(\gamma_1) + \exp(\eta_{BC} + \gamma_2)),$$

$$p_2^{(3)} = \exp(\gamma_1)/(\exp(\eta_{AC}) + \exp(\gamma_1) + \exp(\eta_{BC} + \gamma_2)),$$

$$p_3^{(3)} = \exp(\eta_{BC} + \gamma_2)/(\exp(\eta_{AC}) + \exp(\gamma_1) + \exp(\eta_{BC} + \gamma_2));$$

for $g = 4$:

$$p_1^{(4)} = \exp(\eta_{AC})/(\exp(\eta_{AC}) + \exp(\gamma_1 + \eta_{BC}) + \exp(\gamma_2)),$$

$$p_2^{(4)} = \exp(\gamma_1 + \eta_{BC})/(\exp(\eta_{AC}) + \exp(\gamma_1 + \eta_{BC}) + \exp(\gamma_2)),$$

$$p_3^{(4)} = \exp(\gamma_2)/(\exp(\eta_{AC}) + \exp(\gamma_1 + \eta_{BC}) + \exp(\gamma_2));$$

for $g = 5$:

$$p_1^{(5)} = \exp(\eta_{BC}) / (\exp(\eta_{BC}) + \exp(\gamma_1) + \exp(\eta_{AC} + \gamma_2)),$$

$$p_2^{(5)} = \exp(\gamma_1) / (\exp(\eta_{BC}) + \exp(\gamma_1) + \exp(\eta_{AC} + \gamma_2)),$$

$$p_3^{(5)} = \exp(\eta_{AC} + \gamma_2) / (\exp(\eta_{BC}) + \exp(\gamma_1) + \exp(\eta_{AC} + \gamma_2));$$

for $g = 6$:

$$p_1^{(6)} = \exp(\eta_{BC}) / (\exp(\eta_{BC}) + \exp(\gamma_1 + \eta_{AC}) + \exp(\gamma_2)),$$

$$p_2^{(6)} = \exp(\gamma_1 + \eta_{AC}) / (\exp(\eta_{BC}) + \exp(\gamma_1 + \eta_{AC}) + \exp(\gamma_2)),$$

$$p_3^{(6)} = \exp(\gamma_2) / (\exp(\eta_{BC}) + \exp(\gamma_1 + \eta_{AC}) + \exp(\gamma_2)).$$

Problem 9.2. Under model (9.1), show that the ratio of mean frequencies $RM_{AC} (= \exp(\eta_{AC}))$ between treatments A and C can be expressed as those equations given in (9.2). (Hint: Use the results found in Problem 9.1.)

Problem 9.3. Show that an estimated asymptotic variance for the WLS estimator $\hat{\eta}_{AC}^{(WLS)}$ (9.3) is given by $\widehat{Var}\left(\hat{\eta}_{AC}^{(WLS)}\right) = 1 / \left(4 \sum_{k=1}^{3} W_k\right)$.

Problem 9.4. Show that the ratio of mean frequencies $RM_{BC} (= \exp(\eta_{BC}))$ between treatments B and C under model (9.1) can be expressed as those equations given in (9.5).

Problem 9.5. Show that the ratio of mean frequencies $RM_{BA} (= \exp(\eta_{BC} - \eta_{AC}))$ between treatments B and A under model (9.1) can be expressed as those equations given in (9.8).

Problem 9.6. Show that an estimated asymptotic covariance between $\hat{\eta}_{AC}^{(WLS)}$ (9.3) and $\hat{\eta}_{BC}^{(WLS)}$ (9.6) is given by (9.20).

Problem 9.7. Show that the ratio of mean frequencies $RM_{21} (= \exp(\gamma_1))$ between periods 2 and 1 can be expressed as those equations given in (9.37) under model (9.1).

Problem 9.8. Show that the ratio of mean frequencies $RM_{31} (= \exp(\gamma_{31}))$ between periods 3 and 1 can be expressed as those equations given in (9.38).

Problem 9.9. Under model (9.44), show that OR_i (for $i = 1, 2, 3$) can be expressed as those equations given in (9.45).

Problem 9.10. Under model (9.44), show that OR_i^* (for $i = 1, 2, 3$) can be expressed as those equations given in (9.47).

Problem 9.11. Following similar ideas as for deriving test procedures (9.46) and (9.48), discuss how to derive the procedure for testing $H_0 : \nu_{11} - \nu_{21} = \nu_{12} - \nu_{22} = 0$.

10

Three-treatment (incomplete block) crossover design in continuous and dichotomous data

When patients are required to take each treatment in a crossover design with three or more treatments under comparison, the duration of a crossover trial can be much longer than that of a parallel groups design. The longer the duration of a trial, the more difficult it is to recruit patients, keep patients from dropping out, and ensure patients closely follow the protocol of a trial. To alleviate these concerns, we may assign each patient to receive only a subset of treatments rather than all treatments (Koch *et al.*, 1989; Senn, 2002). For example, consider the data in Table 10.1 (Senn, 2002, p. 213) taken from a double-blind placebo controlled crossover trial comparing 12 and 24 μg of formoterol solution aerosol with a placebo. For practical reasons, it was decided that each patient could receive only two of the three treatments: the placebo, 12 μg of formoterol solution, and 24 μg of formoterol solution. When patients receive only a subset of treatments under investigation, we call this an incomplete block crossover design (Senn, 2002).

In this chapter, we focus our attention on the crossover design, in which each patient receives two out of three treatments under comparison in both continuous and dichotomous data. Under a random effects linear additive risk model (Grizzle, 1965) for continuous data (Lui, 2015b) and a random effects logistic regression model for binary data (Lui and Chang, 2015a), we consider use of the WLS approach to do hypothesis testing and estimation (Fleiss, 1981; Senn, 2002). We discuss testing non-equality between either of the two experimental treatments and a placebo. We further

Crossover Designs: Testing, Estimation, and Sample Size, First Edition. Kung-Jong Lui.
© 2016 John Wiley & Sons, Ltd. Published 2016 by John Wiley & Sons, Ltd.
Companion website: www.wiley.com/go/lui/crossover

Table 10.1   The FEV_1 (in liters) taken at two periods on
24 patients under a crossover trial comparing (treatment A =)
12 µg and (treatment B =) 24 µg with a placebo.

Treatment-receipt sequence	Period I	Period II
P-A	2.500	3.500
	1.600	2.650
	1.750	2.190
	0.640	0.840
A-P	3.400	2.500
	2.250	1.925
	1.460	1.260
	1.480	0.880
	2.050	2.100
P-B	2.100	3.100
	2.300	2.700
	1.030	1.870
	0.810	0.940
B-P	1.750	1.350
	2.525	2.150
	1.080	0.840
	3.120	2.310
A-B	2.500	2.450
	1.750	1.725
	1.370	1.120
B-A	2.700	2.250
	0.900	0.925
	1.270	1.010
	2.150	2.100

discuss testing non-inferiority of either experimental treatment to an active control treatment in binary data. We address interval estimation of the relative effect between treatments. As an alternative approach to the WLS method, we include the SAS codes of PROC GLM, PROC MIXED, and PROC GLIMMIX in (SAS Institute, 2009) and compare the results using various methods. Also, we outline in exercises the derivation of an exact interval estimator for the relative treatment effect when the underlying patient response is dichotomous (Lui, 2015c).

Consider comparing two experimental treatments A and B with an active control treatment (or a placebo) C under a two-period crossover design. We let X-Y denote the treatment-receipt sequence in which a patient receives treatment X at the first period and then crosses over to receive treatment Y at the second period. Suppose that we randomly assign n_g patients to group $g = 1$ with C-A treatment-receipt sequence; = 2 with A-C treatment-receipt sequence; = 3 with C-B treatment-receipt sequence; = 4 with B-C treatment-receipt sequence; = 5 with A-B treatment-receipt sequence; and = 6 with B-A treatment-receipt sequence. With an adequate washout period, we assume that there are no carry-over effects due to the treatment administered at an earlier period.

10.1   Continuous data

For patient i (= 1, 2, $\cdots$, n_g) assigned to group g (= 1, 2, 3, 4, 5, 6), we let $Y_{iz}^{(g)}$ denote the patient response at period z (= 1, 2). Following Grizzle (1965), we assume the following random effects linear additive risk model for the patient response:

$$Y_{iz}^{(g)} = \mu_i^{(g)} + \eta_{AC} X_{iz1}^{(g)} + \eta_{BC} X_{iz2}^{(g)} + \gamma 1_i^{(g)} (z=2) + \varepsilon_{iz}^{(g)}, \qquad (10.1)$$

where $\mu_i^{(g)}$ denotes the random effect due to the ith patient in group g, and $\mu_i^{(g)}$'s are assumed to independently follow an unspecified probability density function $f_g(\mu)$; $X_{iz1}^{(g)}$ denotes the indicator function of treatment-receipt for treatment A, and $X_{iz1}^{(g)} = 1$ if the ith patient in group g at period z receives treatment A, and = 0 otherwise; $X_{iz2}^{(g)}$ denotes the indicator function of treatment-receipt for treatment B, and $X_{iz2}^{(g)} = 1$ if the corresponding patient at period z receives treatment B, and = 0 otherwise; $1_i^{(g)}(z=2)$ represents the indicator function for period $z=2$, and $1_i^{(g)}(z=2) = 1$ for period $z=2$, and = 0 otherwise; and the random errors $\varepsilon_{iz}^{(g)}$'s are assumed to be independent and identically distributed as the normal distribution with mean 0 and variance σ_e^2, as well as all $\varepsilon_{iz}^{(g)}$'s are assumed to be independent of $\mu_i^{(g)}$. Note that parameters η_{AC} and η_{BC} denote the respective effect of treatments A and B versus an active control treatment (or a placebo) C, as well as γ represents the effect of period 2 versus period 1. When there is no difference in effects between treatments A and C, the parameter η_{AC} is equal to 0. When treatment A tends to increase the patient response as compared with treatment C, the parameter η_{AC} is greater than 0. When treatment A tends to decrease the patient response as compared with treatment C, η_{AC} is less than 0. Similar interpretations as those for η_{AC} are applicable to η_{BC} and γ. Note that the mean difference in responses between treatments B and A under model (10.1) for a fixed period on a given patient is $\eta_{BA} = \eta_{BC} - \eta_{AC}$. When there is no difference in effects between treatments B and A, η_{BA} equals 0.

For patient i (= 1, 2, 3, $\cdots$, n_g) assigned to group g (= 1, 2, 3, $\cdots$, 6), we define $d_i^{(g)} = Y_{i2}^{(g)} - Y_{i1}^{(g)}$, representing the difference in responses between periods 2 and 1. Note that the difference $d_i^{(g)}$ does not depend on the random effect $\mu_i^{(g)}$ under model (10.1). We define $\bar{d}^{(g)} = \sum_{i=1}^{n_g} d_i^{(g)} / n_g$ as the average of the response difference between periods 2 and 1 over patients in group g. Under model (10.1), we can easily show that an unbiased consistent estimator for η_{AC} is given by (Problem 10.1)

$$\hat{\eta}_{AC} = \left(\bar{d}^{(1)} - \bar{d}^{(2)}\right)/2, \tag{10.2}$$

with variance

$$Var(\hat{\eta}_{AC}) = \sigma_d^2(1/n_1 + 1/n_2)/4, \tag{10.3}$$

where $\sigma_d^2 = 2\sigma_e^2$.

Similarly, we obtain an unbiased consistent estimator for η_{BC} as

$$\hat{\eta}_{BC} = \left(\bar{d}^{(3)} - \bar{d}^{(4)}\right)/2, \tag{10.4}$$

with variance

$$Var(\hat{\eta}_{BC}) = \sigma_d^2(1/n_3 + 1/n_4)/4. \tag{10.5}$$

Also, we can show that an unbiased consistent estimator for $\eta_{BA}(=\eta_{BC}-\eta_{AC})$ is given by

$$\hat{\eta}_{BA} = \left(\bar{d}^{(5)} - \bar{d}^{(6)}\right)/2, \tag{10.6}$$

with variance

$$Var(\hat{\eta}_{BA}) = \sigma_d^2(1/n_5 + 1/n_6)/4. \tag{10.7}$$

Note that $E(\hat{\eta}_{BC} - \hat{\eta}_{BA}) = \eta_{BC}-(\eta_{BC}-\eta_{AC}) = \eta_{AC}$. Thus, we can also obtain an unbiased estimator for η_{AC} indirectly based on the data from groups $g = 3, 4, 5,$ and 6, as

$$\hat{\eta}_{AC}^* = \hat{\eta}_{BC} - \hat{\eta}_{BA}, \tag{10.8}$$

with variance

$$Var\left(\hat{\eta}_{AC}^*\right) = \sigma_d^2(1/n_3 + 1/n_4 + 1/n_5 + 1/n_6)/4. \tag{10.9}$$

On the basis of the two unbiased estimators $\hat{\eta}_{AC}$ (10.2) and $\hat{\eta}_{AC}^*$ (10.8), we obtain the WLS estimator for η_{AC} (Fleiss, 1981; Senn, 2002) as

$$\hat{\eta}_{AC}^{(WLS)} = \left[W_{AC}\hat{\eta}_{AC} + (1-W_{AC})\hat{\eta}_{AC}^*\right], \tag{10.10}$$

where $W_{AC} = (1/n_1 + 1/n_2)^{-1}/\left[(1/n_1 + 1/n_2)^{-1} + (1/n_3 + 1/n_4 + 1/n_5 + 1/n_6)^{-1}\right]$.

Note that $\hat{\eta}_{AC}^{(WLS)}$ (10.10) is an unbiased estimator for η_{AC} as well. Furthermore, the variance of $\hat{\eta}_{AC}^{(WLS)}$ is given by (Problem 10.2)

$$Var\left(\hat{\eta}_{AC}^{(WLS)}\right) = \sigma_d^2/\left\{4\left[(1/n_1 + 1/n_2)^{-1} + (1/n_3 + 1/n_4 + 1/n_5 + 1/n_6)^{-1}\right]\right\}, \tag{10.11}$$

which is smaller than both $Var(\hat{\eta}_{AC})$ (10.3) and $Var(\hat{\eta}_{AC}^*)$ (10.9).

When estimating η_{BC}, we note that $E(\hat{\eta}_{AC} + \hat{\eta}_{BA}) = \eta_{AC} + (\eta_{BC} - \eta_{AC}) = \eta_{BC}$. Thus, we define

$$\hat{\eta}_{BC}^* = \hat{\eta}_{AC} + \hat{\eta}_{BA}, \tag{10.12}$$

which is an unbiased estimator for η_{BC}. On the basis of $\hat{\eta}_{BC}$ (10.4) and $\hat{\eta}_{BC}^*$ (10.12), we obtain the WLS estimator for η_{BC} as

$$\hat{\eta}_{BC}^{(WLS)} = \left[W_{BC}\hat{\eta}_{BC} + (1 - W_{BC})\hat{\eta}_{BC}^* \right], \tag{10.13}$$

where $W_{BC} = (1/n_3 + 1/n_4)^{-1} / \left[(1/n_3 + 1/n_4)^{-1} + (1/n_1 + 1/n_2 + 1/n_5 + 1/n_6)^{-1} \right]$.

Again, $\hat{\eta}_{BC}^{(WLS)}$ is an unbiased estimator for η_{BC}. The variance of the WLS estimator $\hat{\eta}_{BC}^{(WLS)}$ (10.13) is equal to

$$Var\left(\hat{\eta}_{BC}^{(WLS)}\right) = \sigma_d^2 / \left\{ 4\left[(1/n_3 + 1/n_4)^{-1} + (1/n_1 + 1/n_2 + 1/n_5 + 1/n_6)^{-1} \right] \right\}. \tag{10.14}$$

Note that the two WLS estimators $\hat{\eta}_{AC}^{(WLS)}$ (10.11) and $\hat{\eta}_{BC}^{(WLS)}$ (10.13) are correlated. We can show that the covariance between these two estimators $\hat{\eta}_{AC}^{(WLS)}$ and $\hat{\eta}_{BC}^{(WLS)}$ under model (10.1) is given by (Problem 10.3)

$$Cov\left(\hat{\eta}_{AC}^{(WLS)}, \hat{\eta}_{BC}^{(WLS)}\right) = W_{AC}(1 - W_{BC})Var(\hat{\eta}_{AC}) + (1 - W_{AC})(W_{BC})Var(\hat{\eta}_{BC})$$
$$- (1 - W_{AC})(1 - W_{BC})Var(\hat{\eta}_{BA}). \tag{10.15}$$

Note that $Var\left(\hat{\eta}_{AC}^{(WLS)}\right)$ (10.11), $Var\left(\hat{\eta}_{BC}^{(WLS)}\right)$ (10.14), and $Cov\left(\hat{\eta}_{AC}^{(WLS)}, \hat{\eta}_{BC}^{(WLS)}\right)$ (10.15) are all functions of unknown σ_d^2. However, we can estimate σ_d^2 by the pooled unbiased sample variance (Problem 10.4)

$$\hat{\sigma}_d^2 = \sum_{g=1}^{6} \sum_{i=1}^{n_g} \left(d_i^{(g)} - \bar{d}^{(g)} \right)^2 / (n_+ - 6), \tag{10.16}$$

where $n_+ = \sum_{g=1}^{6} n_g$ denotes the total number of patients in the trial. Therefore, when substituting $\hat{\sigma}_d^2$ (10.16) for σ_d^2 in $Var\left(\hat{\eta}_{AC}^{(WLS)}\right)$ (10.11), $Var\left(\hat{\eta}_{BC}^{(WLS)}\right)$ (10.14), and $Cov\left(\hat{\eta}_{AC}^{(WLS)}, \hat{\eta}_{BC}^{(WLS)}\right)$ (10.15), we obtain $\widehat{Var}\left(\hat{\eta}_{AC}^{(WLS)}\right)$, $\widehat{Var}\left(\hat{\eta}_{BC}^{(WLS)}\right)$, and $\widehat{Cov}\left(\hat{\eta}_{AC}^{(WLS)}, \hat{\eta}_{BC}^{(WLS)}\right)$, respectively.

10.1.1   Testing non-equality of treatments

Suppose that we wish to study whether there is a difference in mean responses between patients receiving either treatment A or B and patients receiving treatment C, while we are not interested in comparing experimental treatment A with treatment B (Dunnett, 1964; Fleiss, 1986a). This leads us to test the null hypothesis $H_0 : \eta_{AC} = \eta_{BC} = 0$ versus the alternative hypothesis $H_a : \eta_{AC} \neq 0$ or $\eta_{BC} \neq 0$. We first consider the test procedure by employing the univariate t-test based on $\hat{\eta}_{AC}^{(WLS)}$ (10.10) and $\hat{\eta}_{BC}^{(WLS)}$ (10.13) together with using Bonferroni's inequality to adjust the inflation due to multiple tests in Type I error. We will reject $H_0 : \eta_{AC} = \eta_{BC} = 0$ at the α-level if either of the following two inequalities holds:

$$|\hat{\eta}_{AC}^{(WLS)}| / \sqrt{\widehat{\text{var}}\left(\hat{\eta}_{AC}^{(WLS)}\right)} > t_{\alpha/4, n_+ - 6} \text{ or } |\hat{\eta}_{BC}^{(WLS)}| / \sqrt{\widehat{\text{var}}\left(\hat{\eta}_{BC}^{(WLS)}\right)} > t_{\alpha/4, n_+ - 6}, \quad (10.17)$$

where $t_{\alpha, n_+ - 6}$ is the upper $100(\alpha)$th percentile of the student t-distribution with $n_+ - 6$ degrees of freedom. Note that the test procedure (10.17) does not account for the dependence between $\hat{\eta}_{AC}^{(WLS)}$ (10.10) and $\hat{\eta}_{BC}^{(WLS)}$ (10.13) and hence may lose power.

To incorporate the covariance $\widehat{Cov}\left(\hat{\eta}_{AC}^{(WLS)}, \hat{\eta}_{BC}^{(WLS)}\right)$ into the test procedure, we may employ the following bivariate test based on the F-distribution (Problem 10.5). We will reject $H_0 : \eta_{AC} = \eta_{BC} = 0$ at the α-level if

$$\left(\hat{\eta}_{AC}^{(WLS)}, \hat{\eta}_{BC}^{(WLS)}\right) \hat{\underline{\Sigma}}^{-1} \begin{pmatrix} \hat{\eta}_{AC}^{(WLS)} \\ \hat{\eta}_{BC}^{(WLS)} \end{pmatrix} > 2F_{\alpha, 2, n_+ - 6}, \quad (10.18)$$

where $\hat{\underline{\Sigma}}$ is the estimated covariance matrix with diagonal elements equal to $\widehat{Var}\left(\hat{\eta}_{AC}^{(WLS)}\right)$ and $\widehat{Var}\left(\hat{\eta}_{BC}^{(WLS)}\right)$, the off-diagonal element equal to $\widehat{Cov}\left(\hat{\eta}_{AC}^{(WLS)}, \hat{\eta}_{BC}^{(WLS)}\right)$, and $F_{\alpha, 2, n_+ - 6}$ is the upper $100(\alpha)$th percentile of the central F-distribution with 2 and $n_+ - 6$ degrees of freedom.

When treatments A and B represent two different doses of a treatment and treatment C represents a placebo, the effects due to the low and high doses of a treatment on the patient response are likely to fall in the same relative direction to placebo. Thus, we may wish to account for this information to improve power by considering a weighted average $w\hat{\eta}_{AC}^{(WLS)} + (1-w)\hat{\eta}_{BC}^{(WLS)}$, where w $(0 < w < 1)$ is the weight reflecting the relative importance of patient response at the low dose to that of the high dose and can be assigned by clinicians based on their subjective knowledge. If we have no prior preference to assign the weight, we may set w equal to 0.50. This leads us to consider the following summary test procedure.v We will reject $H_0 : \eta_{AC} = \eta_{BC} = 0$ at the α-level if

$$\left|\hat{\eta}_{AC}^{(WLS)} + \hat{\eta}_{BC}^{(WLS)}\right| / \sqrt{\widehat{Var}\left(\hat{\eta}_{AC}^{(WLS)} + \hat{\eta}_{BC}^{(WLS)}\right)} > t_{\alpha/2, n_+ - 6}, \quad (10.19)$$

where $\widehat{Var}\left(\hat{\eta}_{AC}^{(WLS)}+\hat{\eta}_{BC}^{(WLS)}\right)=\widehat{Var}\left(\hat{\eta}_{AC}^{(WLS)}\right)+\widehat{Var}\left(\hat{\eta}_{BC}^{(WLS)}\right)+2\widehat{Cov}\left(\hat{\eta}_{AC}^{(WLS)},\hat{\eta}_{BC}^{(WLS)}\right)$.

Note that we can set, as for the WLS estimator, w equal to the optimal weight to minimize the variance of $w\hat{\eta}_{AC}^{(WLS)}+(1-w)\hat{\eta}_{BC}^{(WLS)}$. Under the balanced design (i.e., $n_1=n_2=\cdots=n_6$), this optimal weight is equal to ½ under model (10.1) (see Problem 10.6).

Using Monte Carlo simulation, Lui (2015b) noted that all test procedures (10.17)–(10.19) could perform well with respect to Type I error in a variety of situations. Lui also noted that when one of treatments A and B relative to treatment C was close to 0 and the other was different from 0, the bivariate test procedure (10.18) outperformed the other two test procedures with respect to power. When both of treatment effects η_{AC} and η_{BC} were in the same direction relative to treatment C and were approximately of equal magnitude away from 0, the test procedure (10.19) could be preferable to the others. When one of the two experimental treatments had a relatively large effect over treatment C, the test procedure (10.17) using Bonferroni's inequality could be of use.

Example 10.1 Consider the data in Table 10.1 regarding FEV_1 at the two periods for patients taken from a double-blind placebo controlled crossover trial comparing the two doses of formoterol solution aerosol at 12 µg (treatment A) and 24 µg (treatment B) with a placebo (Senn, 2002, p. 213). For practical reasons, it was decided that patients could visit only four times in the trial. Because it was required to evaluate general medical conditions of each patient before each treatment day, patients could only receive treatments at visits 2 and 4. To nullify the carry-over effect due to treatments administered at visit 2 (or at period 1), a washout period of approximately one week was used between visits 2 and 3. When applying test procedures (10.17)–(10.19) to study whether there is a difference between either dose of formoterol and placebo on FEV_1, we test $H_0 : \eta_{AC}=\eta_{BC}=0$ and obtain all the p-values less than 0.001. Thus, there is strong evidence that taking 12 or 24 µg of formoterol can significantly affect the readings of FEV_1 as compared with the placebo.

10.1.2   Testing non-equality between experimental treatments (or non-nullity of dose effects)

We may be interested in studying whether there is a dose effect when experimental treatments A and B represent two different doses of a drug. Thus, we may consider testing $H_0 : \eta_{BA}(=\eta_{BC}-\eta_{AC})=0$ versus $H_a : \eta_{BA}\neq 0$.

We define

$$\hat{\eta}_{BA}^{*}=\hat{\eta}_{BC}-\hat{\eta}_{AC}, \tag{10.20}$$

which is an unbiased consistent estimator for η_{BA}. When estimating η_{BA}, we may again consider the WLS estimator based on $\hat{\eta}_{BA}$ (10.6) and $\hat{\eta}_{BA}^{*}$ (10.20) as

$$\hat{\eta}_{BA}^{(WLS)}=\left[W_{BA}\hat{\eta}_{BA}+(1-W_{BA})\hat{\eta}_{BA}^{*}\right], \tag{10.21}$$

where $W_{BA} = (1/n_5 + 1/n_6)^{-1} / \left[(1/n_5 + 1/n_6)^{-1} + (1/n_1 + 1/n_2 + 1/n_3 + 1/n_4)^{-1} \right]$.

Thus, we will reject $H_0 : \eta_{BA} = 0$ at the α-level if

$$|\hat{\eta}_{BA}^{(WLS)}| / \sqrt{\widehat{Var}\left(\hat{\eta}_{BA}^{(WLS)}\right)} > t_{\alpha/2, n_+ -6}, \tag{10.22}$$

where $\widehat{Var}\left(\hat{\eta}_{BA}^{(WLS)}\right) = \hat{\sigma}_d^2 / \left\{ 4\left[(1/n_5 + 1/n_6)^{-1} + (1/n_1 + 1/n_2 + 1/n_3 + 1/n_4)^{-1} \right] \right\}$.

10.1.3   Interval estimation of the mean difference

When assessing the magnitude of the relative effect on the patient response between treatment A (or treatment B) and a placebo, we may wish to obtain an interval estimator for η_{AC} (or η_{BC}). On the basis of $\hat{\eta}_{AC}^{(WLS)}$ (10.10) and $\widehat{Var}\left(\hat{\eta}_{AC}^{(WLS)}\right)$, we obtain a $100(1 - \alpha)\%$ confidence interval for η_{AC} as given by

$$\left[\hat{\eta}_{AC}^{(WLS)} - t_{\alpha/2, n_+ -6} \sqrt{\widehat{Var}\left(\hat{\eta}_{AC}^{(WLS)}\right)}, \hat{\eta}_{AC}^{(WLS)} + t_{\alpha/2, n_+ -6} \sqrt{\widehat{Var}\left(\hat{\eta}_{AC}^{(WLS)}\right)} \right]. \tag{10.23}$$

Similarly, we obtain a $100(1 - \alpha)\%$ confidence interval for η_{BC} on the basis of $\hat{\eta}_{BC}^{(WLS)}$ (10.13) and $\widehat{Var}\left(\hat{\eta}_{BC}^{(WLS)}\right)$ as given by

$$\left[\hat{\eta}_{BC}^{(WLS)} - t_{\alpha/2, n_+ -6} \sqrt{\widehat{Var}\left(\hat{\eta}_{BC}^{(WLS)}\right)}, \hat{\eta}_{BC}^{(WLS)} + t_{\alpha/2, n_+ -6} \sqrt{\widehat{Var}\left(\hat{\eta}_{BC}^{(WLS)}\right)} \right]. \tag{10.24}$$

Furthermore, if we are interested in assessing the relative effect between treatments B and A, we obtain a $100(1 - \alpha)\%$ confidence interval for η_{BA} based on $\hat{\eta}_{BA}^{(WLS)}$ (10.21) and $\widehat{Var}\left(\hat{\eta}_{BA}^{(WLS)}\right)$ as given by

$$\left[\hat{\eta}_{BA}^{(WLS)} - t_{\alpha/2, n_+ -6} \sqrt{\widehat{Var}\left(\hat{\eta}_{BA}^{(WLS)}\right)}, \hat{\eta}_{BA}^{(WLS)} + t_{\alpha/2, n_+ -6} \sqrt{\widehat{Var}\left(\hat{\eta}_{BA}^{(WLS)}\right)} \right]. \tag{10.25}$$

Note that interval estimators (10.23)–(10.25) are not for simultaneous $100(1 - \alpha)\%$ confidence intervals. If we know the number K of confidence intervals of interest, we may employ Bonferroni's inequality and use $t_{\alpha/(2K), n_+ -6}$ instead of $t_{\alpha/2, n_+ -6}$ in use of interval estimators (10.23)–(10.25). For example, if we want to obtain simultaneous $100(1 - \alpha)\%$ confidence intervals for the three treatment effects η_{AC}, η_{BC}, and η_{BA}, we may replace $t_{\alpha/2, n_+ -6}$ with $t_{\alpha/6, n_+ -6}$ in use of (10.23)–(10.25). On the other hand, if we have no clear idea about how many interval estimators will be made in advance or the number K of confidence intervals of interest is quite large, we may apply Scheffe's method (Graybill, 1976, pp. 224–225) to obtain simultaneous $100(1 - \alpha)\%$ confidence intervals for all possible linear combinations $l_1\eta_{AC} + l_2\eta_{BC}$ as given by (Problem 10.7)

$$\left[l_1\hat{\eta}_{AC}^{(WLS)} + l_2\hat{\eta}_{BC}^{(WLS)} - \sqrt{2F_{\alpha,2,n_+-6}}\sqrt{\widehat{Var}\left(l_1\hat{\eta}_{AC}^{(WLS)} + l_2\hat{\eta}_{BC}^{(WLS)}\right)}, \right.$$

$$\left. l_1\hat{\eta}_{AC}^{(WLS)} + l_2\hat{\eta}_{BC}^{(WLS)} + \sqrt{2F_{\alpha,2,n_+-6}}\sqrt{\widehat{Var}\left(l_1\hat{\eta}_{AC}^{(WLS)} + l_2\hat{\eta}_{BC}^{(WLS)}\right)} \right], \quad (10.26)$$

$$\widehat{Var}\left(l_1\hat{\eta}_{AC}^{(WLS)} + l_2\hat{\eta}_{BC}^{(WLS)}\right) = l_1^2\widehat{Var}\left(\hat{\eta}_{AC}^{(WLS)}\right) + l_2^2\widehat{Var}\left(\hat{\eta}_{BC}^{(WLS)}\right) + 2l_1 l_2\widehat{Cov}\left(\hat{\eta}_{AC}^{(WLS)}, \hat{\eta}_{BC}^{(WLS)}\right).$$

Note that parameters η_{AC}, η_{BC}, and η_{BA} are special cases of $l_1\eta_{AC} + l_2\eta_{BC}$ when the vector $(l_1, l_2) = (1, 0)$, $(0, 1)$, and $(-1, 1)$.

Example 10.2   Given the data in Table 10.1, we obtain $\hat{\eta}_{AC}^{(WLS)} = 0.52$ (SE = 0.091) and $\hat{\eta}_{BC}^{(WLS)} = 0.54$ (SE = 0.094), where SE represents the estimated standard error of the parameter estimate. Thus, taking either 12 or 24 μg of formoterol can increase the mean of FEV$_1$ by approximately 0.50 *liters*. Furthermore, when using interval estimators (10.23) and (10.24), we obtain 95% confidence intervals for η_{AC} and η_{BC} as [0.328, 0.712] and [0.342, 0.738], respectively. Because both of these resulting lower limits fall above 0, there is evidence that taking either a dose of 12 or 24 μg can significantly increase FEV$_1$ as compared with the placebo. This is consistent with the previous result based on hypothesis testing found in Example 10.1. When assessing whether there is dose effect on FEV$_1$, we obtain $\hat{\eta}_{BA}^{(WLS)} = 0.02$ (SE = 0.097) and the 95% confidence interval for η_{BA} as [−0.185, 0.225]. Note that this resulting 95% confidence interval includes $\eta_{BA} = 0$. Thus, the mean response of FEV$_1$ for taking the high dose (24 μg) of the formoterol is only slightly larger than that for taking the low dose (12 μg), but this increase is not significant at the 0.05 level.

When the normal assumption for the random errors $\varepsilon_{iz}^{(g)}$'s holds, all test procedures (10.17)–(10.19) and interval estimators (10.23)–(10.25) are valid for use despite the number n ($= n_1 = n_2 = \cdots = n_6$) of patients per group. When the normality assumption for these random errors is violated, the test procedures and interval estimators may still perform well due to their robustness properties (Lui, 2015b). Also, it is possible that the variance of responses can vary between treatments. Lui (2015b) found that test procedures (10.17)–(10.19) and interval estimators (10.23)–(10.25) can be used if the assumed homogeneity of variances is not too seriously violated. When the variance of patient responses varies substantially between treatments, however, we may wish to incorporate this information into test procedures or interval estimators (Problem 10.8) to improve accuracy.

When a treatment has the same effect as a placebo, we may reasonably assume that this treatment has no different carry-over effect from the placebo as well. Thus, in testing $H_0: \eta_{AC} = \eta_{BC} = 0$, all Type I errors for (10.17)–(10.19) remain unchanged, and thereby these test procedures are valid for use. If there are differential carry-over effects between treatments, however, we can show that $\hat{\eta}_{AC}^{(WLS)}$ (10.2), $\hat{\eta}_{BC}^{(WLS)}$ (10.4), and $\hat{\eta}_{BA}^{(WLS)}$ (10.6) are all biased. Therefore, all interval estimators (10.23)–(10.25) based on these estimators can lose accuracy with respect to the coverage probability, especially when the number of patients n_g is large. Koch *et al.* (1989) noted that the relative treatment effect can be estimated with accounting for simple carry-over effects from within-patient information under the incomplete block crossover design considered here, but the loss of efficiency can be substantial due to the adjustment of carry-over effects. This may raise the question against the choice of employing a crossover design instead of a parallel groups design in the presence of carry-over effects, because the dropping-out rate, logistics support, and time length in the former are larger or longer than those in the latter. Thus, it is essentially important that we have a carefully thought out and well-planned protocol that includes use of a washout period to nullify carry-over effects when employing a crossover design. Note that one can easily apply the WLS method to do hypothesis testing and interval estimation for the period effect γ under model (10.1). For brevity, we include the discussion on studying the period effect in Problem 10.9. Note also that the WLS approach presented here actually originates from Senn's heuristic arguments (Senn, 2002, pp. 211–217). Although we can easily redefine the sets of strata and derive other WLS estimators to reduce the variance of the WLS estimators considered in the above, this reduction in variance is likely to be minimal in practice (Problem 10.10). This is because we commonly assign patients with equal probability to groups with different treatment-receipt sequences, and hence the numbers of patients assigned to different groups are expected to approximately equal one another in most crossover designs. When designing an incomplete block crossover design, we note that a recent discussion on sample size determination (Lui and Chang, 2015b) for testing non-equality of either treatment A or treatment B versus a placebo can be of use.

10.1.4   SAS codes for fixed effects and mixed effects models

When treating effects $\mu_i^{(g)}$ due to patients as fixed, we may employ SAS PROC GLM (SAS Institute, 2009) to obtain ordinal least squares estimates of the relative treatment and period effects (Jones and Kenward, 1989). We present the SAS codes applying PROC GLM to the data in Table 10.1 in the following box.

```
data step1;
ls = 120;
input patient treatment period resp;
cards;
    1    1    1   2.50
    1    2    2   3.50
    2    1    1   1.60
    2    2    2   2.65
 . . .
;;;
```

```
proc glm data=step1;
  class patient period treatment;
  model resp=patient period treatment;
  estimate "treatment effect A versus P" treatment -1 1 0;
  estimate "treatment effect B versus P" treatment -1 0 1;
  estimate "treatment effect B versus A" treatment 0 -1 1;
  estimate "period effect" period -1 1;
run;
```

To allow readers to compare the results between using the WLS method and using PROC GLM, we present in the following box the partial outputs of using PROC GLM.

Parameter	Estimate	Standard Error	t Value	Pr > |t|
treatment effect A versus P	0.50406852	0.09140275	5.51	<.0001
treatment effect B versus P	0.54429947	0.09453174	5.76	<.0001
treatment effect B versus A	0.04023095	0.09732160	0.41	0.6835
period effect	0.03101248	0.06666973	0.47	0.6466

We can see that both doses 12 µg (treatment A) and 24 µg (treatment B) of formoterol can significantly increase the mean of FEV_1 by approximately 0.50 liters; both the p-values < 0.0001. Furthermore, these resulting parameter estimates and their estimated standard errors are essentially similar to those found previously in Examples 10.1 and 10.2.

When regarding patient effects as random variables independently following a normal distribution, we may employ PROC MIXED or PROC GLIMMIX. We present the SAS codes of applying PROC MIXED to the data in Table 10.1 and the corresponding outputs in the following two boxes, respectively.

```
data step1;
ls = 120;
input patient treatment period resp;
cards;
    1    1    1   2.50
    1    2    2   3.50
    2    1    1   1.60
    2    2    2   2.65
```

```
. . .
;;;
proc print;
proc mixed data=step1;
  class patient period treatment;
  model resp=period treatment/solution;
  random patient;
  estimate "treatment effect A versus P" treatment -1 1 0;
  estimate "treatment effect B versus P" treatment -1 0 1;
  estimate "treatment effect B versus A" treatment 0 -1 1;
  estimate "period effect" period -1 1;
run;
```

Label	Estimate	Standard Error	DF	tValue	Pr>|t|
treatment effect A versus P	0.4932	0.09072	21	5.44	<.0001
treatment effect B versus P	0.5289	0.09372	21	5.64	<.0001
treatment effect B versus A	0.03570	0.09639	21	0.37	0.7148
period effect	0.03037	0.06666	21	0.46	0.6533

Again, we can see that the above results are similar to those obtained by using the WLS methods focused on here as well as those obtained by using PROC GLM with assuming the fixed effects model.

10.2   Dichotomous data

For patient i (= 1, 2, $\cdots$, n_g) assigned to group g (= 1, 2, 3, 4, 5, 6), we let $Y_{iz}^{(g)}$ denote the patient response at period z (= 1, 2), and $Y_{iz}^{(g)} = 1$ for positive, and = 0 otherwise. We assume that the probability of a positive response $Y_{iz}^{(g)} = 1$ for patient i (= 1, 2, $\cdots$, n_g) assigned to group g (= 1, 2, 3, 4, 5, 6) at period z (= 1, 2) is given by the following random effects logistic regression model (Lui and Chang, 2015a):

$$P\left(Y_{iz}^{(g)} = 1 | X_{iz1}^{(g)} = x_{iz1}^{(g)}, X_{iz2}^{(g)} = x_{iz2}^{(g)}, 1_{i1}^{(g)}\right) = \frac{\exp\left(\mu_i^{(g)} + \eta_{AC}x_{iz1}^{(g)} + \eta_{BC}x_{iz2}^{(g)} + \gamma 1_{iz}^{(g)}\right)}{1 + \exp\left(\mu_i^{(g)} + \eta_{AC}x_{iz1}^{(g)} + \eta_{BC}x_{iz2}^{(g)} + \gamma 1_{iz}^{(g)}\right)},$$

$$(10.27)$$

where $\mu_i^{(g)}$ denotes the random effect due to the ith patient assigned to group g and $\mu_i^{(g)}$'s are assumed to independently follow an unspecified probability density function $f_g(\mu)$; $X_{iz1}^{(g)}$ denotes the indicator function of treatment-receipt for treatment A, and = 1 if the patient at period z receives treatment A, and = 0 otherwise; $X_{iz2}^{(g)}$ denotes the indicator function of treatment-receipt for treatment B, and = 1 if the patient at period z receives treatment B, and = 0 otherwise; $1_{iz}^{(g)}$ denotes the indicator function of period 2, and = 1 for the patient response at period 2, and = 0 otherwise; η_{AC} and η_{BC} denote the respective effect of treatments A and B relative to treatment C; and γ represents the effect of period 2 versus period 1. On the basis of model (10.27), the OR of a positive response for a given fixed period on the same patient between treatments A and C is equal to $\varphi_{AC} = \exp(\eta_{AC})$. When there is no difference in effects between treatments A and C, we have $\varphi_{AC} = 1$ (or $\eta_{AC} = 0$). When treatment A increases the probability of a positive response as compared with treatment C, we have $\varphi_{AC} > 1$ (or $\eta_{AC} > 0$). When treatment A decreases the probability of a positive response as compared with treatment C, we have $\varphi_{AC} < 1$ (or $\eta_{AC} < 0$). The ORs of a positive response for a given fixed period on the same patient between treatments B and C and that between treatments B and A are given by $\varphi_{BC} = \exp(\eta_{BC})$ and $\varphi_{BA} = \exp(\eta_{BC} - \eta_{AC})$, respectively. Similar interpretations as those for φ_{AC} are applicable to φ_{BC} and φ_{BA}. Let $n_{rs}^{(g)}$ denote the number of patients in group g (= 1, 0) with the vector of responses ($Y_{i1}^{(g)} = r$, $Y_{i2}^{(g)} = s$), where $r = 1, 0, s = 1, 0$, among n_g patients. The set of random frequencies $\{n_{rs}^{(g)} \mid r = 1, 0, s = 1, 0\}$ follows the quadrinomial distribution with parameters n_g and $\{\pi_{rt}^{(g)} \mid r = 1, 0, s = 1\}$, where $\pi_{rs}^{(g)}$ denotes the cell probability that a randomly selected patient i from group g has the vector of responses ($Y_{i1}^{(g)} = r$, $Y_{i2}^{(g)} = s$). We can estimate $\pi_{rs}^{(g)}$ by the unbiased consistent sample proportion estimator $\hat{\pi}_{rs}^{(g)} = n_{rs}^{(g)}/n_g$. We can show that the OR (= φ_{AC}) of a positive response between treatments A and C for a fixed period on a given patient under model (10.27) is equal to (Problem 10.11)

$$\varphi_{AC} = \left[\left(\pi_{01}^{(1)} \pi_{10}^{(2)} \right) / \left(\pi_{10}^{(1)} \pi_{01}^{(2)} \right) \right]^{1/2} \tag{10.28}$$

regardless of any given probability density function $f_g(\alpha)$. Similarly, we can show that the OR of a positive response between treatments B and C for a fixed period on a given patient under model (10.27) is equal to (Problem 10.12)

$$\varphi_{BC} = \left[\left(\pi_{01}^{(3)} \pi_{10}^{(4)} \right) / \left(\pi_{10}^{(3)} \pi_{01}^{(4)} \right) \right]^{1/2}. \tag{10.29}$$

Furthermore, we can show that the OR of a positive response between treatments B and A for a fixed period on a given patient under model (10.27) is equal to (Problem 10.13)

$$\varphi_{BA}(=\exp(\eta_{BC}-\eta_{AC})) = \left[\left(\pi_{01}^{(5)}\pi_{10}^{(6)}\right)/\left(\pi_{10}^{(5)}\pi_{01}^{(6)}\right)\right]^{1/2}. \tag{10.30}$$

When substituting $\hat{\pi}_{rs}^{(g)}$ for $\pi_{rs}^{(g)}$ in (10.28), we obtain a consistent estimator for $\eta_{AC}(=\log(\varphi_{AC}))$ as

$$\hat{\eta}_{AC} = \left(\frac{1}{2}\right)\log\left(\left(n_{01}^{(1)}n_{10}^{(2)}\right)/\left(n_{10}^{(1)}n_{01}^{(2)}\right)\right). \tag{10.31}$$

Using the delta method (Agresti, 1990; Lui, 2004), we further obtain an estimated asymptotic variance of $\hat{\eta}_{AC}$ (10.31) as (Problem 10.14)

$$\widehat{Var}(\hat{\eta}_{AC}) = \left(\frac{1}{4}\right)\left(1/n_{01}^{(1)} + 1/n_{10}^{(1)} + 1/n_{10}^{(2)} + 1/n_{01}^{(2)}\right). \tag{10.32}$$

Following similar ideas as those for deriving (10.31) and (10.32), we obtain a consistent estimator for $\eta_{BC}(=\log(\varphi_{BC}))$ as

$$\hat{\eta}_{BC} = \left(\frac{1}{2}\right)\log\left(\left(n_{01}^{(3)}n_{10}^{(4)}\right)/\left(n_{10}^{(3)}n_{01}^{(4)}\right)\right), \tag{10.33}$$

and its estimated asymptotic variance given by

$$\widehat{Var}(\hat{\eta}_{BC}) = \left(\frac{1}{4}\right)\left(1/n_{01}^{(3)} + 1/n_{10}^{(3)} + 1/n_{10}^{(4)} + 1/n_{01}^{(4)}\right). \tag{10.34}$$

Also, when substituting $\hat{\pi}_{rs}^{(g)}$ for $\pi_{rs}^{(g)}$ in (10.30) and employing the delta method, we obtain the following consistent estimator for $\eta_{BA}(=\log(\varphi_{BA})=\eta_{BC}-\eta_{AC})$ as

$$\hat{\eta}_{BA} = \left(\frac{1}{2}\right)\log\left(\left(n_{01}^{(5)}n_{10}^{(6)}\right)/\left(n_{10}^{(5)}n_{01}^{(6)}\right)\right), \tag{10.35}$$

and its estimated asymptotic variance

$$\widehat{Var}(\hat{\eta}_{BA}) = \left(\frac{1}{4}\right)\left(1/n_{01}^{(5)} + 1/n_{10}^{(5)} + 1/n_{10}^{(6)} + 1/n_{01}^{(6)}\right). \tag{10.36}$$

Whenever we fail to apply (10.31)–(10.36) due to $n_{rs}^{(g)}=0$ for some (r, s) in group g, we may use the ad hoc adjustment procedure for sparse data by adding 0.50 to all cells involved in calculation of the particular corresponding estimate.

Note that because $\eta_{BC}-(\eta_{BC}-\eta_{AC})=\eta_{AC}$, we can obtain an alternative consistent estimator for η_{AC} indirectly based on the data from groups $g=3$, 4, 5, and 6, as

$$\hat{\eta}_{AC}^{*} = \hat{\eta}_{BC}-\hat{\eta}_{BA}, \tag{10.37}$$

and its estimated variance of $\hat{\eta}_{AC}^{*}$ given by $\widehat{Var}(\hat{\eta}_{AC}^{*}) = \widehat{Var}(\hat{\eta}_{BC}) + \widehat{Var}(\hat{\eta}_{BA})$.

Based on $\hat{\eta}_{AC}$ (10.31) and $\hat{\eta}_{AC}^*$ (10.37), we obtain the WLS estimator for η_{AC} as

$$\hat{\eta}_{AC}^{(WLS)} = \left[W_{AC}\hat{\eta}_{AC} + (1 - W_{AC})\hat{\eta}_{AC}^* \right], \tag{10.38}$$

where $W_{AC} = \left(\widehat{Var}(\hat{\eta}_{AC}) \right)^{-1} / \left[\left(\widehat{Var}(\hat{\eta}_{AC}) \right)^{-1} + \left(\widehat{Var}(\hat{\eta}_{AC}^*) \right)^{-1} \right]$. An estimated asymptotic variance of $\hat{\eta}_{AC}^{(WLS)}$ (10.38) is approximately given by (Problem 10.15)

$$\widehat{Var}\left(\hat{\eta}_{AC}^{(WLS)} \right) = 1 / \left[\left(\widehat{Var}(\hat{\eta}_{AC}) \right)^{-1} + \left(\widehat{Var}(\hat{\eta}_{AC}^*) \right)^{-1} \right], \tag{10.39}$$

which is smaller than both $\widehat{Var}(\hat{\eta}_{AC})$ and $\widehat{Var}(\hat{\eta}_{AC}^*)$, the variances of its two components $\hat{\eta}_{AC}$ and $\hat{\eta}_{AC}^*$ in (10.38).

Because $\eta_{AC} + (\eta_{BC} - \eta_{AC}) = \eta_{BC}$, we may also obtain a consistent estimator of η_{BC} indirectly based on the data from group $g = 1, 2, 5$, and 6 as

$$\hat{\eta}_{BC}^* = \hat{\eta}_{AC} + \hat{\eta}_{BA}, \tag{10.40}$$

and its estimated asymptotic variance $\widehat{Var}(\hat{\eta}_{BC}^*) = \widehat{Var}(\hat{\eta}_{AC}) + \widehat{Var}(\hat{\eta}_{BA})$. On the basis of $\hat{\eta}_{BC}$ (10.33) and $\hat{\eta}_{BC}^*$ (10.40), we obtain the WLS estimator for η_{BC} as

$$\hat{\eta}_{BC}^{(WLS)} = \left[W_{BC}\hat{\eta}_{BC} + (1 - W_{BC})\hat{\eta}_{BC}^* \right], \tag{10.41}$$

where $W_{BC} = \left(\widehat{Var}(\hat{\eta}_{BC}) \right)^{-1} / \left[\left(\widehat{Var}(\hat{\eta}_{BC}) \right)^{-1} + \left(\widehat{Var}(\hat{\eta}_{BC}^*) \right)^{-1} \right]$. The estimated asymptotic variance of $\hat{\eta}_{BC}^{(WLS)}$ (10.41) is given by

$$\widehat{Var}\left(\hat{\eta}_{BC}^{(WLS)} \right) = 1 / \left[\left(\widehat{Var}(\hat{\eta}_{BC}) \right)^{-1} + \left(\widehat{Var}(\hat{\eta}_{BC}^*) \right)^{-1} \right]. \tag{10.42}$$

Note that the two WLS estimators $\hat{\eta}_{AC}^{(WLS)}$ (10.38) and $\hat{\eta}_{BC}^{(WLS)}$ (10.41) are correlated. We can show that an estimated asymptotic covariance between these two estimators $\hat{\eta}_{AC}^{(WLS)}$ and $\hat{\eta}_{BC}^{(WLS)}$ is (Problem 10.16)

$$\widehat{Cov}\left(\hat{\eta}_{AC}^{(WLS)}, \hat{\eta}_{BC}^{(WLS)} \right) = W_{AC}(1 - W_{BC})\widehat{Var}(\hat{\eta}_{AC}) + (1 - W_{AC})(W_{BC})\widehat{Var}(\hat{\eta}_{BC})$$

$$- (1 - W_{AC})(1 - W_{BC})\widehat{Var}(\hat{\eta}_{BA}). \tag{10.43}$$

10.2.1 Testing non-equality of treatments

Suppose that we want to study whether there is a difference in responses between patients receiving either treatment A or treatment B and patients receiving treatment

C. This leads us to consider testing the null hypothesis $H_0 : \eta_{AC} = \eta_{BC} = 0$ versus the alternative hypothesis $H_a : \eta_{AC} \neq 0$ or $\eta_{BC} \neq 0$. As the number of patients n_g is large, we may consider use of the univariate z-test based on $\hat{\eta}_{AC}^{(WLS)}$ (10.38) and $\hat{\eta}_{BC}^{(WLS)}$ (10.41) and Bonferroni's inequality to adjust the inflation in Type I error due to multiple tests. We will reject $H_0 : \eta_{AC} = \eta_{BC} = 0$ at the α-level if either of the following two inequalities holds (Lui and Chang, 2015a):

$$|\hat{\eta}_{AC}^{(WLS)}|/\sqrt{\widehat{Var}\left(\hat{\eta}_{AC}^{(WLS)}\right)} > Z_{\alpha/4} \text{ or } |\hat{\eta}_{BC}^{(WLS)}|/\sqrt{\widehat{Var}\left(\hat{\eta}_{BC}^{(WLS)}\right)} > Z_{\alpha/4}, \qquad (10.44)$$

where Z_α is the upper $100(\alpha)$th percentile of the standard normal distribution. To incorporate $\widehat{Cov}\left(\hat{\eta}_{AC}^{(WLS)}, \hat{\eta}_{BC}^{(WLS)}\right)$ into the test procedure to improve power, we consider the following bivariate test procedure. We will reject $H_0 : \eta_{AC} = \eta_{BC} = 0$ at the α-level if

$$\left(\hat{\eta}_{AC}^{(WLS)}, \hat{\eta}_{BC}^{(WLS)}\right) \hat{\underline{\Sigma}}^{-1} \begin{pmatrix} \hat{\eta}_{AC}^{(WLS)} \\ \hat{\eta}_{BC}^{(WLS)} \end{pmatrix} > \chi_\alpha^2(2), \qquad (10.45)$$

where $\hat{\underline{\Sigma}}$ is the estimated covariance matrix with diagonal elements equal to $\widehat{Var}\left(\hat{\eta}_{AC}^{(WLS)}\right)$ (10.39) and $\widehat{Var}\left(\hat{\eta}_{BC}^{(WLS)}\right)$ (10.42), and the off-diagonal element equal to $\widehat{Cov}\left(\hat{\eta}_{AC}^{(WLS)}, \hat{\eta}_{BC}^{(WLS)}\right)$ (10.43), and $\chi_\alpha^2(2)$ is the upper $100(\alpha)$th percentile of the central χ^2-distribution with two degrees of freedom (Lui and Chang, 2015a).

When treatments A and B represent two different doses of a treatment and treatment C represents placebo, the effects due to the low and high doses of a treatment on the patient response are most likely to fall in the same direction relative to placebo C. Thus, we may account for this information to improve power by using a summary test statistic $w\hat{\eta}_{AC}^{(WLS)} + (1-w)\hat{\eta}_{BC}^{(WLS)}$, where w $(0 < w < 1)$ is a weight reflecting the relative importance of responses at the low dose to that at the high dose and is assigned by clinicians based on their subjective knowledge. This leads us to consider the following test procedure. We will reject $H_0 : \eta_{AC} = \eta_{BC} = 0$ at the α-level if

$$\left| w\hat{\eta}_{AC}^{(WLS)} + (1-w)\hat{\eta}_{BC}^{(WLS)} \right| / \sqrt{\widehat{Var}\left(w\hat{\eta}_{AC}^{(WLS)} + (1-w)\hat{\eta}_{BC}^{(WLS)}\right)} > Z_{\alpha/2}, \qquad (10.46)$$

where $\widehat{Var}\left(w\hat{\eta}_{AC}^{(WLS)} + (1-w)\hat{\eta}_{BC}^{(WLS)}\right) = w^2\widehat{Var}\left(\hat{\eta}_{AC}^{(WLS)}\right) + (1-w)^2\widehat{Var}\left(\hat{\eta}_{BC}^{(WLS)}\right) + 2w(1-w)\widehat{Cov}\left(\hat{\eta}_{AC}^{(WLS)}, \hat{\eta}_{BC}^{(WLS)}\right)$. If we have no prior preference to assign the weight w or feel equally important between responses at the two doses, we may set w equal to 0.50.

10.2.2   Testing non-equality between experimental treatments (or non-nullity of dose effects)

We may sometimes want to find out whether there is a difference in effects between the two experimental treatments A and B, especially when treatments A and B represent the low and high doses of a treatment. Thus, we want to test $H_0 : \eta_{BA} (= \eta_{BC} - \eta_{AC}) = 0$ versus $H_a : \eta_{BA} \neq 0$. We define

$$\hat{\eta}_{BA}^* = \hat{\eta}_{BC} - \hat{\eta}_{AC}. \tag{10.47}$$

The estimated asymptotic variance for $\hat{\eta}_{BA}^*$ (10.47) is $\widehat{Var}(\hat{\eta}_{BA}^*) = \widehat{Var}(\hat{\eta}_{BC}) + \widehat{Var}(\hat{\eta}_{AC})$. When estimating η_{BA}, we may employ the same ideas as before and consider the WLS estimator based on $\hat{\eta}_{BA}$ (10.35) and $\hat{\eta}_{BA}^*$ (10.47) as

$$\hat{\eta}_{BA}^{(WLS)} = \left[W_{BA} \hat{\eta}_{BA} + (1 - W_{BA}) \hat{\eta}_{BA}^* \right], \tag{10.48}$$

where $W_{BA} = \left(\widehat{Var}(\hat{\eta}_{BA}) \right)^{-1} / \left[\left(\widehat{Var}(\hat{\eta}_{BA}) \right)^{-1} + \left(\widehat{Var}(\hat{\eta}_{BA}^*) \right)^{-1} \right]$. Thus, we will reject $H_0 : \eta_{BA} = 0$ at the α-level if

$$|\hat{\eta}_{BA}^{(WLS)}| / \sqrt{\widehat{Var}\left(\hat{\eta}_{BA}^{(WLS)} \right)} > Z_{\alpha/2}, \tag{10.49}$$

where $\widehat{Var}\left(\hat{\eta}_{BA}^{(WLS)} \right) = 1 / \left[\left(\widehat{Var}(\hat{\eta}_{BA}) \right)^{-1} + \left(\widehat{Var}(\hat{\eta}_{BA}^*) \right)^{-1} \right]$.

10.2.3   Testing non-inferiority of either experimental treatment to an active control treatment

When treatment C represents an active control treatment, we can be interested in studying whether either experimental treatment A or B is non-inferior to treatment C. Suppose that the higher the probability of a positive response, the better the treatment. Thus, we want to test $H_0 : \varphi_{AC} \leq \varphi_l$ and $\varphi_{BC} \leq \varphi_l$ versus $H_a : \varphi_{AC} > \varphi_l$ or $\varphi_{BC} > \varphi_l$, where φ_l $(0 < \varphi_l < 1)$ denotes the maximum clinically acceptable non-inferior margin of the OR for treatment A (or treatment B) and can be regarded as non-inferior to treatment C if $\varphi_{AC} > \varphi_l$ (or $\varphi_{BC} > \varphi_l$) holds. Some discussions on how to determine the choice of φ_l appear elsewhere (Wiens, 2002; D'Agostino, Massaro, and Sullivan, 2003; Hung et al., 2003; Brittain and Hu, 2009).

Because the function log(x) increases over the range x > 0, testing $H_0 : \varphi_{AC} \leq \varphi_l$ and $\varphi_{BC} \leq \varphi_l$ is equivalent to testing $H_0 : \eta_{AC} \leq \log(\varphi_l)$ and $\eta_{BC} \leq \log(\varphi_l)$. Thus, we will reject $H_0 : \varphi_{AC} \leq \varphi_l$ and $\varphi_{BC} \leq \varphi_l$ at the α-level and claim that either treatment A or B is non-inferior to treatment C if

$$\left(\hat{\eta}_{AC}^{(WLS)} - \log(\varphi_l)\right)/\sqrt{\widehat{Var}\left(\hat{\eta}_{AC}^{(WLS)}\right)} > Z_{\alpha/2} \text{ or } \left(\hat{\eta}_{BC}^{(WLS)} - \log(\varphi_l)\right)/\sqrt{\widehat{Var}\left(\hat{\eta}_{BC}^{(WLS)}\right)} > Z_{\alpha/2}.$$

$$(10.50)$$

If treatments A and B represent the low x_l and high x_u doses of an experimental treatment, we may consider testing non-inferiority of an experimental treatment at a dose x_0 falling between the low and high doses (i.e., $x_l < x_0 < x_u$). When employing the linear interpolation on the log-scale, we want to test $H_0 : w_0\eta_{AC} + (1-w_0)\eta_{BC} \le \log(\varphi_l)$ versus $H_a : w_0\eta_{AC} + (1-w_0)\eta_{BC} > \log(\varphi_l)$, where $w_0 = (x_u-x_0)/(x_u-x_l)$. We will reject $H_0 : w_0\eta_{AC} + (1-w_0)\eta_{BC} \le \log(\varphi_l)$ at the α-level if

$$\left(w_0\hat{\eta}_{AC}^{(WLS)} + (1-w_0)\hat{\eta}_{BC}^{(WLS)} - \log(\varphi_l)\right)/\sqrt{\widehat{Var}\left(w_0\hat{\eta}_{AC}^{(WLS)} + (1-w_0)\hat{\eta}_{BC}^{(WLS)}\right)} > Z_{\alpha}.$$

$$(10.51)$$

10.2.4   Interval estimation of the odds ratio

When assessing the magnitude of the relative treatment effect, we want to obtain an interval estimator for η_{AC} (or η_{BC}). Based on $\hat{\eta}_{AC}^{(WLS)}$ (10.38) and $\widehat{Var}\left(\hat{\eta}_{AC}^{(WLS)}\right)$ (10.39), we obtain an asymptotic $100(1 - \alpha)\%$ confidence interval for η_{AC} as

$$\left[\hat{\eta}_{AC}^{(WLS)} - Z_{\alpha/2}\sqrt{\widehat{Var}\left(\hat{\eta}_{AC}^{(WLS)}\right)}, \hat{\eta}_{AC}^{(WLS)} + Z_{\alpha/2}\sqrt{\widehat{Var}\left(\hat{\eta}_{AC}^{(WLS)}\right)}\right].$$

$$(10.52)$$

To obtain an asymptotic $100(1 - \alpha)\%$ confidence interval for the OR $\varphi_{AC}(= \exp(\eta_{AC}))$, we can simply apply the antilogarithmic transformation on the confidence limits given in (10.52).

Similarly, we may obtain an asymptotic $100(1 - \alpha)\%$ confidence interval for η_{BC} on the basis of $\hat{\eta}_{BC}^{(WLS)}$ (10.41) and $\widehat{Var}\left(\hat{\eta}_{BC}^{(WLS)}\right)$ (10.42) as

$$\left[\hat{\eta}_{BC}^{(WLS)} - Z_{\alpha/2}\sqrt{\widehat{Var}\left(\hat{\eta}_{BC}^{(WLS)}\right)}, \hat{\eta}_{BC}^{(WLS)} + Z_{\alpha/2}\sqrt{\widehat{Var}\left(\hat{\eta}_{BC}^{(WLS)}\right)}\right].$$

$$(10.53)$$

Also, to assess the magnitude of a weighted average of effects due to treatments A and B versus treatment C, we may obtain an asymptotic $100(1 - \alpha)\%$ confidence interval for $w\eta_{AC} + (1-w)\eta_{BC}$ as given by

$$\left[w\hat{\eta}_{AC}^{(WLS)} + (1-w)\hat{\eta}_{BC}^{(WLS)} - Z_{\alpha/2}\sqrt{\widehat{Var}\left(w\hat{\eta}_{AC}^{(WLS)} + (1-w)\hat{\eta}_{BC}^{(WLS)}\right)},\right.$$
$$\left. w\hat{\eta}_{AC}^{(WLS)} + (1-w)\hat{\eta}_{BC}^{(WLS)} + Z_{\alpha/2}\sqrt{\widehat{Var}\left(w\hat{\eta}_{AC}^{(WLS)} + (1-w)\hat{\eta}_{BC}^{(WLS)}\right)}\right].$$

$$(10.54)$$

Note that the interval estimator (10.54) includes interval estimators (10.52) and (10.53) as special cases for $w = 1$ and $w = 0$, respectively. Similarly, on the basis of $\hat{\eta}_{BA}^{(WLS)}$ (10.48) and $\widehat{Var}\left(\hat{\eta}_{BA}^{(WLS)}\right)$, we obtain an asymptotic $100(1 - \alpha)\%$ confidence interval for η_{BA} as given by

$$\left[\hat{\eta}_{BA}^{(WLS)} - Z_{\alpha/2}\sqrt{\widehat{Var}\left(\hat{\eta}_{BA}^{(WLS)}\right)}, \hat{\eta}_{BA}^{(WLS)} + Z_{\alpha/2}\sqrt{\widehat{Var}\left(\hat{\eta}_{BA}^{(WLS)}\right)}\right]. \tag{10.55}$$

Interval estimators (10.52)–(10.55) are not for simultaneous $100(1 - \alpha)\%$ confidence intervals. If we wish to obtain simultaneous interval estimators, we can employ Bonferroni's inequality as discussed before for the continuous cases. We can also employ Scheffe's method and replace $Z_{\alpha/2}$ with $\sqrt{\chi_{\alpha,2}^2}$ in (10.54) to obtain approximately simultaneous $100(1 - \alpha)\%$ confidence intervals for $w\eta_{AC} + (1 - w)\eta_{BC}$ (Lui and Chang, 2015a).

Example 10.3   For the purpose of illustration only, we consider in Table 10.2 the data obtained by collapsing the original data according to responses based on the first two periods (Table 7.1) from a crossover trial comparing the low and high doses of analgesic and placebo for the relief (yes = 1, no = 0) of primary dysmenorrhea (Jones and Kenward, 1987). A washout period of one month was applied to separate for each of the treatment periods. Note that treatments A and B here actually represent the low and high doses of the analgesic, respectively. When employing test procedures (10.44)–(10.46), we obtain the p-values 0.001, 0.001, and 0.000, respectively. All these small p-values suggest that there should be a difference in the relief rates of primary dysmenorrhea between use of either dose of analgesic and placebo. When employing the WLS point estimators (10.38) and (10.41) as well as interval estimators (10.52) and (10.53), we obtain $\hat{\eta}_{AC}^{(WLS)} = 1.526$ and $\hat{\eta}_{BC}^{(WLS)} = 2.027$ together with

Table 10.2   Frequency of patients with response vector ($Y_{i1}^{(g)} = r$, $Y_{i2}^{(g)} = s$), where r and $s = 1$ for relief, = 0 otherwise, at two periods in each treatment-receipt sequence group.

Response pattern ($Y_{i1}^{(g)} = r$, $Y_{i2}^{(g)} = s$)		(1,1)	(1,0)	(0,1)	(0,0)	Total
P–A	($g = 1$)	2	0	11	2	15
A–P	($g = 2$)	1	9	4	1	15
P–B	($g = 3$)	4	1	9	2	16
B–P	($g = 4$)	2	7	2	3	14
A–B	($g = 5$)	9	1	1	1	12
B–A	($g = 6$)	4	8	1	1	14

A, lower dose of the analgesic; B, higher dose of the analgesic; P, placebo.

their corresponding asymptotic 95% confidence intervals as [0.280, 2.771] and [0.896, 3.158]. These lead us to obtain the point estimates for the OR of relief between the low dose and the placebo, as well as that between the high dose and placebo as 4.600 (= exp(1.526)) and 7.591 (= exp(2.027)), respectively. Furthermore, using the antilogarithmic transformation, we obtain the corresponding asymptotic 95% confidence intervals for φ_{AC} and φ_{BC} as [1.323, 15.975] and [2.450, 23.524]. Because both the lower limits of these resulting confidence intervals for φ_{AC} and φ_{BC} fall above 1, we may conclude that there is significant evidence at the 5% level to support that either dose of analgesic may increase the relief of dysmenorrhea as compared with the placebo. This is consistent with the findings based on test procedures (10.44)–(10.46). Furthermore, when studying whether there is a difference in the relief rates between the low and high doses, we employ the point estimator (10.48) and interval estimator (10.55) and obtain $\hat{\eta}_{BA}^{(WLS)} = 0.502$ (> 0) together with the 95% confidence interval for η_{BA} as [−0.808, 1.811]. These lead us to obtain the point estimate for the OR of relief between the high and low doses as 1.652 (= exp(0.502)) and an asymptotic 95% confidence interval for φ_{BA} given by [0.446, 6.117]. Because this resulting interval includes 1, although taking the high dose may increase the relief rate as compared with the low dose, there is no significant evidence that the high dose can increase the relief rate as compared with the low dose at the 5% level.

10.2.5   SAS codes for the likelihood-based approach

If we are willing to assume random effects $\mu_i^{(g)}$'s due to patients under model (10.27) to independently follow a normal distribution, we may consider use of PROC NLMIXED or PROC GLIMMIX to obtain estimates for the relative treatment and period effects based on the likelihood-based approach (Ezzet and Whitehead, 1992). For example, we present the SAS codes in use of PROC GLIMMIX to the data in Table 10.2 in the following box.

```
option ls = 70;
data step1;
input patid treatment period n pos;
cards;
    1    1    1    1    1
    1    2    2    1    1
    2    1    1    1    1
    2    2    2    1    1
 . . .
;;;;
proc glimmix data=step1;
  class patid treatment period;
    model pos/n=treatment period/ solution;
```

```
      random intercept /subject=patid;
      estimate "treatment A versus p" treatment -1 1 0;
      estimate "treatment B versus p" treatment -1 0 1;
      estimate "treatment B versus A" treatment 0 -1 1;
      estimate "period 2 versus period 1" period -1 1;
   run;
```

We present the partial outputs of using PROC GLIMMIX in the following box.

Label	Estimate	Standard Error	DF	t Value	Pr > |t|
treatment A versus p	1.7569	0.4089	83	4.30	<.0001
treatment B versus p	2.3104	0.4374	83	5.28	<.0001
treatment B versus A	0.5535	0.4336	83	1.28	0.2054
period 2 versus period 1	0.07053	0.3463	83	0.20	0.8391

We can see that both treatments A (low dose) and B (high dose) can significantly improve the relief of primary dysmenorrhea. The above estimates 1.757 and 2.310 for the relative treatment effects are similar to those of 1.526 and 2.027 obtained previously in Example 10.3. Furthermore, there is no evidence that the rates of relief between treatments B and A are different from each other at the 5% level, although using the former can increase the rate of relief as compared with using the latter. We would like to note that we have applied PROC GLIMMIX with use of "method = quad" (Jones and Kenward, 2014) or PROC NLMIXED to the data in Table 10.2. We have obtained essentially identical results to those shown in the above box.

When the number of patients is small, the above test procedures and interval estimators derived from large-sample theory are theoretically invalid. In this case, the exact test and interval estimator for the relative effect between treatments under an incomplete block design in binary data can be of use (Lui, 2015c; Lui and Chang, 2016). For brevity, we outline the derivation of exact interval estimators in Problems 10.17 and 10.18.

Exercises

Problem 10.1. Show that $\hat{\eta}_{AC} = \left(\bar{d}^{(1)} - \bar{d}^{(2)}\right)/2$ is an unbiased estimator for η_{AC} under model (10.1) and its variance $Var(\hat{\eta}_{AC}) = \sigma_d^2(1/n_1 + 1/n_2)/4$, where $\sigma_d^2 = 2\sigma_e^2$.

Problem 10.2. Show that the variance of $\hat{\eta}_{AC}^{(WLS)}$ (10.10) is given by $Var\left(\hat{\eta}_{AC}^{(WLS)}\right) = \sigma_d^2 / \left\{4\left[(1/n_1 + 1/n_2)^{-1} + (1/n_3 + 1/n_4 + 1/n_5 + 1/n_6)^{-1}\right]\right\}$.

Problem 10.3. Show that the covariance between the two estimators $\hat{\eta}_{AC}^{(WLS)}$ and $\hat{\eta}_{BC}^{(WLS)}$ under model (10.1) is given by (Lui, 2015b)

$$Cov\left(\hat{\eta}_{AC}^{(WLS)},\hat{\eta}_{BC}^{(WLS)}\right) = W_{AC}(1-W_{BC})Var(\hat{\eta}_{AC}) + (1-W_{AC})(W_{BC})Var(\hat{\eta}_{BC})$$
$$- (1-W_{AC})(1-W_{BC})Var(\hat{\eta}_{BA}).$$

Problem 10.4. Show that the pooled sample variance $\hat{\sigma}_d^2 = \sum_{g=1}^{6}\sum_{i=1}^{n_g}\left(d_i^{(g)}-\bar{d}^{(g)}\right)^2/(n_+-6)$, where $n_+ = \sum_{g=1}^{6}n_g$ denotes the total sample size of the trial, is an unbiased estimator for σ_d^2.

Problem 10.5. Show that under $H_0 : \eta_{AC} = \eta_{BC} = 0$, the test statistic (Lui, 2015b)

$$\left(\hat{\eta}_{AC}^{(WLS)},\hat{\eta}_{BC}^{(WLS)}\right)\hat{\Sigma}^{-1}\begin{pmatrix}\hat{\eta}_{AC}^{(WLS)}\\\hat{\eta}_{BC}^{(WLS)}\end{pmatrix}/2$$ follows the central F-distribution with 2 and

n_+-6 degrees of freedom, where $\hat{\Sigma}$ is the estimated covariance matrix with diagonal elements equal to $\widehat{Var}\left(\hat{\eta}_{AC}^{(WLS)}\right)$ and $\widehat{Var}\left(\hat{\eta}_{BC}^{(WLS)}\right)$, and the off-diagonal element equal to $\widehat{Cov}\left(\hat{\eta}_{AC}^{(WLS)},\hat{\eta}_{BC}^{(WLS)}\right)$.

Problem 10.6. Show that under the balanced design (i.e., $n_1 = n_2 = \cdots = n_6$), the optimal weight to minimize the variance of the linear weighted average $w\hat{\eta}_{AC}^{(WLS)} + (1-w)\hat{\eta}_{BC}^{(WLS)}$ is 1/2.

Problem 10.7. Show that we can apply interval estimator (10.26) to obtain simultaneous $100(1-\alpha)\%$ confidence intervals for all possible linear combinations $l_1\eta_{AC} + l_2\eta_{BC}$ (Graybill, 1976, pp. 224–225).

Problem 10.8. Assume that the variance of random errors $\varepsilon_{iz}^{(g)}$'s depends on the treatment patients received under model (10.1). Let σ_{eA}^2, σ_{eB}^2, and σ_{eC}^2 denote the variance of $\varepsilon_{iz}^{(g)}$ when a patient receives treatment A, treatment B, and treatment C, respectively.

(a) Note that the variance $Var(\hat{\eta}_{AC}) = \sigma_{AC}^2(1/n_1 + 1/n_2)/4$, where $\sigma_{AC}^2 = \sigma_{eA}^2 + \sigma_{eC}^2$. Show that $\hat{\sigma}_{AC}^2 = \sum_{g=1}^{2}\sum_{i=1}^{n_g}\left(d_i^{(g)}-\bar{d}^{(g)}\right)^2/(n_1+n_2-2)$ is an unbiased estimator for σ_{AC}^2.

(b) Note that $Var(\hat{\eta}_{AC}^*) = \sigma_{BC}^2(1/n_3 + 1/n_4)/4 + \sigma_{BA}^2(1/n_5 + 1/n_6)/4$, where $\sigma_{BC}^2 = \sigma_{eB}^2 + \sigma_{eC}^2$ and $\sigma_{BA}^2 = \sigma_{eB}^2 + \sigma_{eA}^2$. Show that $\hat{\sigma}_{BC}^2 = \sum_{g=3}^{4}\sum_{i=1}^{n_g}\left(d_i^{(g)}-\bar{d}^{(g)}\right)^2/(n_3+n_4-2)$ and $\hat{\sigma}_{BA}^2 = \sum_{g=5}^{6}\sum_{i=1}^{n_g}\left(d_i^{(g)}-\bar{d}^{(g)}\right)^2/(n_5+n_6-2)$ are unbiased estimators for σ_{BC}^2 and σ_{BA}^2, respectively.

(c) Show that an unbiased variance estimator for $W_{AC}\hat{\eta}_{AC} + (1 - W_{AC})\hat{\eta}^*_{AC}$ (which is unbiased for η_{AC} but is no longer the WLS estimator) is $\widehat{Var}(W_{AC}\hat{\eta}_{AC} + (1 - W_{AC})\hat{\eta}^*_{AC}) = W^2_{AC}\hat{\sigma}^2_{AC}(1/n_1 + 1/n_2)/4 + (1 - W_{AC})^2 [\hat{\sigma}^2_{BC}(1/n_3 + 1/n_4)/4 + \hat{\sigma}^2_{BA}(1/n_5 + 1/n_6)/4]$. Thus, we can apply the test statistic $(W_{AC}\hat{\eta}_{AC} + (1 - W_{AC})\hat{\eta}^*_{AC} - \eta_{AC})/\sqrt{\widehat{Var}(W_{AC}\hat{\eta}_{AC} + (1 - W_{AC})\hat{\eta}^*_{AC})}$, which approximately follows the t-distribution with the degrees of freedom given by Satterthwaite's approximation (Satterthwaite, 1946; Fleiss, 1986a, p. 30), to do hypothesis testing and interval estimator relevant to η_{AC}.

Problem 10.9.   Under model (10.1), derive the WLS estimator for the period effect γ and its estimated variance. (Hint: Note that $\left(\bar{d}^{(1)} + \bar{d}^{(2)}\right)/2$, $\left(\bar{d}^{(3)} + \bar{d}^{(4)}\right)/2$, and $\left(\bar{d}^{(5)} + \bar{d}^{(6)}\right)/2$ are all unbiased estimators for γ).

Problem 10.10.

(a) Under model (10.1), show that the expectations $E\left(\bar{d}^{(3)} - \bar{d}^{(5)}\right) = E\left(\bar{d}^{(6)} - \bar{d}^{(4)}\right) = \eta_{AC}$, as well as variances $Var\left(\bar{d}^{(3)} - \bar{d}^{(5)}\right) = \sigma^2_d(1/n_3 + 1/n_5)$ and $Var\left(\bar{d}^{(6)} - \bar{d}^{(4)}\right) = \sigma^2_d(1/n_6 + 1/n_4)$. These together with estimator $\hat{\eta}_{AC}$ (10.2) and its variance $Var(\hat{\eta}_{AC})$ (10.3) lead to produce the WLS estimator for η_{AC} to be $W^{(1)}_{AC}\hat{\eta}_{AC} + W^{(2)}_{AC}\left(\bar{d}^{(3)} - \bar{d}^{(5)}\right) + W^{(3)}_{AC}\left(\bar{d}^{(6)} - \bar{d}^{(4)}\right)$ with optimal weights given by $W^{(1)}_{AC} \propto 4(1/n_1 + 1/n_2)^{-1}$, $W^{(2)}_{AC} \propto (1/n_3 + 1/n_5)^{-1}$, and $W^{(3)}_{AC} \propto (1/n_6 + 1/n_4)^{-1}$.

(b) Consider the data in Table 10.1. Show that the variance of this WLS estimator is $0.0793 \ \sigma^2_d$, which is slightly less than the value $0.0795 \ \sigma^2_d$ for $Var\left(\hat{\eta}^{(WLS)}_{AC}\right)$ (10.11).

(c) When $n_1 = n_2 = \ldots = n_6 = n$, show that the variance of the new WLS estimator defined in this exercise and $Var\left(\hat{\eta}^{(WLS)}_{AC}\right)$ (10.11) are both equal to $\sigma^2_d/(3n)$.

Problem 10.11.   Show that the OR of a positive response between treatments A and C for a fixed period on a given patient under model (10.27) is equal to (Lui and Chang, 2015a) $\varphi_{AC} = \left[\left(\pi^{(1)}_{01}\pi^{(2)}_{10}\right)/\left(\pi^{(1)}_{10}\pi^{(2)}_{01}\right)\right]^{1/2}$ despite any given probability density function $f_g(\alpha)$.

Problem 10.12.   Show that the OR of a positive response between treatments B and C for a fixed period on a given patient under model (10.27) is equal to $\varphi_{BC} = \left[\left(\pi^{(3)}_{01}\pi^{(4)}_{10}\right)/\left(\pi^{(3)}_{10}\pi^{(4)}_{01}\right)\right]^{1/2}$.

Problem 10.13.   Show that the OR of a positive response between treatments B and A for a fixed period on a given patient under model (10.27) is equal to $\varphi_{BA}(=\exp(\eta_{BC}-\eta_{AC}))=\left[\left(\pi_{01}^{(5)}\pi_{10}^{(6)}\right)/\left(\pi_{10}^{(5)}\pi_{01}^{(6)}\right)\right]^{1/2}$.

Problem 10.14.   Show that an estimated asymptotic variance of $\hat{\eta}_{AC}$ (10.31) with use of the delta method is given by $\widehat{Var}(\hat{\eta}_{AC})=\left(\dfrac{1}{4}\right)\left(1/n_{01}^{(1)}+1/n_{10}^{(1)}+1/n_{10}^{(2)}+1/n_{01}^{(2)}\right)$.

Problem 10.15.   Show that an estimated asymptotic variance of $\hat{\eta}_{AC}^{(WLS)}$ (10.38) is approximately given by $\widehat{Var}\left(\hat{\eta}_{AC}^{(WLS)}\right)=1/\left[\left(\widehat{Var}(\hat{\eta}_{AC})\right)^{-1}+\left(\widehat{Var}(\hat{\eta}_{AC}^{*})\right)^{-1}\right]$.

Problem 10.16.   Show that an estimated asymptotic covariance between these two estimators $\hat{\eta}_{AC}^{(WLS)}$ and $\hat{\eta}_{BC}^{(WLS)}$ is approximately given by $\widehat{Cov}\left(\hat{\eta}_{AC}^{(WLS)},\hat{\eta}_{BC}^{(WLS)}\right)=$
$W_{AC}(1-W_{BC})\widehat{Var}(\hat{\eta}_{AC})+(1-W_{AC})(W_{BC})\widehat{Var}(\hat{\eta}_{BC})-(1-W_{AC})(1-W_{BC})\widehat{Var}(\hat{\eta}_{BA})$.

Problem 10.17.   Show that the conditional distribution of $n_{01}^{(g)}$, given $n_{dis}^{(g)}=n_{01}^{(g)}+n_{10}^{(g)}$ fixed, follows the binomial distribution with parameters $n_{dis}^{(g)}$ and $\pi_{01}^{(g)}/\left(\pi_{10}^{(g)}+\pi_{01}^{(g)}\right)$, where $\pi_{01}^{(1)}/\left(\pi_{10}^{(1)}+\pi_{01}^{(1)}\right)=\exp(\eta_{AC}+\gamma)/(1+\exp(\eta_{AC}+\gamma))$; $\pi_{01}^{(2)}/\left(\pi_{10}^{(2)}+\pi_{01}^{(2)}\right)=$
$\exp(-\eta_{AC}+\gamma)/(1+\exp(-\eta_{AC}+\gamma))$; $\pi_{01}^{(3)}/\left(\pi_{10}^{(3)}+\pi_{01}^{(3)}\right)=\exp(\eta_{BC}+\gamma)/$
$(1+\exp(\eta_{BC}+\gamma))$; $\pi_{01}^{(4)}/\left(\pi_{10}^{(4)}+\pi_{01}^{(4)}\right)=\exp(-\eta_{BC}+\gamma)/(1+\exp(-\eta_{BC}+\gamma))$;
$\pi_{01}^{(5)}/\left(\pi_{10}^{(5)}+\pi_{01}^{(5)}\right)=\exp((\eta_{BC}-\eta_{AC})+\gamma)/(1+\exp((\eta_{BC}-\eta_{AC})+\gamma))$;   and
$\pi_{01}^{(6)}/\left(\pi_{10}^{(6)}+\pi_{01}^{(6)}\right)=\exp(-(\eta_{BC}-\eta_{AC})+\gamma)/(1+\exp(-(\eta_{BC}-\eta_{AC})+\gamma))$.

Problem 10.18.   For simplicity in notation, we define $a_g=n_{01}^{(g)}$ and $t_g=n_{dis}^{(g)}$ for $g=1$, 2, 3, 4, 5, 6. We further define $a_+^{(i,j)}=a_i+a_j$ for $i\neq j$ $(i,j=1, 2, 3, 4, 5, 6)$. We let $\underline{t}$ denote the random vector $(t_1, t_2, t_3, t_4, t_5, t_6)$.

(a) Given the results in Problem 10.17, show that the joint conditional probability mass function for $\underline{a}= (a_1, a_3, a_6)$, given $a_+^{(1,2)}, a_+^{(3,5)}, a_+^{(4,6)}$ and $\underline{t}$ fixed, is given by (Lui, 2015c)

$$f\left(\underline{a}|a_+^{(1,2)},a_+^{(3,5)},a_+^{(4,6)},\underline{t},\varphi>_{AC}\right)=\left[\binom{t_1}{a_1}\binom{t_2}{a_+^{(1,2)}-a_1}\varphi_{AC}^{2a_1}\bigg/\sum_x\binom{t_1}{x}\binom{t_2}{a_+^{(1,2)}-x}\varphi_{AC}^{2x}\right]$$
$$\times\left[\binom{t_3}{a_3}\binom{t_5}{a_+^{(3,5)}-a_3}\varphi_{AC}^{a_3}\bigg/\sum_u\binom{t_3}{u}\binom{t_5}{a_+^{(3,5)}-u}\varphi_{AC}^{u}\right]$$
$$\times\left[\binom{t_4}{a_+^{(4,6)}-a_6}\binom{t_6}{a_6}\varphi_{AC}^{a_6}\bigg/\sum_v\binom{t_4}{a_+^{(4,6)}-v}\binom{t_6}{v}\varphi_{AC}^{v}\right],$$

where $\varphi_{AC} = \exp(\eta_{AC})$, and the summations in the denominators are over ranges $\max\left\{0, a_+^{(1,2)} - t_2\right\} \le x \le \min\left\{t_1, a_+^{(1,2)}\right\}$, $\max\left\{0, a_+^{(3,5)} - t_5\right\} \le u \le \min\left\{t_3, a_+^{(3,5)}\right\}$, and $\max\left\{a_+^{(4,6)} - t_4, 0\right\} \le v \le \min\left\{t_6, a_+^{(4,6)}\right\}$.

(b) Define $S = 2a_1 + a_3 + a_6$. Show that the CMLE $\hat{\varphi}_{AC}^{(CMLE)}$ for φ_{AC}, given an observed value $(S=)s_0$, is the solution satisfying $s_0 = E\left(S | a_+^{(1,2)}, a_+^{(3,5)}, a_+^{(4,6)}, \underline{t}, \hat{\varphi}_{AC}^{(CMLE)}\right)$, where $E\left(S | a_+^{(1,2)}, a_+^{(3,5)}, a_+^{(4,6)}, \underline{t}, \hat{\varphi}^{AC(CMLE)}\right)$ denotes the conditional expectation of S, given $a_+^{(1,2)}, a_+^{(3,5)}, a_+^{(4,6)}$ and $\underline{t}$ fixed.

(c) Using the observed information matrix and the delta method (Agresti, 1990; Lui, 2004), show that an estimated asymptotic variance for $\log\left(\hat{\varphi}_{AC}^{(CMLE)}\right)$ is $\widehat{Var}\left(\log\left(\hat{\varphi}_{AC}^{(CMLE)}\right)\right) = 1/Var\left(S | a_+^{(1,2)}, a_+^{(3,5)}, a_+^{(4,6)}, \underline{t}, \hat{\varphi}_{AC}^{(CMLE)}\right)$, where $Var\left(S | a_+^{(1,2)}, a_+^{(3,5)}, a_+^{(4,6)}, \underline{t}, \hat{\varphi}_{AC}^{(CMLE)}\right)$ denotes the conditional variance of S with φ_{AC} replaced by the CMLE $\hat{\varphi}_{AC}^{(CMLE)}$, given $a_+^{(1,2)}, a_+^{(3,5)}, a_+^{(4,6)}$ and $\underline{t}$ fixed, and is actually the sum of conditional variances given by $Var\left(2a_1 | a_+^{(1,2)}, t_1, t_2, \hat{\varphi}_{AC}^{(CMLE)}\right) + Var\left(a_3 | a_+^{(3,5)}, t_3, t_5, \hat{\varphi}_{AC}^{(CMLE)}\right) + Var\left(a_6 | a_+^{(4,6)}, t_4, t_6, \hat{\varphi}_{AC}^{(CMLE)}\right)$. Thus, we may obtain an approximate $100(1-\alpha)\%$ confidence interval for φ_{AC} using Wald's method as $\left[\hat{\varphi}^{AC(CMLE)} \exp\left(-Z_{\alpha/2}\sqrt{\widehat{Var}\left(\log\left(\hat{\varphi}_{AC}^{(CMLE)}\right)\right)}\right), \hat{\varphi}_{AC}^{(CMLE)} \exp\left(Z_{\alpha/2}\sqrt{\widehat{Var}\left(\log\left(\hat{\varphi}_{AC}^{(CMLE)}\right)\right)}\right)\right]$. Note that the conditional probability mass function for S, given $a_+^{(1,2)}$, $a_+^{(3,5)}, a_+^{(4,6)}$ and $\underline{t}$ fixed, is given by $P(S=s|\varphi_{AC}) = \sum_{\underline{a} \in G} f\left(\underline{a} | a_+^{(1,2)}, a_+^{(3,5)}, a_+^{(4,6)}, \underline{t}, \varphi_{AC}\right)$, where $G = \left\{\underline{a} | S = 2a_1 + a_3 + a_6 = s, \max\left\{0, a_+^{(1,2)} - t_2\right\} \le a_1 \le \min\left\{t_1, a_+^{(1,2)}\right\}, \max\left\{0, a_+^{(3,5)} - t_5\right\} \le a_3 \le \min\left\{t_3, a_+^{(3,5)}\right\}$, and $\max\left\{a_+^{(4,6)} - t_4, 0\right\} \le a_6 \le \min\left\{t_6, a_+^{(4,6)}\right\}\right\}$.

(d) For an observed value s_0, discuss how to find an exact $100(1-\alpha)\%$ confidence interval for φ_{AC} based on the probability mass function $P(S=s|\varphi_{AC})$ (Casella and Berger, 1990). Following similar arguments as above, we can derive the CMLE $\hat{\varphi}_{BC}^{(CMLE)}$ and $\hat{\varphi}_{BA}^{(CMLE)}$, as well as the corresponding asymptotic and exact interval estimators for φ_{BC} and φ_{BA}.

Problem 10.19.   Using the data in Table 10.2, (a) what are the CMLE $\hat{\varphi}_{AC}^{(CMLE)}$, $\hat{\varphi}_{BC}^{(CMLE)}$, and $\hat{\varphi}_{BA}^{(CMLE)}$, as well as their corresponding asymptotic 95% confidence intervals using Wald's method for φ_{AC}, φ_{BC}, and φ_{BA}? (b) What are the exact 95% confidence intervals for φ_{AC}, φ_{BC}, and φ_{BA}?

References

Agresti, A. (1980). Generalized odds ratios for ordinal data. *Biometrics*, **36**, 59–67.

Agresti, A. (1990). *Categorical Data Analysis*. John Wiley & Sons, Inc., New York.

Anderson, S. and Hauck, W.W. (1990). Consideration of individual bioequivalence. *Journal of Pharmacokinetics and Biopharmaceutics*, **18**, 259–274.

Balaam, L.N. (1968). A two-period design with t^2 experimental units. *Biometrics*, **24**, 61–73.

Breslow, N.E. and Day, N.E. (1980). *Statistical Methods in Cancer Research*. Vol. 1, *The Analysis of Case–Control Studies*. International Agency for Research on Cancer, Lyon, France.

Bristol, D.R. (1993). Probabilities and sample sizes for the two one-sided test procedures. *Communications in Statistics, Theory and Methods*, **22**, 1953–1961.

Brittain, E. and Hu, Z. (2009). Noninferiority trial design and analysis with an ordered three-level categorical endpoint. *Journal of Biopharmaceutical Statistics*, **19**, 685–699.

Brown, B.W. Jr. (1980). The crossover experiment for clinical trials. *Biometrics*, **36**, 69–79.

Casella, G. and Berger, R.L. (1990). *Statistical Inference*. Duxbury Press, Belmont, CA.

Chassan, J.B. (1964). On the analysis of simple cross-overs with unequal numbers of replicates. *Biometrics*, **20**, 206–208.

Chen, J.J., Tsong, Y., and Kang, S.-H. (2000). Tests for equivalence or noninferiority between two proportions. *Drug Information Journal*, **34**, 569–578.

Chow, S.C. and Liu, J.P. (2009). *Design and Analysis of Bioavailability and Bioequivalence Studies*, 3rd ed. Chapman & Hall/CRC, Taylor and Francis, Boca Raton, FL.

Clayton, D.G. (1974). Some odds ratio statistics for the analysis of ordered categorical data. *Biometrika*, **61**, 525–531.

Clayton, D. and Cuzick, J. (1985). Multivariate generalizations of the proportional hazards model. *Journal of the Royal Statistical Society, Series A*, **148**, 82–117.

Cleophas, T.J.M. (1991). The performance of the two-stage analysis of two-treatment, two-period crossover trials. *Statistics in Medicine*, **10**, 489–491 (letter).

Cochran, W.G. (1977). *Sampling Techniques*, 3rd ed. John Wiley & Sons, Inc., New York.

Cornell, R.G. (1980). Evaluation of bioavailability data using non-parametric statistics, in *Drug Absorption and Disposition: Statistical Considerations* (ed. K.S. Albert), American Pharmaceutical Association, Washington, DC, pp. 51–57.

Cox, D.R. and Snell, E.J. (1989). *Analysis of Binary Data*, 2nd ed. Chapman and Hall, London.

Crossover Designs: Testing, Estimation, and Sample Size, First Edition. Kung-Jong Lui.
© 2016 John Wiley & Sons, Ltd. Published 2016 by John Wiley & Sons, Ltd.
Companion website: www.wiley.com/go/lui/crossover

D'Agostino, R.B. Sr., Massaro, J.M., and Sullivan, L.M. (2003). Non-inferiority trials: design concepts and issues – the encounters of academic consultants in statistics. *Statistics in Medicine*, **22**, 169–186.

Dunnett, C.W. (1964). New tables for multiple comparisons with a control. *Biometrics*, **20**, 482–491.

Dunnett, C.W. and Gent, M. (1977). Significance testing to establish equivalence between treatments, with special reference to data in the form of 2×2 tables. *Biometrics*, **33**, 593–602.

Ebbutt, A.F. (1984). Three-period crossover designs for two treatments. *Biometrics*, **40**, 219–224.

Edwardes, M.D. and Baltzan, M. (2000). The generalization of the odds ratio, risk ratio and risk difference to $r \times k$ tables. *Statistics in Medicine*, **19**, 1901–1914.

Ejigou, A. and McHugh, R. (1984). Testing the homogeneity of the relative risk under multiple matching. *Biometrika*, **71**, 408–411.

Ezzet, F. and Whitehead, J. (1991). A random effects model for ordinal responses from a cross-over trial. *Statistics in Medicine*, **10**, 901–907.

Ezzet, F. and Whitehead, J. (1992). A random effects model for ordinal responses from a crossover trial. *Applied Statistics*, **41**, 117–126.

Ezzet, F. and Whitehead, J. (1993). A random effects model for ordinal responses from a cross-over trial. *Statistics in Medicine*, **12**, 2150–2151 (authors' reply).

Fava, G.M. and Patel, H.I. (1986). A survey of crossover designs used in industry. Unpublished manuscript.

FDA (1997). Guidance for Industry. Evaluating Clinical Studies of Antimicrobials in the Division of Anti-infective Drug Products. FDA, Silver Spring, MD, p. 87, 17 February.

Fleiss, J.L. (1981). *Statistical Methods for Rates and Proportion*, 2nd ed. John Wiley & Sons, Inc., New York.

Fleiss, J.L. (1986a). *The Design and Analysis of Clinical Experiments*. John Wiley & Sons, Inc., New York.

Fleiss, J.L. (1986b). On multiperiod crossover studies. *Biometrics*, **42**, 449–450 (correspondence).

Fleiss, J.L. (1989). A critique of recent research on the two-treatment crossover design. *Controlled Clinical Trials*, **10**, 237–243.

Fleiss, J.L., Levin, B., and Paik, M.C. (2003). *Statistical Methods for Rates and Proportions*, 3rd ed. John Wiley & Sons, Inc., Hoboken, NJ.

Freeman, P. (1989). The performance of the two-stage analysis of two-treatment, two-period trials. *Statistics in Medicine*, **8**, 1421–1432.

Freeman, P. (1991). The performance of the two-stage analysis of two-treatment, two-period trials. *Statistics in Medicine*, **10**, 491 (letter reply).

Garcia, R., Benet, M., Arnau, C., and Cobo, E. (2004). Efficiency of the cross-over design: an empirical estimation. *Statistics in Medicine*, **23**, 3773–3780.

Garrett, A.D. (2003). Therapeutic equivalence: fallacies and falsification. *Statistics in Medicine*, **22**, 741–762.

Gart, J.J. (1969). An exact test for comparing matched proportions in crossover designs. *Biometrika*, **56**, 75–80.

Gart, J.J. (1970). Point and interval estimation of the common odds ratio in the combination of 2×2 tables with fixed marginals. *Biometrika*, **57**, 471–475.

Gart, J.J. and Thomas, D.G. (1972). Numerical results on approximate confidence limits for the odds ratio. *Journal of Royal Statistical Society B*, **34**, 441–447.

Graybill, F.A. (1976). *Theory and Application of the Linear Model*. Duxbury Press, North Scituate, MA.

Grizzle, J.E. (1965). The two-period change-over design and its use in clinical trials. *Biometrics*, **21**, 467–480.

Hauck, W.W. and Anderson, S. (1986). A proposal for interpreting and reporting negative studies. *Statistics in Medicine*, **5**, 203–209.

Hauck, W.W. and Anderson, S. (1991). Individual bioequivalence – what matters to the patient. *Statistics in Medicine*, **10**, 959–960.

Hauck, W.W. and Anderson, S. (1992). Types of bioequivalence and related statistical considerations. *International Journal of Clinical Pharmacology and Therapeutics*, **30**, 181–187.

Hauschke, D., Steinijans, V.W., and Diletti, E. (1990). A distribution-free procedure for the statistical analysis of bioequivalence studies. *International Journal of Clinical Pharmacology, Therapy, and Toxicology*, **28**, 72–78.

Hills, M. and Armitage, P. (1979). The two-period cross-over clinical trial. *British Journal of Clinical Pharmacology*, **8**, 7–20.

Hollander, M. and Wolfe, D.A. (1973). *Nonparametric Statistical Methods*. John Wiley & Sons, Inc., New York.

Hosmer, D.W. and Lemeshow, S. (2000). *Applied Logistic Regression*. John Wiley & Sons, Inc., New York.

Hung, H.M.J., Wang, S.-J., Tsong, Y., Lawrence, J., and O'Neill, R.T. (2003). Some fundamental issues with noninferiority testing in active control trials. *Statistics in Medicine*, **22**, 213–225.

Jones, B. and Donev, A.N. (1996). Modelling and design of cross-over trials. *Statistics in Medicine*, **15**, 1435–1446.

Jones, B. and Kenward, M.G. (1987). Modelling binary data from a three-period cross-over trial. *Statistics in Medicine*, **6**, 555–564.

Jones, B. and Kenward, M.G. (1989). *Design and Analysis of Cross-Over Trials*. Chapman and Hall, London.

Jones, B. and Kenward, M.G. (2003). *Design and Analysis of Cross-Over Trials*, 2nd ed. Chapman and Hall/CRC, Boca Raton, FL.

Jones, B. and Kenward, M.G. (2014). *Design and Analysis of Cross-Over Trials*, 3rd ed. Chapman & Hall/CRC, Taylor and Francis, Boca Raton, FL.

Kenward, M.G. and Jones, B. (1987). A log-linear model for binary data. *Applied Statistics*, **36**, 192–204.

Kenward, M.G. and Jones, B. (1991). The analysis of categorical data from cross-over trials using a latent variable model. *Statistics in Medicine*, **10**, 1607–1619.

Kenward, M.G. and Jones, B. (1992). Alternative approaches to the analysis of binary and categorical repeated measurements. *Journal of Biopharmaceutical Statistics*, **2**, 137–170.

Kershner, R.P. and Federer, W.T. (1981). Two-treatment crossover designs for estimating a variety of effects. *Journal of the American Statistical Association*, **80**, 612–619.

Koch, G.G. (1972). The use of non-parametric methods in the statistical analysis of the two-period change-over design. *Biometrics*, **28**, 577–584.

Koch, G.G., Amara, I.A., Brown, B.W. Jr., Colton, T., and Gillings, D.B. (1989). A two-period crossover design for the comparison of two active treatments and placebo. *Statistics in Medicine*, **8**, 487–504.

Laska, E.M. and Meisner, M. (1985). A variational approach to optimal two-treatment crossover designs: applications to carryover effect models. *Journal of the American Statistical Association*, **80**, 704–710.

Laska, E.M., Meisner, M., and Kushner, H.B. (1983). Optimal crossover designs in the presence of carryover effects. *Biometrics*, **39**, 1087–1091.

Layard, M.W. and Arveson, J.N. (1978). Analysis of Poisson data in crossover experimental designs. *Biometrics*, **34**, 421–428.

Lehmacher, W. (1991). Analysis of the crossover design in the presence of residual effects. *Statistics in Medicine*, **10**, 891–899.

Lehmann, E.L. (1975). *Nonparametrics*. Holden-Day, Oakland, CA.

Lemanske, R.F. Jr., Mauger, D.T., Sorkness, C.A., Jackson, D.J., Boehmer, S.J., Martinez, F. D., Strunk, R.C., Szefler, S.J., Zeiger, R.S., Bacharier, L.B., Covar, R.A., Guilbert, T.W., Larsen, G., Morgan, W.J., Moss, M.H., Spahn, J.D., and Taussig, L.M. (2010). Step-up therapy for children with uncontrolled asthma receiving inhaled corticosteroids. *New England Journal of Medicine*, **362**, 975–985.

Liu, J.P. and Chow, S.C. (1992). Sample size determination for the two one-sided tests procedure in bioequivalence. *Journal of Pharmacokinetics and Biopharmaceutics*, **20**, 101–104.

Liu, J. P. and Chow, S.C. (1993). On assessment of bioequivalence of drugs with negligible plasma levels. *Biometrical Journal*, **35**, 109–123.

Liu, J.P., Fan, H.-Y. and Ma, M.-C. (2005). Tests for equivalence based on odds ratio for matched-pair design. *Journal of Biopharmaceutical Statistics*, **15**, 889–901.

Lucas, H.L. (1957). Extra-period Latin square changeover designs. *Journal of Dairy Science*, **4**, 225–239.

Lui, K.-J. (2002a). Notes on estimation of the general odds ratio and the general risk difference for paired-sample data. *Biometrical Journal*, **44**, 957–968.

Lui, K.-J. (2002b). Interval estimation of generalized odds ratio in data with repeated measurements. *Statistics in Medicine*, **21**, 3107–3117.

Lui, K.-J. (2004). *Statistical Estimation of Epidemiological Risk*. John Wiley & Sons, Inc., Hoboken, NJ.

Lui, K.-J. (2013). Sample size determination for testing equality in Poisson frequency data under an AB/BA crossover trial. *Pharmaceutical Statistics*, **12**, 74–81.

Lui, K.-J. (2015a). Notes on estimation of the intraclass correlation under the AB/BA crossover trial. *Journal of Applied Statistics*, **42**, 1374–1381.

Lui, K.-J. (2015b). Test equality between three treatments under an incomplete block crossover design. *Journal of Biopharmaceutical Statistics*, **25**, 795–811.

Lui, K.-J. (2015c) Estimation of the treatment effect under an incomplete block crossover design in binary data – a conditional likelihood approach. *Statistical Methods in Medical Research*, doi: 10.1177/0962280215595434.

Lui, K.-J. (2015d). Notes on estimation of the proportion ratio in the presence of carryover effects under the AB/BA crossover trial. *Communications in Statistics, Simulation and Computation*, doi: 10.1080/03610918.2014.977920.

Lui, K.-J. (2015e). Notes on crossover design. *Enliven: Biostatistics and Metrics*, **1**, 002.

Lui, K.-J. (2016). Comments on "Test non-inferiority (and equivalence) based on the odds ratio under a simple crossover trial." *Statistics in Medicine*, in press (letter to the editor).

Lui, K.-J. and Chang, K.-C. (2011). Test non-inferiority (and equivalence) based on the odds ratio under a simple crossover trial. *Statistics in Medicine*, **30**, 1230–1242.

Lui, K.-J. and Chang, K.-C. (2012a). Estimation of the proportion ratio under a simple crossover trial. *Computational Statistics and Data Analysis*, **56**, 522–530.

Lui, K.-J. and Chang, K.-C. (2012b). Exact sample-size determination in testing non-inferiority under a simple crossover trial. *Pharmaceutical Statistics*, **11**, 129–134.

Lui, K.-J. and Chang, K.-C. (2012c). Hypothesis testing and estimation in ordinal data under a simple crossover design. *Journal of Biopharmaceutical Statistics*, **22**, 1137–1147.

Lui, K.-J. and Chang, K.-C. (2012d) Analysis of Poisson frequency data under a simple crossover trial. *Statistical Methods in Medical Research*, doi: 10.1177/0962280212455753.

Lui, K.-J. and Chang, K.-C. (2012e) A semi-parametric approach to the frequency of occurrence under a simple crossover trial. *Statistical Methods in Medical Research*, doi: 10.1177/0962280212438157.

Lui, K.-J. and Chang, K.-C. (2013a). Notes on interval estimation of the generalized odds ratio under stratified random sampling. *Journal of Biopharmaceutical Statistics*, **23**, 513–525.

Lui, K.-J. and Chang, K.-C. (2013b). Notes on testing noninferiority in ordinal data under the parallel groups design. *Journal of Biopharmaceutical Statistics*, **23**, 1294–1307.

Lui, K.-J. and Chang, K.-C. (2014). Notes on testing equality and interval estimation in Poisson frequency data under a three-treatment three-period crossover trial. *Statistical Methods in Medical Research*, doi: 10.1177/0962280213519249.

Lui, K.-J. and Chang, K.-C. (2015a). Test and estimation in binary data analysis under an incomplete block crossover design. *Computational Statistics and Data Analysis*, **81**, 130–138.

Lui, K.-J. and Chang, K.-C. (2015b). Sample size determination for testing nonequality under a three-treatment two-period incomplete block crossover trial. *Biometrical Journal*, **57**, 410–421.

Lui, K.-J. and Chang, K.-C. (2016). Exact tests in binary data under an incomplete block crossover design. *Statistical Methods in Medical Research*, doi: 10.1177/0962280216638382.

Lui, K.-J., Chang, K.-C., and Lin, C.-D. (2015). Testing equality and interval estimation of the generalized odds ratio in ordinal data under a three-period crossover design. *Statistical Methods in Medical Research*, doi: 10.1177/0962280215569623.

Lui, K.-J., and Cumberland, W.G. (2001). A test procedure of equivalence in ordinal data with matched pairs. *Biometrical Journal*, **43**, 977–983.

Lui, K.-J., Cumberland, W.G., and Chang, K.-C. (2014). Notes on testing equality in binary data under a three-period crossover design. *Computational Statistics and Data Analysis*, **80**, 89–98.

Lui, K.-J. and Lin, C.-D. (2003). A revisit on comparing the asymptotic interval estimators of odds ratio in a single 2×2 table. *Biometrical Journal*, **45**, 226–237.

Mainland, D. (1963). *Elementary Medical Statistics*, 2nd ed. Saunders, Philadelphia, PA.

McCulloch, C.E. and Neuhaus, J.M. (2011). Misspecifying the shape of a random effects distribution: why getting it wrong may not matter. *Statistical Science*, **26**, 388–402.

McNair, D.M. (1971). Antianxiety drugs and human performance. *Archives of General Psychiatry, Chicago*, **29**, 611–617.

Mills, E.J., Chan, A.-W., Wu, P., Vail, A., Guyatt, G.H. and Altman, D.G. (2009). Design, analysis, and presentation of crossover trials. *Trials*, **10**, 27.

Mosteller, F. (1968). Association and estimation in contingency tables. *Journal of the American Statistical Association*, **63**, 1–28.

Munzel, U. and Hauschke, D. (2003). A nonparametric test for proving noninferiority in clinical trials with ordered categorical data. *Pharmaceutical Statistics*, **2**, 31–37.

National Asthma Educational Program (1991). *Executive Summary: Guidelines for the Diagnosis and Management of Asthma*. US Department of Health and Human Services, National Institutes of Health, Bethesda, MD.

Nicholson, K.G., Nguyen-Van-Tam, J.S., Ahmed, A.H., Wiselka, M.J., Leese, J., Ayres, J., Campbell, J.H., Ebden, P., Eiser, N.M., Hutchcroft, B.J., Pearson, J.C.G., Willey, R.F., Wolstenholme, R.J., and Woodhead, M.A. (1998). Randomised placebo-controlled crossover trial on effect of inactivated influenza vaccine on pulmonary function in asthma. *Lancet*, **351**, 326–331.

Patterson, H.D. and Lucas, H.L. (1959). Extra-period changeover designs. *Biometrics*, **15**, 116–132.

Prescott, R.J. (1981). The comparison of success rates in cross-over trials in the presence of an order effect. *Applied Statistics*, **30**, 9–15.

Rhind, G.B., Connaughton, J.J., McFie, J., Douglas, N.J. and Flenley, D.C. (1985). Sustained release choline theophyllinate in nocturnal asthma. *British Medical Journal* **291**, 1605–1607.

Robins, J., Breslow, N., and Greenland, S. (1986). Estimators of the Mantel–Haenszel variance consistent in both sparse data and large-strata limiting models. *Biometrics*, **42**, 311–323.

Rousson, V. and Seifert, B. (2008). A mixed approach for proving non-inferiority in clinical trials with binary endpoints. *Biometrical Journal*, **50**, 190–204.

SAS Institute (2009). *SAS/STAT 9.2 User's Guide*, 2nd ed. SAS Institute, Cary, NC.

Satterthwaite, F.E. (1946). An approximate distribution of estimates of variance components. *Biometrics*, **2**, 110–114.

Schall, R. and Luus, H.G. (1993). On population and individual bioequivalence. *Statistics in Medicine*, **12**, 1109–1124.

Schouten, H. and Kester, A. (2010). A simple analysis of a simple crossover trial with a dichotomous outcome measure. *Statistics in Medicine*, **29**, 193–198.

Schuirmann, D.J. (1987). A comparison of the two one-sided tests procedure and the power approach for assessing the equivalence of average bioavailability. *Journal of Pharmacokinetics and Biopharmaceutics*, **15**, 657–680.

Senn, S.J. (1988). Cross-over trials, carry-over effects and the art of self-delusion. *Statistics in Medicine*, **7**, 1099–1101 (letter).

Senn, S.J. (1991). Problems with the two stage analysis of crossover trials. *British Journal of Clinical Pharmacology*, **32**, 133 (letter).

Senn, S.J. (1992). Is the simple carry-over model useful? *Statistics in Medicine*, **11**, 715–726.

Senn, S.J. (1993). A random effects model for ordinal responses from a crossover trial. *Statistics in Medicine*, **12**, 2147–2150 (letter to the editor).

Senn, S.J. (1996). The AB/BA cross-over: how to perform the two-stage analysis if you can't be persuaded that you shouldn't, in *Liber Amicorum Roel van Strik*, (eds. B. Hansen and M. de Ridder), Erasmus University, Rotterdam, pp. 93–100.

Senn, S.J. (1997). The case for cross-over trials in phase III. *Statistics in Medicine*, **16**, 2021–2022 (letter to the editor).

Senn, S.J. (2000). Consensus and controversy in pharmaceutical statistics (with discussion). *Journal of the Royal Statistical Society, Series D*, **49**, 135–176.

Senn, S.J. (2002). *Cross-over Trials in Clinical Research*, 2nd ed. John Wiley & Sons, Ltd, Chichester.

Senn S.J. (2004). Carry-over in cross-over trials in bioequivalence: theoretical concerns and empirical evidence. *Pharmaceutical Statistics*, **3**, 133–142.

Senn, S.J. (2006). Cross-over trials in *Statistics in Medicine*: the first "25" years. *Statistics in Medicine*, **25**, 3430–3442.

Senn, S.J. and Auclair, P. (1990). The graphical representation of clinical trials with particular reference to measurements over time. *Statistics in Medicine*, **9**, 1287–1302. Erratum (1991). *Statistics in Medicine*, **10**, 487.

Senn, S., D'Angelo, G., and Potvin, D. (2004). Carry-over in cross-over trials in bioequivalence: theoretical concepts and empirical evidence. *Pharmaceutical Statistics*, **3**, 133–142.

Senn, S.J. and Hildebrand, H. (1991). Crossover trials, degrees of freedom, the carryover problem and its dual. *Statistics in Medicine*, **10**, 1361–1374.

Senn, S. and Lee, S. (2004). The analysis of the AB/BA cross-over trial in the medical literature. *Pharmaceutical Statistics*, **3**, 123–131.

Sheiner, L.B. (1992). Bioequivalence revisited. *Statistics in Medicine*, **11**, 1777–1788.

Smith, S.J., Markandu, N.D., Sagnella, G.A., and MacGregor, G.A. (1985). Moderate potassium chloride supplementation in essential hypertension: is it additive to moderate sodium restriction? *British Medical Journal*, **290**, 110–113.

Steinijans, V.W. (1989) Pharmacokinetic characteristics of controlled release products and their biostatistical analysis, in *Oral Controlled Release Products – Therapeutic and Biopharmaceutic Assessment* (eds U. Gundert-Remy and H. Moeller), Wissenschaftliche Verlagsgesellschaft mbH, Stuttgart, pp. 99–115.

Steinijans, V.W., Sauter, R., Jonkman, J.H.G., Schulz, H.U., Stricker, H., and Blume, H. (1989). Bioequivalence studies: single vs. multiple dose. *International Journal of Clinical Pharmacology, Therapy, and Toxicology*, **27**, 261–266.

Taylor, D.R., Town, G.I., Herbison, G.P., *et al.* (1998). Asthma control during long term treatment with regular inhaled salbutamol and salmeterol. *Thorax*, **53**, 744–752.

Taylor, D.R., Drazen, J.M., Herbison, G.P., Yandava, C.N., Hancox, R.J., and Town, G.I. (2000). Asthma exacerbations during long term β agonist use: influence of β_2 adrenoceptor polymorphism. *Thorax*, **55**, 762–767.

Tsong, Y., Zhang, J., and Wang, S.J. (2004). Group sequential design and analysis of clinical equivalence assessment for generic nonsystematic drug products. *Journal of Biopharmaceutical Statistics*, **14**, 359–373.

Tsoy, A.N., Cheltzov, O.V., Zaseyeva, V., Shilinish, L.A., and Yashina, L.A. (1990). Preventive effect of formoterol aerosol in exercise-induced bronchoconstriction. *European Respiratory Journal*, **3**, 235s.

Tu, D. (1998). On the use of the ratio or the odds ratio of cure rates in establishing therapeutic equivalence of non-systemic drugs with binary clinical endpoints. *Journal of Biopharmaceutical Statistics*, **8**, 263–282.

Tu, D. (2001). Statistical procedures in therapeutic equivalence clinical trials with ordinal categorical clinical endpoints. *Journal of Statistical Research*, **35**, 65–77.

Tu, D. (2003). Odds ratio, in *Encyclopedia of Biopharmaceutical Statistics* (ed. S.C. Chow), Taylor & Francis Group, Dekker, New York, pp. 917–921.

Wang, H., Chow, S.C., and Li, G. (2002). On sample size calculation based on odds ratio in clinical trials. *Journal of Biopharmaceutical Statistics*, **12**, 471–483.

Weng, C.S. and Liu, J.P. (1994). Some pitfalls in sample size estimation for anti-infective study. Proceedings of Biopharmaceutical Section of American Statistical Association, pp. 56–60.

Westlake, W.J. (1988). Bioavailability and bioequivalence of pharmaceutical formulations, in *Biopharmaceutical Statistics for Drug Development* (ed K.E. Peace), Dekker, New York, pp. 329–352.

Wiens, B.L. (2002). Choosing an equivalence limit for noninferiority or equivalence studies. *Controlled Clinical Trials*, **23**, 2–14.

Wilding, P., Clark, M., Coon, J.T., Lewis, S., Rushton, L., Bennett, J., Oborne, J., Cooper, S., and Tatterfield, A.E. (1997). Effect of long-term treatment with salmeterol on asthma control: a double blind, randomized crossover study. *British Medical Journal*, **314**, 1441–1446.

Willan, A.R. and Pater, J.L. (1986). Carryover and the two-period crossover clinical trial. *Biometrics*, **42**, 593–599.

Zelen, M. (1971). The analysis of several 2 × 2 contingency tables. *Biometrika*, **58**, 129–137.

Zimmermann, H. and Rahlfs, V. (1978). Test hypotheses in the two-period change-over with binary data. *Biometrical Journal*, **20**, 133–141.

Index

Crossover Designs: Testing, Estimation, and Sample Size, First Edition. Kung-Jong Lui.
© 2016 John Wiley & Sons, Ltd. Published 2016 by John Wiley & Sons, Ltd.
Companion website: www.wiley.com/go/lui/crossover

Statistics in practice

Human and Biological Sciences

Berger – Selection Bias and Covariate Imbalances in Randomized Clinical Trials

Berger and Wong – An Introduction to Optimal Designs for Social and Biomedical Research

Brown, Gregory, Twelves, and Brown – A Practical Guide to Designing Phase II Trials in Oncology

Brown and Prescott – Applied Mixed Models in Medicine, Second Edition

Campbell and Walters – How to Design, Analyse and Report Cluster Randomised Trials in Medicine and Health Related Research

Carpenter and Kenward – Multiple Imputation and Its Application

Carstensen – Comparing Clinical Measurement Methods

Chevret (Ed.) – Statistical Methods for Dose-Finding Experiments

Cooke – Uncertainty Modeling in Dose Response: Bench Testing Environmental Toxicity

Eldridge – A Practical Guide to Cluster Randomised Trials in Health Services Research

Ellenberg, Fleming, and DeMets – Data Monitoring Committees in Clinical Trials: A Practical Perspective

Gould (Ed.) – Statistical Methods for Evaluating Safety in Medical Product Development

Hauschke, Steinijans, and Pigeot – Bioequivalence Studies in Drug Development: Methods and Applications

Källén – Understanding Biostatistics

Lawson, Browne, and Vidal Rodeiro – Disease Mapping with Win-BUGS and MLwiN

Lesaffre, Feine, Leroux, and Declerck – Statistical and Methodological Aspects of Oral Health Research

Lesaffre and Lawson – Bayesian Biostatistics

Lui – Binary Data Analysis of Randomized Clinical Trials with Noncompliance

Lui – Statistical Estimation of Epidemiological Risk

Lui – Crossover Designs: Testing, Estimation and Sample Size

Marubini and Valsecchi – Analysing Survival Data from Clinical Trials and Observation Studies

Millar – Maximum Likelihood Estimation and Inference: With Examples in R, SAS and ADMB

Molenberghs and Kenward – Missing Data in Clinical Studies

Morton, Mengersen, Playford, and Whitby – Statistical Methods for Hospital Monitoring with R

O'Hagan, Buck, Daneshkhah, Eiser, Garthwaite, Jenkinson, Oakley, and Rakow – Uncertain Judgements: Eliciting Expert's Probabilities

O'Kelly and Ratitch – Clinical Trials with Missing Data: A Guide for Practitioners

Parmigiani – Modeling in Medical Decision Making: A Bayesian Approach

Pintilie – Competing Risks: A Practical Perspective

Senn – Cross-over Trials in Clinical Research, Second Edition

Senn – Statistical Issues in Drug Development, Second Edition

Spiegelhalter, Abrams, and Myles – Bayesian Approaches to Clinical Trials and Health-Care Evaluation

Walters – Quality of Life Outcomes in Clinical Trials and Health-Care Evaluation

Welton, Sutton, Cooper, and Ades – Evidence Synthesis for Decision Making in Healthcare

Whitehead – Design and Analysis of Sequential Clinical Trials, Revised Second Edition

Whitehead – Meta-Analysis of Controlled Clinical Trials

Willan and Briggs – Statistical Analysis of Cost Effectiveness Data

Winkel and Zhang – Statistical Development of Quality in Medicine

Zhou, Zhou, Lui, and Ding – Applied Missing Data Analysis in the Health Sciences

Earth and Environmental Sciences

Buck, Cavanagh, and Litton – Bayesian Approach to Interpreting Archaeological Data

Chandler and Scott – Statistical Methods for Trend Detection and Analysis in the Environmental Statistics

Christie, Cliffe, Dawid, and Senn (Eds.) – Simplicity, Complexity and Modelling

Gibbons, Bhaumik, and Aryal – Statistical Methods for Groundwater Monitoring, 2nd Edition

Haas – Improving Natural Resource Management: Ecological and Political Models

Haas – Introduction to Probability and Statistics for Ecosystem Managers

Helsel – Nondetects and Data Analysis: Statistics for Censored Environmental Data

Illian, Penttinen, Stoyan, and Stoyan – Statistical Analysis and Modelling of Spatial Point Patterns

Mateu and Muller (Eds.) – Spatio-Temporal Design: Advances in Efficient Data Acquisition

McBride – Using Statistical Methods for Water Quality Management

Ofungwu – Statistical Applications for Environmental Analysis and Risk Assessment

Okabe and Sugihara – Spatial Analysis Along Networks: Statistical and Computational Methods

Webster and Oliver – Geostatistics for Environmental Scientists, Second Edition

Wymer (Ed.) – Statistical Framework for Recreational Water Quality Criteria and Monitoring

Industry, Commerce, and Finance

Aitken – Statistics and the Evaluation of Evidence for Forensic Scientists, Second Edition

Balding – Weight-of-Evidence for Forensic DNA Profiles

Brandimarte – Numerical Methods in Finance and Economics: A MATLAB-Based Introduction, Second Edition

Brandimarte and Zotteri – Introduction to Distribution Logistics

Chan – Simulation Techniques in Financial Risk Management

Coleman, Greenfield, Stewardson, and Montgomery (Eds) – Statistical Practice in Business and Industry

Frisen (Ed.) – Financial Surveillance

Fung and Hu – Statistical DNA Forensics

Gusti Ngurah Agung – Time Series Data Analysis Using EViews

Jank and Shmueli – Modeling Online Auctions

Jank and Shmueli (Ed.) – Statistical Methods in e-Commerce Research

Lloyd – Data Driven Business Decisions

Kenett (Ed.) – Operational Risk Management: A Practical Approach to Intelligent Data Analysis

Kenett (Ed.) – Modern Analysis of Customer Surveys: With Applications Using R

Kenett and Zacks – Modern Industrial Statistics: With Applications in R, MINITAB and JMP, Second Edition

Kruger and Xie – Statistical Monitoring of Complex Multivariate Processes: With Applications in Industrial Process Control

Lehtonen and Pahkinen – Practical Methods for Design and Analysis of Complex Surveys, Second Edition

Mallick, Gold, and Baladandayuthapani – Bayesian Analysis of Gene Expression Data

Ohser and Mücklich – Statistical Analysis of Microstructures in Materials Science

Pasiouras (Ed.) – Efficiency and Productivity Growth: Modelling in the Financial Services Industry

Pfaff – Financial Risk Modelling and Portfolio Optimization with R

Pourret, Naim, and Marcot (Eds) – Bayesian Networks: A Practical Guide to Applications

Rausand – Risk Assessment: Theory, Methods, and Applications

Ruggeri, Kenett, and Faltin – Encyclopedia of Statistics and Reliability

Taroni, Biedermann, Bozza, Garbolino, and Aitken – Bayesian Networks for Probabilistic Inference and Decision Analysis in Forensic Science, Second Edition

Taroni, Bozza, Biedermann, Garbolino, and Aitken – Data Analysis in Forensic Science